Technical Aspects of Oncologic Hepatic Surgery

Editor

CLIFFORD S. CHO

SURGICAL CLINICS
OF NORTH AMERICA

www.surgical.theclinics.com

Consulting Editor
RONALD F. MARTIN

April 2016 • Volume 96 • Number 2

ELSEVIER

1600 John F. Kennedy Boulevard • Suite 1800 • Philadelphia, Pennsylvania, 19103-2899

http://www.surgical.theclinics.com

SURGICAL CLINICS OF NORTH AMERICA Volume 96, Number 2

April 2016 ISSN 0039–6109, ISBN-13: 978-0-323-41773-0

Editor: John Vassallo, j.vassallo@elsevier.com

Developmental Editor: Colleen Viola

Surgical Clinics of North America (ISSN 0039–6109) is published bimonthly by Elsevier Inc., 360 Park Avenue South, New York, NY 10010-1710. Months of publication are February, April, June, August, October, and December. Business and Editorial Offices: 1600 John F. Kennedy Blvd., Suite 1800, Philadelphia, PA 19103-2899. Periodicals postage paid at New York, NY and additional mailing offices. Subscription prices are $375.00 per year for US individuals, $707.00 per year for US institutions, $100.00 per year for US students and residents, $455.00 per year for Canadian individuals, $895.00 per year for Canadian institutions, $510.00 for international individuals, $895.00 per year for international institutions and $250.00 per year for Canadian and foreign students/residents. To receive student/resident rate, orders must be accompanied by name of affiliated institution, date of term, and the *signature* of program/residency coordinator on institution letterhead. Orders will be billed at individual rate until proof of status is received. Foreign air speed delivery is included in all *Clinics* subscription prices. All prices are subject to change without notice. POSTMASTER: Send address changes to *Surgical Clinics*, Elsevier Health Sciences Division, Subscription Customer Service, 3251 Riverport Lane, Maryland Heights, MO 63043. **Customer Service (orders, claims, online, change of address): Telephone: 1-800-654-2452 (U.S. and Canada); 314-447-8871 (outside U.S. and Canada). Fax: 314-447-8029. E-mail: journalscustomerservice-usa@elsevier.com (for print support); journalsonlinesupport-usa@elsevier.com (for online support).**

Reprints. For copies of 100 or more, of articles in this publication, please contact the Commercial Reprints Department, Elsevier Inc., 360 Park Avenue South, New York, New York 10010-1710. Tel. 212-633-3874, Fax: 212-633-3820, E-mail: reprints@elsevier.com.

The Surgical Clinics of North America is also published in Spanish by McGraw-Hill Interamericana Editores S.A., P.O. Box 5-237 06500 Mexico D.F. Mexico; and in Portuguese by Interlivros Edicoes Ltda., Rua Comandante Coelho 1085, CEP 21250, Rio de Janeiro, Brazil; and in Greek by Paschalidis Medical Publications, Athens Greece.

The Surgical Clinics of North America is covered in *MEDLINE/PubMed (Index Medicus), EMBASE/Excerpta Medica, Current Contents/Clinical Medicine, Current Contents/Life Sciences, Science Citation Index*, and *ISI/BIOMED*.

Contributors

CONSULTING EDITOR

RONALD F. MARTIN, MD, FACS
Lead Surgeon, York Hospital System, York, Maine; Colonel (ret.), United States Army Reserve

EDITOR

CLIFFORD S. CHO, MD, FACS
Associate Professor, Chief, Division of Surgical Oncology, Department of Surgery, University of Wisconsin School of Medicine and Public Health; Co-Director, Gastrointestinal Disease-Oriented Working Group, University of Wisconsin Carbone Cancer Center, Madison, Wisconsin

AUTHORS

THOMAS A. ALOIA, MD
Associate Professor of Surgical Oncology, HPB Surgery Section, Department of Surgical Oncology, UT-MD Anderson Cancer Center, Houston, Texas

JENNIFER BERUMEN, MD
Assistant Professor, Division of Transplantation and Hepatobiliary Surgery, University of California San Diego, California

NEAL BHUTIANI, MD
Division of Surgical Oncology, Department of Surgery, University of Louisville, Louisville, Kentucky

MARK BLOOMSTON, MD, FACS
Division of Surgical Oncology, 21st Century Oncology, Inc., Ft Myers, Florida

CHRISTOPHER L. BRACE, PhD
Associate Professor, Departments of Radiology and Biomedical Engineering, University of Wisconsin School of Medicine and Public Health, Madison, Wisconsin

MICHAEL I. D'ANGELICA, MD, FACS
Enid A. Haupt Chair in Surgery, Attending Surgeon, Memorial Sloan Kettering Cancer Center; Professor of Surgery, Weill Cornell University School of Medicine, New York, New York

GARETH EESON, MD, MSc
Clinical Fellow, Hepatobiliary, Pancreatic and Gastrointestinal Surgical Oncology; Department of Surgical Oncology, Sunnybrook Health Sciences Centre, University of Toronto, Toronto, Canada

CECILIA G. ETHUN, MD
Katz Foundation Research Fellow, Division of Surgical Oncology, Department of Surgery, Winship Cancer Institute, Emory University, Atlanta, Georgia

DAVID P. FOLEY, MD
Department of Surgery, University of Wisconsin School of Medicine and Public Health; Veterans Administration Surgical Services, William S. Middleton Memorial Veterans Hospital, Madison, Wisconsin

YUMAN FONG, MD
Professor and Chairman, Department of Surgery, City of Hope National Medical Center, Duarte, California

T. CLARK GAMBLIN, MD, MS
Division of Surgical Oncology, Medical College of Wisconsin, Milwaukee, Wisconsin

HERMIEN HARTOG, MD, PhD
HPB and transplant surgeon, Division of HPB and Transplant Surgery, Department of Surgery, Erasmus MC, Rotterdam, The Netherlands

ALAN HEMMING, MD
Professor and Chief, Division of Transplantation and Hepatobiliary Surgery, University of California San Diego, San Diego, California

J. LOUIS HINSHAW, MD
Professor, Department of Radiology, University of Wisconsin School of Medicine and Public Health, Madison, Wisconsin

JAN N.M. IJZERMANS, MD, PhD
Professor of HPB and Transplant Surgery, Division of HPB and Transplant Surgery, Department of Surgery, Erasmus MC, Rotterdam, The Netherlands

PAUL J. KARANICOLAS, MD, PhD
Assistant Professor of Surgery, Department of Surgical Oncology, Sunnybrook Health Sciences Centre, University of Toronto, Toronto, Canada

T. PETER KINGHAM, MD, FACS
Department of Surgery, Memorial Sloan Kettering Cancer Center, New York, New York

BAS GROOT KOERKAMP, MD, PhD
HPB Surgeon, Division of HPB and Transplant Surgery, Department of Surgery, Erasmus MC, Rotterdam, The Netherlands

FRED T. LEE Jr, MD
Professor, Departments of Radiology and Biomedical Engineering, University of Wisconsin School of Medicine and Public Health, Madison, Wisconsin

LUNG-YI LEE, MD
Department of Surgery, University of Wisconsin School of Medicine and Public Health, Madison, Wisconsin

HEATHER L. LEWIS, MD
Surgical Oncology Fellow, Division of Surgical Oncology, The Ohio State University Wexner Medical Center, Columbus, Ohio

MICHAEL C. LOWE, MD
Surgical Oncology Fellow, Memorial Sloan Kettering Cancer Center, New York, New York

MEGHAN G. LUBNER, MD
Associate Professor, Department of Radiology, University of Wisconsin School of Medicine and Public Health, Madison, Wisconsin

SHISHIR K. MAITHEL, MD, FACS
Associate Professor of Surgery, Division of Surgical Oncology, Department of Surgery, Winship Cancer Institute, Emory University, Atlanta, Georgia

ROBERT C.G. MARTIN II, MD, PhD, FACS
Professor of Surgery; Director, Division of Surgical Oncology; Director, Upper Gastrointestinal and Hepato-Pancreatico-Biliary Clinic, Academic Advisory Dean, Department of Surgery, University of Louisville, Louisville, Kentucky

LEE M. OCUIN, MD
Division of Surgical Oncology, Department of Surgery, University of Pittsburgh Medical Center, Pittsburgh, Pennsylvania

MOTAZ QADAN, MD, PhD
Department of Surgery, Memorial Sloan Kettering Cancer Center, New York, New York

RAHUL RAJEEV, MBBS
Division of Surgical Oncology, Medical College of Wisconsin, Milwaukee, Wisconsin

GAGANDEEP SINGH, MD
Clinical Professor of Surgery, Head, Hepatobiliary and Pancreatic Surgery, Chief, Division of Surgical Oncology, Department of Surgery, City of Hope National Medical Center, Duarte, California

PRAGATHEESHWAR THIRUNAVUKARASU, MD
Fellow, HPB Surgery Section, Department of Surgical Oncology, UT-MD Anderson Cancer Center, Houston, Texas

ALLAN TSUNG, MD
Division of Hepatobiliary and Pancreatic Surgery, Department of Surgery, Liver Cancer Center, University of Pittsburgh Medical Center, Pittsburgh, Pennsylvania

KIRAN K. TURAGA, MD, MPH
Division of Surgical Oncology, Medical College of Wisconsin, Milwaukee, Wisconsin

THOMAS M. VAN GULIK, MD, PhD
Professor of Gastrointestinal and HPB Surgery, Department of Surgery, Academic Medical Center, Amsterdam, The Netherlands

SHANE A. WELLS, MD
Assistant Professor, Department of Radiology, University of Wisconsin School of Medicine and Public Health, Madison, Wisconsin

MICHAEL A. WHITE, MD
Fellow, Complex Surgical Oncology, Division of Surgical Oncology, Department of Surgery, City of Hope National Medical Center, Duarte, California

TIMOTHY J. ZIEMLEWICZ, MD
Assistant Professor, Department of Radiology, University of Wisconsin School of Medicine and Public Health, Madison, Wisconsin

Contents

therapy is used to decrease tumor burden and "bridge" patients to liver transplant. Surgical technique during liver transplantation may need to be altered in light of these preoperative therapies used for treating HCC. In this review, we discuss the technical aspects of liver transplantation and how they are impacted in patients with HCC.

address sequencing of regional and systemic therapies. However, HAI is not without complications and requires close monitoring and attention to detail. However, it can offer reasonable control of liver tumor burden when managed jointly between medical and surgical oncologists. Herein we describe the technical aspects of HAI pump placement and review pertinent studies in primary and secondary liver tumors.

Isolated hepatic perfusion uses the unique vascular supply of hepatic malignancies to deliver cytotoxic chemotherapy. The procedure involves vascular isolation of the liver and delivery of chemotherapy via the hepatic artery and extraction from retrohepatic vena cava. Benefits of hepatic perfusion have been observed in hepatic metastases of ocular melanoma and colorectal cancer and primary hepatocellular carcinoma. Percutaneous and prophylactic perfusions are avenues of ongoing research.

Until recently, hepatic arterial therapies (HAT) had been used for colorectal liver metastases after failure of first-, second-, and third-line chemotherapies. HAT has gained greater acceptance in patients with liver-dominant colorectal metastases after failure of surgery or systemic chemotherapy. The current data demonstrate that HAT is a safe and effective option for preoperative downsizing, optimizing the time to surgery, limiting non-tumor-bearing liver toxicity, and improving overall survival after surgery in patients with colorectal liver-only metastases. The aim of this review is to present the current data for HAT in liver-only and liver-dominant colorectal liver metastases.

SURGICAL CLINICS
OF NORTH AMERICA

ISSUE OF RELATED INTEREST

Surgical Oncology Clinics, January 2015 (Vol. 24, Issue 1)
Hepatocellular Cancer, Cholangiocarcinoma, and Metastatic Tumors of the Liver
Lawrence D. Wagman, *Editor*
Available at: www.surgonc.theclinics.com

THE CLINICS ARE AVAILABLE ONLINE!
Access your subscription at:
www.theclinics.com

SURGICAL CLINICS
OF NORTH AMERICA

FORTHCOMING ISSUES

June 2016
Practical Urology for the General Surgeon
Lee T. Skinner and Gloria H. Hansen,
Editors

August 2015
Sleutech and Bariatric Surgery
Ashley C. Day, Editor

October 2015
Management of Sarcoma
Jeffrey M. Farma and Andrea Porpiglia,
Editors

RECENT ISSUES

February 2016
Development of a Surgeon: Medical School
through Retirement
Ronald J. Martin and Paul J. Schenarts,
Editors

December 2015
Inflammatory Bowel Disease
Kerry L. Hammond, Editor

October 2015
Cancer Screening and Genetics
Christopher L. Wedlgang, Editor

August 2015
Simulation in Surgical Training and Practice
Kimberly M. Brown and John T. Paige,
Editor

ISSUE OF RELATED INTEREST

Surgical Oncology Clinics, January 2015 (Vol. 24, Issue 1)
Hepatocellular Cancer, Cholangiocarcinoma, and Metastatic Tumors of the Liver
Lawrence D. Wagman, Editor
Available at: www.surgonc.theclinics.com

THE CLINICS ARE AVAILABLE ONLINE!
Access your subscription at:
www.theclinics.com

Foreword

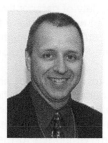

Ronald F. Martin, MD, FACS
Consulting Editor

In just about every textbook of liver surgery that I have seen, there is an image, usually in the front matter or close to it, of some work of art depicting Prometheus chained to the rock. As the legend goes, Prometheus was chained to a rock by an angry Zeus. Every day, an eagle would come and peck at Prometheus' liver, and his liver would grow back. He would suffer this ignominious fate day after day until he was freed by Heracles at some later date. The image is usually included to illustrate some longstanding human knowledge of liver regeneration or perhaps to amaze the readership with the idea that the liver has been mysterious to humans for a very long time. Also, it gives people who write about liver surgery a chance to impress us with their broad knowledge of the fine arts.

Everyday mystery and amazement put aside, the liver remains a most impressive organ. It is second in mass only to skin, is impressively resilient to all kinds of insults, rids us of all manner of microbes and toxins that would otherwise harm us, and does, indeed, regenerate. Whether the Greeks really knew the last part or they just liked stories about immortal beings, I wouldn't hazard a guess.

The liver also demonstrates its importance in one other way—when it fails, people do very badly. Medically, we are pretty good at supporting the failing heart or lungs, very good at supporting or even replacing kidney function, not bad at improving or giving people new marrow. Sometimes we can do without gut, and often we can do fine without whole extremities. Bodies can go on for quite a long time without a functioning central nervous system, though it opens a philosophical debate about the difference between not being dead and being alive. If one loses his or her liver, however, one is in dire straits until one gets a new liver.

Like Prometheus' liver, the knowledge base we have of the management and operative care of liver-related problems keeps getting pecked at and keeps regenerating. It wasn't that long ago when we focused on how much liver we wanted to ablate or how disease volume dictated our course. Today, we have flipped the question to focus on how much liver we have to preserve and what options or combinations of options we have to achieve that. In fact, much of what we held true about the management of liver diseases—especially the neoplastic diseases—is markedly different than even a decade ago, or less.

Surg Clin N Am 96 (2016) xiii–xiv
http://dx.doi.org/10.1016/j.suc.2016.02.013
0039-6109/16/$ – see front matter © 2016 Published by Elsevier Inc.

surgical.theclinics.com

Dr Cho and his colleagues have assembled an impressive and thought-provoking collection of articles about the evaluation and management of liver neoplastic disease. The collection represents a comprehensive view from a wide variety of perspectives about what we can do and how we can combine efforts. It is an excellent place to either start learning or to continue learning about this complicated set of patients and their complicated set of problems. We are indebted to them for adding it to our series.

One thing that is often overlooked about the Prometheus story is what got him chained to the rock in the first place. Most people say it is because he stole fire from the gods and gave it to men—which is partly right. Before the fire incident, Prometheus had already angered Zeus by loving men more than the gods—that and not telling Zeus which of his children would dethrone him. Giving fire to men was perhaps the last straw.

So perhaps as much as the story of Prometheus tells us about the regenerative power of the liver, it also informs us of how much people in power are afraid to lose it and don't like it when the little guy is loved more than they are. Fire and knowledge are both powerful tools that can be used for good or otherwise. Our goal is to disseminate knowledge and inspire passion. I doubt anybody would consider us as Zeus regarded Prometheus. Even if that were to happen, I prefer to think the Prometheus story shows that resilience in the face of seemingly insurmountable odds eventually pays off. We would be in good company anyway.

Ronald F. Martin, MD, FACS
York Hospital
16 Hospital Drive, STE A
York, ME 03909, USA

E-mail address:
rmartin@yorkhospital.com

Preface

Oncologic Hepatic Surgery: Appreciating the Landscape

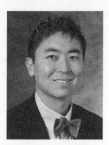

Clifford S. Cho, MD, FACS
Editor

Like mountain ranges and life stories, the field of oncologic hepatic surgery is best understood when viewed from a wide-angle-lens perspective. Consider the dizzying array of biological variables that characterize clinical decision-making for liver cancer. Diseases like gallbladder cancer and fibrolamellar hepatocellular carcinoma disseminate in a lymphotropic manner that encourages portal lymphadenectomy; other diseases do not. Resection of a 2-cm colorectal metastasis located along the periphery of segment VI could result in a negligible loss of functional hepatic parenchyma; resection of an identical 2-cm colorectal metastasis located just a few centimeters over to the left could result in crippling hepatic insufficiency. The difference between resection and transplantation for hepatocellular carcinoma can be separated by millimeters. A single patient with a primary hepatic malignancy can be offered half a dozen different treatment options with relative equanimity—and the menu is growing. Navigating this kind of multilevel and dynamic complexity demands a close and comprehensive appreciation of the entire landscape of liver cancer treatment options. In this issue of *Surgical Clinics of North America*, we have asked a diverse team of renowned surgical oncologists, transplant surgeons, and radiologists to comment on their specific areas of technical expertise. Topics for discussion include preoperative, operative, and nonoperative techniques as applied broadly as well as to specific diseases.

Surg Clin N Am 96 (2016) xv–xvi
http://dx.doi.org/10.1016/j.suc.2016.01.001
0039-6109/16/$ – see front matter © 2016 Published by Elsevier Inc.

surgical.theclinics.com

It is our hope that this issue will provide a panoramic view to inform the contemporary surgical management of liver cancer.

Clifford S. Cho, MD, FACS
Division of Surgical Oncology
Department of Surgery
University of Wisconsin
School of Medicine and Public Health
University of Wisconsin
Carbone Cancer Center
J4/703 Clinical Sciences Center
600 Highland Avenue
Madison, WI 53792, USA

E-mail address:
cho@surgery.wisc.edu

Erratum

In the February 2016 issue (Volume 96, number 1), in the article, "Education and Training to Address Specific Needs During the Career Progression of Surgeons," Dr. Sachdeva should be listed on the title page as "Ajit K. Sachdeva, MD, FRCSC, FACS."

In the same article, on page 118, nine lines from the bottom of the page, the following sentences should read: "The renowned and evidence-based *Surgical Education and Self-Assessment Program (SESAP)* is offered in various formats to support individual goals and learning styles and remains the premier self- assessment program for surgeons. This program includes a unique guided learning model that is aimed at enhancing cognitive skills. The evidence-based *Selected Readings in General Surgery* includes syntheses of the current literature and topical reviews of surgical content."

Also in the February issue, in the article, "Alternative Considerations for Surgical Training and Funding," by Ronald F. Martin, MD, there were two errors. The first full sentence on page 38 should read: "Data provided by the Center for Medicare and Medicaid Services (CMS) state that total US health care expenditures for 2013 reached $2.9 trillion, or approximately 17.4% of the gross domestic product."

In the same article, on page 39, the ninth line from the top, the sentence should read: "Most of the health care in the United States is delivered in medical environments that are not involved in GME training, so none of those facilities would see a direct loss if the federal GME money went away."

Surg Clin N Am 96 (2016) xvii
http://dx.doi.org/10.1016/j.suc.2016.02.016
0039-6109/16/$ – see front matter © 2016 Elsevier Inc. All rights reserved.

surgical.theclinics.com

Determination of Resectability

Cecilia G. Ethun, MD, Shishir K. Maithel, MD*

KEYWORDS

- Liver tumors • Resectability • Oncologic assessment • Liver function

KEY POINTS

- Determining resectability of hepatic malignancies relies on 3 key concepts: oncologic appropriateness, host condition, and technical resectability.
- Oncologic appropriateness is based on tumor biology. Adequately defining the extent of disease and understanding the nature of the tumor in question are critical before pursuing operative intervention.
- Host condition refers a patient's general state of health and his or her ability to tolerate major surgery, or surgical fitness.
- Technical resectability of a liver tumor requires that the future liver remnant be of sufficient quantity and quality, with adequate inflow, outflow, and biliary drainage, in order to sustain function postoperatively.

INTRODUCTION

When determining the resectability of hepatic malignancies, several key considerations must be addressed:

1. Oncologic appropriateness. The surgeon's first responsibility is to determine those patients most likely to benefit from an operation. In malignancy, this is largely measured by the survival benefit of surgery, which is ultimately governed by tumor biology. Thus, it is critical to adequately define the extent of disease and understand the nature of the tumor in question before proceeding with operative intervention.
2. Host condition. This refers to the general health and surgical fitness of a patient. In most patients, this can be successfully evaluated through a careful history and physical examination, as well as any other indicated adjunct workup. Several additional assessment tools may be used to further stratify patients according to risk.

Disclosures: None.
Division of Surgical Oncology, Department of Surgery, Winship Cancer Institute, Emory University, 1365C Clifton Road NE, Building C, 2nd Floor, Atlanta, GA 30322, USA
* Corresponding author.
E-mail address: smaithe@emory.edu

Surg Clin N Am 96 (2016) 163–181
http://dx.doi.org/10.1016/j.suc.2015.12.002
0039-6109/16/$ – see front matter © 2016 Elsevier Inc. All rights reserved.

3. Technical resectability. Before pursuing any degree of hepatic resection, the remnant liver should be determined to have sufficient inflow, outflow, and biliary drainage, and be of adequate quantity and quality.

If surgery is determined to be reasonable from an oncologic perspective; the patient is deemed fit for surgery; and the extent of planned resection leaves an adequate functional liver remnant (FLR), nearly all patients should be candidates for liver resection. This article will elaborate on these 3 concepts within the context of liver tumors, both primary and metastatic, as well as discuss ways by which resectability rates can be potentially increased.

ONCOLOGIC APPROPRIATENESS

Understanding the resectability of a tumor from an oncologic perspective is paramount and should be the first consideration of any surgeon faced with a cancer patient. This is based on the concept of nonmalfeasance, often represented by the phrase, "first, do no harm." When performed with a curative intent, the value of surgery for malignancy is measured by its survival benefit. Tumor biology, however, ultimately dictates patient outcome. Thus, a thorough preoperative evaluation should be performed to assess the extent of spread, which, among other tumor-specific factors, can help predict the nature of disease. Whether a primary or metastatic liver tumor, extrahepatic spread is an indicator of aggressive tumor biology, and, while not always a preclusion of surgery,[1] the benefit of resection in these cases should be questioned strongly. Improvements in imaging technology, and, in appropriately selected patients, diagnostic laparoscopy, have increased surgeons' ability to identify those patients unlikely to benefit from surgery and avoid unnecessary hepatectomy. In certain cases where the oncologic appropriateness of surgery is in question, a trial of preoperative systemic or liver-directed therapy may help biologically select more favorable tumors for resection.

Preoperative Evaluation

Preoperative evaluation of the oncologic appropriateness of liver resection should focus on characterizing the lesion in question, defining the extent of disease, and determining its biologic behavior. Imaging modalities should include a staging chest radiograph or chest computed tomography (CT), and either a CT or MRI of the abdomen and pelvis, with preference depending on the type of tumor being evaluated, institutional expertise, and patient-related factors. In many cases, however, both CT and MRI may be necessary.[2] Positron emission tomography (PET) scan may also be a useful and important tool in evaluating the extent of disease in fluorodeoxyglucose (FDG)-avid tumors.[3–6] Preoperative biopsy for certain tumor types is often not necessary and should only be pursued in select cases where the information gained will alter the treatment plan, such as administering preoperative therapy.

Despite advances in various high-quality imaging modalities, roughly 9% to 36% of patients are still found to have occult metastatic disease at the time of surgery.[7–11] Staging laparoscopy has been advocated by some to identify peritoneal metastases not detected on cross-sectional imaging, thereby avoiding unnecessary laparotomy.[10–14] However, its routine use is subject to debate, and may only be of benefit in patients already identified as high-risk for having unresectable disease.[15–17]

Tumor-Specific Factors

Hepatocellular carcinoma

Hepatocellular carcinoma (HCC) is the most common primary liver tumor and the third most common cause of cancer-related death worldwide.[18] Although various nonoperative treatment options exist, surgery remains first-line therapy, with the choice between resection and transplantation generally dictated by the degree of underlying liver dysfunction and tumor burden.[19,20] From an oncologic perspective, 4 major clinical prognostic indicators have been identified—tumor size, multifocality, vascular invasion, and extrahepatic spread—and serve as the basis for the tumor-node-metastasis (TMN) staging system.[21,22] Since the widespread adoption of the Milan criteria, which creates a selection cut-off using these clinical indicators, the identification of cirrhotic patients for transplantation has been simplified with consistently favorable results.[23,24] Translating these clinical indicators into oncologic criteria for resection, however, has proven difficult.

Several clinical staging systems have been proposed using different clinicopathologic parameters with varying success in applicability, cancer-specific focus, and prognostic value.[25–27] One commonly used system is the Barcelona Clinic Liver Cancer (BCLC) staging system. Based on tumor stage, liver function, and performance status, it stratifies patients with HCC into 4 categories—early, intermediate, advanced, and terminal—and makes treatment recommendations for each.[28,29] According to this staging system, hepatic resection is indicated only in patients with early stage HCC (single tumor ≤5 cm or ≤3 tumors all <3 cm, without vascular invasion or extrahepatic spread; satisfactory liver function; and performance status of 0), with the oncologic appropriateness of resection mirroring that of The Milan criteria.[23,28] The widespread acceptance of the BCLC system in guiding resection, however, has been controversial, as conflicting data regarding the prognostic value of these clinical indicators continues to emerge.[30–36]

Tumor size historically has been an important predictor of outcome following surgery for HCC. It is easy to measure preoperatively and has been shown to be inversely correlated with survival, particularly for tumors larger than 5 cm and 10 cm in diameter.[32,37–40] However, several groups have demonstrated more acceptable and durable long-term survival following resection for large HCCs, questioning the prognostic significance of tumor size alone.[33,36,41–43] Furthermore, when controlling for other factors, such as number of tumors and vascular invasion, size has demonstrated little impact on survival, even in tumors more than 10 cm in diameter.[21,36,44–46] In fact, the current American Join Committee on Cancer (AJCC) 7th edition staging classification no longer uses tumor size alone to stratify patients.[21,22] Increasingly, however, studies focusing on the link between tumor size and vascular invasion have shown that the frequency of microscopic and macroscopic vascular invasion drastically increases as tumor size increases.[34,36,47] This suggests that tumor size, rather than being an independent prognostic indicator, may serve as a surrogate marker for vascular invasion. Thus, while size alone should not dictate treatment, recognizing the link between size and more aggressive tumor biology is critical when discussing the oncologic appropriateness of resection in patients with HCC.

The presence of multiple tumors is another important independent prognostic factor in patients with HCC. The pathogenesis of multifocal HCC is thought to be caused by at least 2 very different biologic mechanisms—multicentric hepatocarcinogenesis, meaning multiple de novo tumors of independent origin, and intrahepatic metastasis, meaning multifocal dissemination of a common clonal origin.[48–50] Although the ability to differentiate between these 2 pathways may have significant implications for understanding tumor biology and guiding management, reliable biomarkers are lacking, and clinical applicability is not yet clear. Still, as a group, multifocal HCC incurs a worse prognosis than equally matched solitary tumors, a fact reflected in the current AJCC staging system.[22,45,46] Although acceptable rates of survival have been shown following resection for multifocal HCCs no more than 5 cm in diameter, the oncologic benefit in patients with larger multifocal HCC is still subject to debate, and a trial of preoperative therapy may be prudent prior to selecting these patients for resection.[21,45,46,51]

Vascular invasion has been shown in multiple studies to be one of the best predictors of outcome following surgery for HCC.[21,29,32–36,45–47] Patients presenting with macroscopic or major vascular invasion, defined as tumor involving a major branch of the portal or hepatic vein, have particularly dismal outcomes, with increased risk of intrahepatic and systemic metastases, and poor overall survival.[21,45,46,52–54] If left untreated, the reported median survival of patients with HCC and major vascular invasion is 9 to 10 weeks.[52,53] Even after hepatic resection for HCC, several studies have reported an overall 5-year survival of only 10% to 11% when major vascular invasion was present.[35,45,55,56] Although a small subset of patients may have more favorable outcomes than those traditionally reported,[35] the benefit of resection in patients with major vascular invasion remains questionable and should be pursued in only highly selected patients. Microscopic vascular invasion has also been shown to be a strong predictor of outcome, with its presence associated with earlier tumor recurrence, metastatic spread, and decreased overall survival.[32–34,36,47] Unfortunately, microscopic vascular invasion is difficult to predict preoperatively, and in isolation it is of little use in determining resectability.

In HCC, extrahepatic spread, which includes regional lymph node involvement and distant metastases, is considered stage IV disease. With few exceptions, it is a contraindication to resection in patients with HCC.[20,22,57]

Intrahepatic cholangiocarcinoma

Intrahepatic cholangiocarcinoma (ICC) is the second most common primary liver tumor, with rising incidence seen in both European and North American countries.[58,59] Despite this, no currently available locoregional or systemic therapies have shown definitive therapeutic benefit, and surgical resection remains the only potentially curative treatment for patients with ICC.[60] Until the current (7th edition) AJCC staging system was developed, TMN staging for ICC was based on that of HCC, which used tumor size, multifocality, vascular invasion, and extrahepatic spread as the major prognostic criteria.[61] However, given the distinct tumor biology, underlying risk factors, and clinical behavior between HCC and ICC, several nomograms and staging systems have been developed in an attempt to identify relevant prognostic indicators and more accurately predict survival in patients with ICC.[62–67]

The applicability of tumor size as a prognostic indicator to stratify patients with ICC has been controversial. Used in previous versions of the AJCC staging system, the prognostic value of tumor size was refuted in one of the earliest proposed staging systems for ICC.[63] This has been supported by several groups, whose authors found no independent association between tumor size and survival in ICC.[62,68–70] Indeed, tumor size is notably absent in the staging system proposed by Nathan and colleagues,[62] as well as in the current and only AJCC staging system addressing ICC independently.[66] The Liver Cancer Study Group of Japan (LCSGJ), on the other hand, found a worse prognosis in patients with ICCs more than 2 cm in diameter, which is used as a cutoff value in their commonly used staging system.[65] Similarly, others have shown a significantly negative effect on recurrence and survival with increasing tumor size, particularly in tumors larger than 5 cm and larger than 7 cm, which is reflected by the fact that tumor size has been incorporated in two of the newer proposed nomograms.[64,67,71–73] More recently, several groups have found that, while not an independent predictor of outcome, increasing tumor size is associated with an increased incidence of nodal involvement, multiple tumors, vascular invasion, and poorly differentiated tumors.[74,75] This suggests that larger tumor size may be indicative of more aggressive tumor biology, and its role in determining resectability, although perhaps subtle, should not be entirely discounted.

Multifocal intrahepatic disease is considered one of the most dominant clinicopathologic factors affecting survival in ICC. Similar to HCC, the pathophysiology of multiple ICC tumors is thought to be due to either satellitosis, multicentric hepatocarcinogenesis, or intrahepatic metastases, although the clinical significance of these is unclear. Still, there is little debate that patients with ICC presenting with multiple tumors face a grim prognosis, particularly with 3 or more tumors.[64,67,69,71–74] Although most patients with multifocal disease never reach resection, the median survival for the few patients who do ranges from 12 to 19 months, with 1 study observing no survival benefit over patients treated nonoperatively.[69,71,73] Thus, in patients with multiple intrahepatic ICC tumors, nonoperative therapies should be the first consideration, with resection reserved for only highly select cases.

The presence of vascular invasion is often cited as an important risk factor for disease recurrence and decreased survival in patients with ICC.[62,64,69,70] Its strength as an independent prognostic indicator, however, is less clear. Indeed, when taking into account other factors, such as positive nodal status and increased tumor number, vascular invasion frequently failed to maintain significance.[68,69,71,74,76] Furthermore, microscopic vascular invasion is difficult to identify on preoperative imaging, giving it little value in determining resectability. Even when faced with major vascular invasion, however, several groups have advocated a more aggressive surgical approach, citing increased resectability rates and comparable or better overall survival when major vascular resection was performed in order to obtain negative margins.[74,76,77] Thus, hepatic resection in the setting of major vascular invasion can be oncologically appropriate in select patients with ICC, particularly after a favorable response to a course of preoperative therapy.

Extrahepatic disease, including regional lymph node involvement, is considered stage IV, and these tumors should be deemed unresectable, except in highly select cases.

Colorectal liver metastases

Colorectal cancer is the most common cancer worldwide and the second most common cause of cancer-related death in the United States.[18] Roughly 25% of patients with colorectal cancer present with metastatic disease, and another 50% to 60% of patients will eventually develop metastases, with the majority being in the liver.[78,79] In patients with metastases confined to the liver, hepatic resection has largely become the standard of care, with a 5-year survival of approximately 50% in most modern series and a 10-year disease-free survival rate reaching nearly 20%.[80,81]

Identifying those patients most likely to achieve these survival benchmarks, however, has been challenging. Several risk factors have been identified and used in various combinations to develop clinical scoring systems and indices in an attempt to predict long-term survival and guide therapy in patients with colorectal liver metastases. These include synchronous liver disease, primary tumor node status and histology, number and size of liver tumors, CEA level, disease-free interval, and the presence of extrahepatic disease.

Although most studies are in agreement as to the general importance of these factors and their cumulative effect on survival, there is little standardization in their individual cut-off values and prognostic strengths, and no single factor has unanimously been shown to affect outcomes.[82–86] In fact, 1 study focusing on patients cured of disease at 10 years showed that well over half of them originally had at least one, and

43% had at least three, of these poor prognostic factors—synchronous disease (7%), node-positive primary (51%), CEA greater than 200 (7%), disease-free interval less than 12 months (37%), multiple hepatic tumors (40%), and size of hepatic tumor greater than 5 cm (36%).[81] Even in the setting of extrahepatic disease, a scenario traditionally considered a contraindication to resection, acceptable 5-year survival rates up to 28% have been shown in select patients undergoing hepatic resection.[87–89] Certainly, there is little question that patients with many risk factors do worse than patients with few to no risk factors. However, the line that separates the biologically resectable from the biologically unresectable patients with colorectal liver metastases continues to be evasive.

HOST CONDITION

Knowing a patient's general health status and his or her ability to tolerate surgery, or surgical fitness, is critical when determining resectability of hepatic malignancies. A thorough history and physical examination, and any other indicated adjunct workup, should be performed preoperatively on all patients. However, because determining the surgical fitness of a patient is often subjective, several risk indices have been developed to aid in patient assessment and decision-making, and provide a more objective way to stratify patients according to risk. Those commonly used by anesthesiologists and surgeons include the American Society of Anesthesiologists (ASA) scale, the Eastern Cooperative Oncology Group (ECOG) Performance Status, the Charlson Comorbidity Index (CCI), and the Revised Cardiac Risk Index (RCRI).[90–93] More recently, the concept of frailty has been introduced as an important surgical risk assessment tool and has formed the basis of the Hopkins Frailty Score, which was later validated in a large multidisciplinary prospective study examining outcomes of patients undergoing major intra-abdominal surgery.[94,95]

TECHNICAL RESECTABILITY

In liver surgery, the technical resectability of a tumor is defined not only by what can be removed, but more importantly by what is subsequently left behind. Thus, hepatic arterial and portal venous inflow, venous outflow, biliary drainage, and the quantity and quality of the future liver remnant (FLR) should all be deemed adequate to sustain function and support regeneration in the postoperative period. Patients with underlying liver dysfunction pose a unique challenge when considering hepatic resection, and understanding the degree of dysfunction and its effect on prognosis is crucial. In select patients, the use of remnant optimizing techniques and staged procedures can increase resectability, and should be considered whenever possible.

Vascular Inflow/Outflow and Biliary Drainage

One of the major dilemmas in determining the technical resectability of liver tumors is balancing the appropriate operation required in order to completely remove the tumor and obtain negative margins while maintaining adequate vascular inflow, outflow, and biliary drainage of the FLR. Thus, mapping out the tumor location in relation to the patient's hepatic vascular and biliary anatomy is critical. In most patients, this can be done successfully with a CT scan, MRI, or both. Even with centrally located tumors, which more frequently involve major vascular structures close to the hilum, improvements in high-quality cross-sectional imaging have allowed for better visualization and characterization of tissue planes. When biliary obstruction is suspected, cholangiography may additionally help delineate biliary involvement, and can be done endoscopically, percutaneously, or using MRI.

Historically, tumor involvement of the portal vein or inferior vena cava (IVC) has been considered a contraindication to surgery, as resection of these tumors incurred significant perioperative morbidity and mortality risk. However, improvements in surgical technique and perioperative management have expanded the definition of resectability and led many centers to adopt a more aggressive surgical policy. Indeed, several studies have demonstrated that in select patients, hepatectomy combined with major vascular resection or thrombectomy can be safe, with low postoperative morbidity and mortality, and that major vascular or biliary involvement should not necessarily preclude resection.[35,77,96–100] In highly select patients whose tumor involves the IVC, the hilum, or the confluence of the IVC and hepatic veins, and would otherwise be considered unresectable by any other resection techniques, ex vivo resection and autotransplantation may be an option.[101–105] However, as data regarding this approach are sparse and limited to case reports and institutional series, understanding of the survival benefit continues to evolve.

Future Liver Remnant Quantity and Quality

Volumetric assessment of the liver

Because of the liver's tremendous capacity for functional compensation and regeneration, healthy livers without cirrhosis can tolerate resections of up to 80% of their parenchymal volume. However, the segmental distribution of the liver's functional capacity is not uniform and varies from person to person, making it difficult to estimate the volume of the FLR needed to sustain function based on traditional anatomic nomenclature.[106] Thus, preoperative volumetric analysis is an important tool to assess the actual volume and predict the function of the FLR, particularly when considering major and extended hepatic resections.

In general, the FLR is standardized to total liver volume (TLV) and is expressed as the percentage of the TLV that is to be left unresected. Various methods for measuring liver volume have been proposed. One such method is using CT and 3-dimensional CT volumetry, which has been shown to be accurate and reproducible in calculating TLV and FLR values.[107–109] However, direct measurement of TLV on imaging may be problematic, as large tumors, biliary dilatation, and underlying liver disease may alter TLV. In addition, accurately measuring TLV requires that the tumor volume be excluded or subtracted, which can be particularly difficult in the setting of multiple tumors, and can lead to user discrepancies and mathematical error.

An alternative approach is to estimate the TLV using a mathematical formula based on body surface area (TLV $[cm^3] = -794.41 + 1267.28 \times$ body surface area $[m^2]$), which has been validated in a meta-analysis and found to be the most superior compared with other similar formulas.[110,111] An FLR volume of 20% or less has been found to be the strongest independent predictor of postoperative liver insufficiency, and a significant risk factor for postoperative liver failure and death.[112–114] Thus, an FLR volume greater than 20% has been proposed as a cutoff for safe hepatic resection in healthy, noncirrhotic livers.

Problems arise, however, when faced with patients without healthy livers. Although the exact pathogenesis is not entirely understood, liver injury is a known risk of chemotherapy, and increasing duration of preoperative treatment has been shown to increase the risk of postoperative complications.[115–121] Furthermore, longer durations of preoperative chemotherapy (>12 weeks) have been associated with higher rates of liver injury and postoperative hepatic insufficiency.[119,122] In patients who receive short-duration preoperative chemotherapy, it has been suggested that an FLR of at least 20% to 30% is sufficient to undergo hepatic resection.[122,123] However, those receiving long-duration (>12 weeks) preoperative chemotherapy should have an

FLR volume of at least 30%, although some suggest as high as 44% in these patients.[122,124,125] In patients with hepatic fibrosis or cirrhosis, the FLR volume is suggested to be at least 40% to 50% of TLV.[126,127]

Functional assessment of the liver

Preoperative evaluation of liver function is one of the most important assessments when determining resectability of liver malignancies. Indeed, the perioperative morbidity and mortality risk has been shown to proportionally increase with worsening degree of hepatocellular compromise in cirrhotic patients undergoing hepatic resection.[128–131] Although a long list of functional studies, imaging techniques, and serum markers exists, the multiple and diverse functions of the liver make comprehensive evaluation difficult, and no single study has been consistently proven to be the best measurement of preoperative liver function or predictor of postoperative hepatic insufficiency and failure prior to resection.

The model for end-stage liver disease (MELD) is one of two major clinical scoring systems frequently used to evaluate liver function in cirrhotic patients, and it is based on a patient's bilirubin, international normalized ratio (INR), and creatinine.[132] Traditionally used to predict survival in cirrhotic patients awaiting liver transplantation, the utility of the MELD score has been expanded to a variety of clinical settings, including the assessment of patients being considered for hepatectomy.[132–135] In cirrhotic patients undergoing hepatic resection, a MELD score of at least 9 has been shown to be an independent predictor of perioperative complications and mortality.[134,135] Thus, a MELD score less than 9 can be considered safe for hepatic resection.

The Child-Turcotte-Pugh (CTP) score is another frequently used clinical scoring system to predict liver-related mortality in cirrhotic patients, and takes into account both clinical measures and laboratory values, including presence of ascites, encephalopathy, total serum bilirubin, INR, and serum albumin.[136] An elevated CTP score has been associated with increased morbidity and mortality following liver resection.[129,131,137] In fact, a Child B classification (score 7–9) is considered a relative contraindication to resection, particularly for major hepatectomy, while a Child C is an absolute contraindication, even for most minor resections.[138] In addition, the presence of encephalopathy, independent of the other factors, is generally considered a contraindication to resection.

An additional method of identifying cirrhotic patients at risk for postoperative complications is to assess for the presence of portal hypertension. Splenomegaly and varices seen on imaging are both reliable signs of portal hypertension; however, they are rarely present in patients being considered for resection, and relying on radiographic evidence of these signs is inadequate. Direct measurement of portal pressure can be done using portal venous wedge pressure; however, routine use of this invasive technique is impractical. Thrombocytopenia, on the other hand, has been shown to be a good surrogate marker for the presence of portal hypertension in patients with underlying liver dysfunction, as it is indicative of increased platelet sequestration due to portal hypertension-induced hypersplenism. Although portal hypertension is not an absolute contraindication to hepatic resection, thrombocytopenia has been associated with increased morbidity and mortality in patients undergoing resection.[139–142] Specifically, a preoperative platelet count of less than 150/nL has been independently associated with major postoperative complications, postoperative hepatic insufficiency, and 60-day mortality in patients with HCC undergoing hepatic resection.[137] In fact, a modified Child score based on these data has been proposed, which replaces encephalopathy in the traditional CTP scoring system with preoperative platelet count. This modified Child score was found to be independently associated with major postoperative complications and 60-day mortality, and the only factor independently associated with postoperative hepatic insufficiency.[137]

Indocyanine green (ICG) clearance is another assessment tool used preoperatively to evaluate liver function in cirrhotic patients being considered for hepatic resection. ICG is an anionic organic dye that is selectively taken up by hepatocytes and excreted in bile. It is usually measured as a percent serum clearance at 15 minutes and indirectly reflects hepatocyte blood flow and functional capacity.[143] An ICG cutoff of less than 10% at 15 minutes has been reported to be safe for extended resection, a cutoff of 10% to 20% for hemi-hepatectomy, 20% to 30% for segmentectomy, and only enucleation for those with greater that 40% ICG clearance.[144] However, the utility of ICG clearance over other well-established functional measures is debated, and it is rarely used in the United States.[140,145]

Increasing Technical Resectability

Portal vein embolization

Portal vein embolization (PVE) is a minimally invasive procedure performed preoperatively in select patients as a means to increase the volume of the anticipated FLR, which has been shown to subsequently improve liver function, thereby decreasing the risk of postoperative complications associated with small FLR size.[146–149] The efficacy of PVE has been well documented, with a reported average increase of 12% plus or minus 5% in FLR volume following PVE.[112,113,124,149] In fact, FLR growth caused by PVE has been shown to increase resectability in roughly 60% of patients who previously would be deemed unresectable owing to inadequate FLR size.[123,150] Furthermore, it has been demonstrated that those patients whose FLR growth following PVE enabled them to undergo resection had no difference in postoperative morbidity and mortality compared with those who underwent resection up front without the need for PVE.[112,150,151] Overall and disease-free survival has also been shown to be similar among these 2 groups in patients undergoing resection for colorectal liver metastases.[124,150]

More recent studies have found the growth rate of the FLR following PVE to be a strong predictor of postoperative liver insufficiency, liver failure, and death.[152,153] Using cutoff values of at least 2% and greater than 2.66% FLR growth per week, patients in this group from both studies had significantly lower postoperative morbidity, and none developed liver failure or suffered liver-related death. This suggests that growth rate of the FLR, rather than standard volumetric measurements, may be a better guide for determining resectability of liver tumors following PVE, although further evaluation is still needed.

Although its application is not standardized, studies have warned against the routine use of PVE, citing a large percentage of patients in whom PVE had no effect on morbidity or mortality following hepatic resection.[123,151] Furthermore, PVE is not entirely without risk. Between 2% and 20% of patients fail to demonstrate remnant hypertrophy following PVE, and roughly 10% of patients suffer adverse events following the procedure.[149,154] Tumor progression following PVE may also be a concern, and has been documented in 17% to 25% of patients with colorectal liver metastases.[150,155]

Therefore, it has been suggested that PVE be indicated for an FLR volume of 20% or less in patients without underlying liver dysfunction.[112,123,150,156] Among patients with or at high risk for liver injury (eg, those who have received extensive preoperative systemic chemotherapy), PVE is recommended for an FLR volume of 30% or less.[112,124,156] In patients with severe hepatic fibrosis or cirrhosis, an FLR of 40% or less is the suggested cutoff value for PVE.[126,127,156]

Two-stage hepatectomy

Initially described by Adam and colleagues[157] in 2000, a 2-stage hepatectomy (TSH) is a potentially curative operative strategy in patients with multiple bilobar colorectal liver metastases that traditionally would be considered unresectable via a single operation, even in conjunction with systemic and local therapies. The first stage of the procedure consists of resection of metastases from only 1 hemiliver, with the intention of inducing compensatory hypertrophy of the remnant liver parenchyma. In select patients, chemotherapy or PVE following the first stage may be appropriate. In the second stage, meant to be potentially curative, all remaining metastases in the contralateral hemiliver are then resected. Although data examining TSHs are limited to single-institution studies with small patient cohorts and widely variable patient selection criteria, a recent meta-analysis found that in select patients with initially unresectable colorectal liver metastases, TSH resulted in low postoperative morbidity and mortality and acceptable survival outcomes.[158] In particular, these patients fared significantly better than their counterparts who received systemic chemotherapy alone. In 1 study examining long-term outcomes following TSH, despite higher postoperative morbidity, comparable 5-year survival was seen between patients undergoing completed TSH and those who underwent a single-stage hepatectomy during the same time period.[159]

Associating liver partition with portal vein ligation for staged hepatectomy

Associating Liver Partition with Portal Vein Ligation for Staged Hepatectomy (ALLPS) is a relatively new 2-stage approach to managing traditionally unresectable liver tumors. More specifically, it was developed to overcome several limitations of PVE, including the ineligibility of certain patients, such as those with portal vein thrombus, the potential for disease progression, and inadequate FLR hypertrophy following PVE. The procedure involves in situ splitting of the liver with right portal vein ligation in the first stage, inducing rapid FLR hypertrophy, followed by a short-interval second stage in which the atrophied contralateral lobe containing the tumor is resected.[160,161] Although several small case series have reported its technical feasibility, complications are high; long-term data are lacking, and its use is highly controversial.[162–168]

SUMMARY

The nuances of determining resectability for liver tumors can be difficult to navigate, owing to the variety of primary and secondary malignancies involving the liver, the range of patient-specific factors to consider, and the hepatic anatomic and functional variability that seems inevitable. The basic principles, however, are simple; if surgery is deemed appropriate from an oncologic standpoint, the patient is in reasonably good health, and the tumor can be safely removed without compromising the integrity of the future remnant, nearly all patients will be candidates for resection. However, as understanding of tumor biology expands, diagnostic and operative techniques evolve, and systemic and local therapies improve, the selection of patients for resection will continue to both expand and simultaneously be refined.

REFERENCES

1. Maithel SK, Ginsberg MS, D'Amico F, et al. Natural history of patients with sub-centimeter pulmonary nodules undergoing hepatic resection for metastatic colorectal cancer. J Am Coll Surg 2010;210(1):31–8.
2. Dewhurst C, Rosen MP, Blake MA, et al. ACR appropriateness criteria pretreatment staging of colorectal cancer. J Am Coll Radiol 2012;9(11):775–81.

3. Ramos E, Valls C, Martinez L, et al. Preoperative staging of patients with liver metastases of colorectal carcinoma. Does PET/CT really add something to multidetector CT? Ann Surg Oncol 2011;18(9):2654–61.
4. Petrowsky H, Wildbrett P, Husarik DB, et al. Impact of integrated positron emission tomography and computed tomography on staging and management of gallbladder cancer and cholangiocarcinoma. J Hepatol 2006;45(1):43–50.
5. Selzner M, Hany TF, Wildbrett P, et al. Does the novel PET/CT imaging modality impact on the treatment of patients with metastatic colorectal cancer of the liver? Ann Surg 2004;240(6):1027–34 [discussion: 1035–26].
6. Wiering B, Krabbe PF, Jager GJ, et al. The impact of fluor-18-deoxyglucose-positron emission tomography in the management of colorectal liver metastases. Cancer 2005;104(12):2658–70.
7. Figueras J, Valls C, Rafecas A, et al. Resection rate and effect of postoperative chemotherapy on survival after surgery for colorectal liver metastases. Br J Surg 2001;88(7):980–5.
8. Jarnagin WR, Conlon K, Bodniewicz J, et al. A clinical scoring system predicts the yield of diagnostic laparoscopy in patients with potentially resectable hepatic colorectal metastases. Cancer 2001;91(6):1121–8.
9. Jarnagin WR, Fong Y, Ky A, et al. Liver resection for metastatic colorectal cancer: assessing the risk of occult irresectable disease. J Am Coll Surg 1999; 188(1):33–42.
10. Rahusen FD, Cuesta MA, Borgstein PJ, et al. Selection of patients for resection of colorectal metastases to the liver using diagnostic laparoscopy and laparoscopic ultrasonography. Ann Surg 1999;230(1):31–7.
11. Goere D, Wagholikar GD, Pessaux P, et al. Utility of staging laparoscopy in subsets of biliary cancers: laparoscopy is a powerful diagnostic tool in patients with intrahepatic and gallbladder carcinoma. Surg Endosc 2006;20(5):721–5.
12. Biondi A, Tropea A, Basile F. Clinical rescue evaluation in laparoscopic surgery for hepatic metastases by colorectal cancer. Surg Laparosc Endosc Percutan Tech 2010;20(2):69–72.
13. Gholghesaei M, van Muiswinkel JM, Kuiper JW, et al. Value of laparoscopy and laparoscopic ultrasonography in determining resectability of colorectal hepatic metastases. HPB (Oxford) 2003;5(2):100–4.
14. Jarnagin WR, Bodniewicz J, Dougherty E, et al. A prospective analysis of staging laparoscopy in patients with primary and secondary hepatobiliary malignancies. J Gastrointest Surg 2000;4(1):34–43.
15. Grobmyer SR, Fong Y, D'Angelica M, et al. Diagnostic laparoscopy prior to planned hepatic resection for colorectal metastases. Arch Surg 2004;139(12): 1326–30.
16. Mann CD, Neal CP, Metcalfe MS, et al. Clinical risk score predicts yield of staging laparoscopy in patients with colorectal liver metastases. Br J Surg 2007; 94(7):855–9.
17. D'Angelica M, Fong Y, Weber S, et al. The role of staging laparoscopy in hepatobiliary malignancy: prospective analysis of 401 cases. Ann Surg Oncol 2003; 10(2):183–9.
18. Jemal A, Bray F, Center MM, et al. Global cancer statistics. CA Cancer J Clin 2011;61(2):69–90.
19. Forner A, Llovet JM, Bruix J. Hepatocellular carcinoma. Lancet 2012;379(9822): 1245–55.
20. Jarnagin W, Chapman WC, Curley S, et al. Surgical treatment of hepatocellular carcinoma: expert consensus statement. HPB (Oxford) 2010;12(5):302–10.

21. Vauthey JN, Lauwers GY, Esnaola NF, et al. Simplified staging for hepatocellular carcinoma. J Clin Oncol 2002;20(6):1527–36.
22. Liver. In: Edge SB, Byrd DR, Compton CC, et al, editors. AJCC cancer staging manual. 7th edition. New York: Springer; 2010. p. 191–200.
23. Mazzaferro V, Regalia E, Doci R, et al. Liver transplantation for the treatment of small hepatocellular carcinomas in patients with cirrhosis. N Engl J Med 1996; 334(11):693–9.
24. Mazzaferro V, Bhoori S, Sposito C, et al. Milan criteria in liver transplantation for hepatocellular carcinoma: an evidence-based analysis of 15 years of experience. Liver Transpl 2011;17(Suppl 2):S44–57.
25. A new prognostic system for hepatocellular carcinoma: a retrospective study of 435 patients: the Cancer of the Liver Italian Program (CLIP) investigators. Hepatology 1998;28(3):751–5.
26. Okuda K, Ohtsuki T, Obata H, et al. Natural history of hepatocellular carcinoma and prognosis in relation to treatment. Study of 850 patients. Cancer 1985;56(4): 918–28.
27. Tateishi R, Yoshida H, Shiina S, et al. Proposal of a new prognostic model for hepatocellular carcinoma: an analysis of 403 patients. Gut 2005;54(3):419–25.
28. Bruix J, Llovet JM. Prognostic prediction and treatment strategy in hepatocellular carcinoma. Hepatology 2002;35(3):519–24.
29. Llovet JM, Fuster J, Bruix J. Prognosis of hepatocellular carcinoma. Hepatogastroenterology 2002;49(43):7–11.
30. Befeler AS, Di Bisceglie AM. Hepatocellular carcinoma: diagnosis and treatment. Gastroenterology 2002;122(6):1609–19.
31. Hassoun Z, Gores GJ. Treatment of hepatocellular carcinoma. Clin Gastroenterol Hepatol 2003;1(1):10–8.
32. Nathan H, Schulick RD, Choti MA, et al. Predictors of survival after resection of early hepatocellular carcinoma. Ann Surg 2009;249(5):799–805.
33. Ng KK, Vauthey JN, Pawlik TM, et al. Is hepatic resection for large or multinodular hepatocellular carcinoma justified? results from a multi-institutional database. Ann Surg Oncol 2005;12(5):364–73.
34. Pawlik TM, Delman KA, Vauthey JN, et al. Tumor size predicts vascular invasion and histologic grade: implications for selection of surgical treatment for hepatocellular carcinoma. Liver Transpl 2005;11(9):1086–92.
35. Pawlik TM, Poon RT, Abdalla EK, et al. Hepatectomy for hepatocellular carcinoma with major portal or hepatic vein invasion: results of a multicenter study. Surgery 2005;137(4):403–10.
36. Pawlik TM, Poon RT, Abdalla EK, et al. Critical appraisal of the clinical and pathologic predictors of survival after resection of large hepatocellular carcinoma. Arch Surg 2005;140(5):450–7 [discussion: 457–58].
37. Predictive factors for long term prognosis after partial hepatectomy for patients with hepatocellular carcinoma in Japan. The Liver Cancer Study Group of Japan. Cancer 1994;74(10):2772–80.
38. Belghiti J, Panis Y, Farges O, et al. Intrahepatic recurrence after resection of hepatocellular carcinoma complicating cirrhosis. Ann Surg 1991;214(2):114–7.
39. Lai EC, Ng IO, Ng MM, et al. Long-term results of resection for large hepatocellular carcinoma: a multivariate analysis of clinicopathological features. Hepatology 1990;11(5):815–8.
40. Minagawa M, Ikai I, Matsuyama Y, et al. Staging of hepatocellular carcinoma: assessment of the Japanese TNM and AJCC/UICC TNM systems in a cohort of 13,772 patients in Japan. Ann Surg 2007;245(6):909–22.

41. Lee NH, Chau GY, Lui WY, et al. Surgical treatment and outcome in patients with a hepatocellular carcinoma greater than 10 cm in diameter. Br J Surg 1998; 85(12):1654–7.
42. Poon RT, Fan ST, Wong J. Selection criteria for hepatic resection in patients with large hepatocellular carcinoma larger than 10 cm in diameter. J Am Coll Surg 2002;194(5):592–602.
43. Zhou XD, Tang ZY, Ma ZC, et al. Surgery for large primary liver cancer more than 10 cm in diameter. J Cancer Res Clin Oncol 2003;129(9):543–8.
44. Kosuge T, Makuuchi M, Takayama T, et al. Long-term results after resection of hepatocellular carcinoma: experience of 480 cases. Hepatogastroenterology 1993;40(4):328–32.
45. Poon RT, Fan ST. Evaluation of the new AJCC/UICC staging system for hepatocellular carcinoma after hepatic resection in Chinese patients. Surg Oncol Clin N Am 2003;12(1):35–50, viii.
46. Lei HJ, Chau GY, Lui WY, et al. Prognostic value and clinical relevance of the 6th edition 2002 American joint committee on cancer staging system in patients with resectable hepatocellular carcinoma. J Am Coll Surg 2006; 203(4):426–35.
47. Tsai TJ, Chau GY, Lui WY, et al. Clinical significance of microscopic tumor venous invasion in patients with resectable hepatocellular carcinoma. Surgery 2000;127(6):603–8.
48. Li Q, Wang J, Juzi JT, et al. Clonality analysis for multicentric origin and intrahepatic metastasis in recurrent and primary hepatocellular carcinoma. J Gastrointest Surg 2008;12(9):1540–7.
49. Morimoto O, Nagano H, Sakon M, et al. Diagnosis of intrahepatic metastasis and multicentric carcinogenesis by microsatellite loss of heterozygosity in patients with multiple and recurrent hepatocellular carcinomas. J Hepatol 2003;39(2): 215–21.
50. Yamamoto T, Kajino K, Kudo M, et al. Determination of the clonal origin of multiple human hepatocellular carcinomas by cloning and polymerase chain reaction of the integrated hepatitis B virus DNA. Hepatology 1999;29(5):1446–52.
51. Cheng CH, Lee CF, Wu TH, et al. Evaluation of the new AJCC staging system for resectable hepatocellular carcinoma. World J Surg Oncol 2011;9:114.
52. Llovet JM, Bustamante J, Castells A, et al. Natural history of untreated nonsurgical hepatocellular carcinoma: rationale for the design and evaluation of therapeutic trials. Hepatology 1999;29(1):62–7.
53. Pawarode A, Voravud N, Sriuranpong V, et al. Natural history of untreated primary hepatocellular carcinoma: a retrospective study of 157 patients. Am J Clin Oncol 1998;21(4):386–91.
54. Vauthey JN, Klimstra D, Franceschi D, et al. Factors affecting long-term outcome after hepatic resection for hepatocellular carcinoma. Am J Surg 1995;169(1):28–34 [discussion: 34–5].
55. Ikai I, Yamamoto Y, Yamamoto N, et al. Results of hepatic resection for hepatocellular carcinoma invading major portal and/or hepatic veins. Surg Oncol Clin N Am 2003;12(1):65–75, ix.
56. Poon RT, Fan ST, Ng IO, et al. Prognosis after hepatic resection for stage IVA hepatocellular carcinoma: a need for reclassification. Ann Surg 2003;237(3): 376–83.
57. Uka K, Aikata H, Takaki S, et al. Clinical features and prognosis of patients with extrahepatic metastases from hepatocellular carcinoma. World J Gastroenterol 2007;13(3):414–20.

58. McGlynn KA, Tarone RE, El-Serag HB. A comparison of trends in the incidence of hepatocellular carcinoma and intrahepatic cholangiocarcinoma in the United States. Cancer Epidemiol Biomarkers Prev 2006;15(6):1198–203.
59. Shaib YH, Davila JA, McGlynn K, et al. Rising incidence of intrahepatic cholangiocarcinoma in the United States: a true increase? J Hepatol 2004;40(3):472–7.
60. Dodson RM, Weiss MJ, Cosgrove D, et al. Intrahepatic cholangiocarcinoma: management options and emerging therapies. J Am Coll Surg 2013;217(4): 736–50.e734.
61. Liver. In: Greene FL, Page DL, Fleming ID, et al, editors. AJCC cancer staging manual. 6th edition. New York: Springer-Verlag; 2002. p. 131–8.
62. Nathan H, Aloia TA, Vauthey JN, et al. A proposed staging system for intrahepatic cholangiocarcinoma. Ann Surg Oncol 2009;16(1):14–22.
63. Okabayashi T, Yamamoto J, Kosuge T, et al. A new staging system for mass-forming intrahepatic cholangiocarcinoma: analysis of preoperative and postoperative variables. Cancer 2001;92(9):2374–83.
64. Wang Y, Li J, Xia Y, et al. Prognostic nomogram for intrahepatic cholangiocarcinoma after partial hepatectomy. J Clin Oncol 2013;31(9):1188–95.
65. Yamasaki S. Intrahepatic cholangiocarcinoma: macroscopic type and stage classification. J Hepatobiliary Pancreat Surg 2003;10(4):288–91.
66. Intrahepatic bile ducts. In: Edge SB, Byrd DR, Compton CC, et al, editors. AJCC cancer staging manual. 7th edition. New York: Springer; 2010. p. 201–10.
67. Hyder O, Marques H, Pulitano C, et al. A nomogram to predict long-term survival after resection for intrahepatic cholangiocarcinoma: an Eastern and Western experience. JAMA Surg 2014;149(5):432–8.
68. Choi SB, Kim KS, Choi JY, et al. The prognosis and survival outcome of intrahepatic cholangiocarcinoma following surgical resection: association of lymph node metastasis and lymph node dissection with survival. Ann Surg Oncol 2009;16(11):3048–56.
69. de Jong MC, Nathan H, Sotiropoulos GC, et al. Intrahepatic cholangiocarcinoma: an international multi-institutional analysis of prognostic factors and lymph node assessment. J Clin Oncol 2011;29(23):3140–5.
70. Inoue K, Makuuchi M, Takayama T, et al. Long-term survival and prognostic factors in the surgical treatment of mass-forming type cholangiocarcinoma. Surgery 2000;127(5):498–505.
71. Endo I, Gonen M, Yopp AC, et al. Intrahepatic cholangiocarcinoma: rising frequency, improved survival, and determinants of outcome after resection. Ann Surg 2008;248(1):84–96.
72. Weber SM, Jarnagin WR, Klimstra D, et al. Intrahepatic cholangiocarcinoma: resectability, recurrence pattern, and outcomes. J Am Coll Surg 2001;193(4):384–91.
73. Spolverato G, Kim Y, Alexandrescu S, et al. Is hepatic resection for large or multifocal intrahepatic cholangiocarcinoma justified? results from a multi-institutional collaboration. Ann Surg Oncol 2015;22(7):2218–25.
74. Ribero D, Pinna AD, Guglielmi A, et al. Surgical approach for long-term survival of patients with intrahepatic cholangiocarcinoma: a multi-institutional analysis of 434 patients. Arch Surg 2012;147(12):1107–13.
75. Spolverato G, Ejaz A, Kim Y, et al. Tumor size predicts vascular invasion and histologic grade among patients undergoing resection of intrahepatic cholangiocarcinoma. J Gastrointest Surg 2014;18(7):1284–91.
76. Konstadoulakis MM, Roayaie S, Gomatos IP, et al. Fifteen-year, single-center experience with the surgical management of intrahepatic cholangiocarcinoma: operative results and long-term outcome. Surgery 2008;143(3):366–74.

77. Ali SM, Clark CJ, Zaydfudim VM, et al. Role of major vascular resection in patients with intrahepatic cholangiocarcinoma. Ann Surg Oncol 2013;20(6): 2023–8.
78. Manfredi S, Lepage C, Hatem C, et al. Epidemiology and management of liver metastases from colorectal cancer. Ann Surg 2006;244(2):254–9.
79. Weiss L, Grundmann E, Torhorst J, et al. Haematogenous metastatic patterns in colonic carcinoma: an analysis of 1541 necropsies. J Pathol 1986;150(3):195–203.
80. House MG, Ito H, Gönen M, et al. Survival after hepatic resection for metastatic colorectal cancer: trends in outcomes for 1,600 patients during two decades at a single institution. J Am Coll Surg 2010;210(5):744–52, 752–5.
81. Tomlinson JS, Jarnagin WR, DeMatteo RP, et al. Actual 10-year survival after resection of colorectal liver metastases defines cure. J Clin Oncol 2007; 25(29):4575–80.
82. Fong Y, Fortner J, Sun RL, et al. Clinical score for predicting recurrence after hepatic resection for metastatic colorectal cancer: analysis of 1001 consecutive cases. Ann Surg 1999;230(3):309–18 [discussion: 318–21].
83. Kato T, Yasui K, Hirai T, et al. Therapeutic results for hepatic metastasis of colorectal cancer with special reference to effectiveness of hepatectomy: analysis of prognostic factors for 763 cases recorded at 18 institutions. Dis Colon Rectum 2003;46(10 Suppl):S22–31.
84. Nordlinger B, Guiguet M, Vaillant JC, et al. Surgical resection of colorectal carcinoma metastases to the liver. A prognostic scoring system to improve case selection, based on 1568 patients. Association Francaise de Chirurgie. Cancer 1996;77(7):1254–62.
85. Rees M, Tekkis PP, Welsh FK, et al. Evaluation of long-term survival after hepatic resection for metastatic colorectal cancer: a multifactorial model of 929 patients. Ann Surg 2008;247(1):125–35.
86. Wei AC, Greig PD, Grant D, et al. Survival after hepatic resection for colorectal metastases: a 10-year experience. Ann Surg Oncol 2006;13(5):668–76.
87. Carpizo DR, Are C, Jarnagin W, et al. Liver resection for metastatic colorectal cancer in patients with concurrent extrahepatic disease: results in 127 patients treated at a single center. Ann Surg Oncol 2009;16(8):2138–46.
88. Elias D, Liberale G, Vernerey D, et al. Hepatic and extrahepatic colorectal metastases: when resectable, their localization does not matter, but their total number has a prognostic effect. Ann Surg Oncol 2005;12(11):900–9.
89. Elias D, Ouellet JF, Bellon N, et al. Extrahepatic disease does not contraindicate hepatectomy for colorectal liver metastases. Br J Surg 2003;90(5):567–74.
90. Saklad M. Grading of patients for surgical procedures. Anesthesiology 1941;2: 281–4.
91. Oken MM, Creech RH, Tormey DC, et al. Toxicity and response criteria of the Eastern cooperative oncology group. Am J Clin Oncol 1982;5(6):649–55.
92. Charlson ME, Pompei P, Ales KL, et al. A new method of classifying prognostic comorbidity in longitudinal studies: development and validation. J Chronic Dis 1987;40(5):373–83.
93. Goldman L, Caldera DL, Nussbaum SR, et al. Multifactorial index of cardiac risk in noncardiac surgical procedures. N Engl J Med 1977;297(16):845–50.
94. Makary MA, Segev DL, Pronovost PJ, et al. Frailty as a predictor of surgical outcomes in older patients. J Am Coll Surg 2010;210(6):901–8.
95. Revenig LM, Canter DJ, Taylor MD, et al. Too frail for surgery? initial results of a large multidisciplinary prospective study examining preoperative variables predictive of poor surgical outcomes. J Am Coll Surg 2013;217(4):665–70.e661.

96. Nuzzo G, Giordano M, Giuliante F, et al. Complex liver resection for hepatic tumours involving the inferior vena cava. Eur J Surg Oncol 2011;37(11):921–7.
97. Hemming AW, Reed AI, Langham MR Jr, et al. Combined resection of the liver and inferior vena cava for hepatic malignancy. Ann Surg 2004;239(5):712–9 [discussion: 719–21].
98. Shi J, Lai EC, Li N, et al. Surgical treatment of hepatocellular carcinoma with portal vein tumor thrombus. Ann Surg Oncol 2010;17(8):2073–80.
99. Wu CC, Hsieh SR, Chen JT, et al. An appraisal of liver and portal vein resection for hepatocellular carcinoma with tumor thrombi extending to portal bifurcation. Arch Surg 2000;135(11):1273–9.
100. Pesi B, Ferrero A, Grazi GL, et al. Liver resection with thrombectomy as a treatment of hepatocellular carcinoma with major vascular invasion: results from a retrospective multicentric study. Am J Surg 2015;210(1):35–44.
101. Gruttadauria S, Marsh JW, Bartlett DL, et al. Ex situ resection techniques and liver autotransplantation: last resource for otherwise unresectable malignancy. Dig Dis Sci 2005;50(10):1829–35.
102. Oldhafer KJ, Lang H, Schlitt HJ, et al. Long-term experience after ex situ liver surgery. Surgery 2000;127(5):520–7.
103. Sugimachi K, Shirabe K, Taketomi A, et al. Successful curative extracorporeal hepatic resection for far-advanced hepatocellular carcinoma in an adolescent patient. Liver Transpl 2010;16(5):685–7.
104. Hemming AW, Cattral MS. Ex vivo liver resection with replacement of the inferior vena cava and hepatic vein replacement by transposition of the portal vein. J Am Coll Surg 1999;189(5):523–6.
105. Lodge JP, Ammori BJ, Prasad KR, et al. Ex vivo and in situ resection of inferior vena cava with hepatectomy for colorectal metastases. Ann Surg 2000;231(4):471–9.
106. Abdalla EK, Denys A, Chevalier P, et al. Total and segmental liver volume variations: implications for liver surgery. Surgery 2004;135(4):404–10.
107. Heymsfield SB, Fulenwider T, Nordlinger B, et al. Accurate measurement of liver, kidney, and spleen volume and mass by computerized axial tomography. Ann Intern Med 1979;90(2):185–7.
108. Saito S, Yamanaka J, Miura K, et al. A novel 3D hepatectomy simulation based on liver circulation: application to liver resection and transplantation. Hepatology 2005;41(6):1297–304.
109. Yamanaka J, Saito S, Fujimoto J. Impact of preoperative planning using virtual segmental volumetry on liver resection for hepatocellular carcinoma. World J Surg 2007;31(6):1249–55.
110. Vauthey JN, Abdalla EK, Doherty DA, et al. Body surface area and body weight predict total liver volume in Western adults. Liver Transpl 2002;8(3):233–40.
111. Johnson TN, Tucker GT, Tanner MS, et al. Changes in liver volume from birth to adulthood: a meta-analysis. Liver Transpl 2005;11(12):1481–93.
112. Abdalla EK, Barnett CC, Doherty D, et al. Extended hepatectomy in patients with hepatobiliary malignancies with and without preoperative portal vein embolization. Arch Surg 2002;137(6):675–80 [discussion: 680–71].
113. Ribero D, Abdalla EK, Madoff DC, et al. Portal vein embolization before major hepatectomy and its effects on regeneration, resectability and outcome. Br J Surg 2007;94(11):1386–94.
114. Vauthey JN, Pawlik TM, Abdalla EK, et al. Is extended hepatectomy for hepatobiliary malignancy justified? Ann Surg 2004;239(5):722–30 [discussion: 730–2].

115. Karoui M, Penna C, Amin-Hashem M, et al. Influence of preoperative chemotherapy on the risk of major hepatectomy for colorectal liver metastases. Ann Surg 2006;243(1):1–7.

116. Nakano H, Oussoultzoglou E, Rosso E, et al. Sinusoidal injury increases morbidity after major hepatectomy in patients with colorectal liver metastases receiving preoperative chemotherapy. Ann Surg 2008;247(1):118–24.

117. Pawlik TM, Olino K, Gleisner AL, et al. Preoperative chemotherapy for colorectal liver metastases: impact on hepatic histology and postoperative outcome. J Gastrointest Surg 2007;11(7):860–8.

118. Vauthey JN, Pawlik TM, Ribero D, et al. Chemotherapy regimen predicts steatohepatitis and an increase in 90-day mortality after surgery for hepatic colorectal metastases. J Clin Oncol 2006;24(13):2065–72.

119. Kishi Y, Zorzi D, Contreras CM, et al. Extended preoperative chemotherapy does not improve pathologic response and increases postoperative liver insufficiency after hepatic resection for colorectal liver metastases. Ann Surg Oncol 2010;17(11):2870–6.

120. Nordlinger B, Sorbye H, Glimelius B, et al. Perioperative chemotherapy with FOLFOX4 and surgery versus surgery alone for resectable liver metastases from colorectal cancer (EORTC Intergroup trial 40983): a randomised controlled trial. Lancet 2008;371(9617):1007–16.

121. Cleary JM, Tanabe KT, Lauwers GY, et al. Hepatic toxicities associated with the use of preoperative systemic therapy in patients with metastatic colorectal adenocarcinoma to the liver. Oncologist 2009;14(11):1095–105.

122. Shindoh J, Tzeng CW, Aloia TA, et al. Optimal future liver remnant in patients treated with extensive preoperative chemotherapy for colorectal liver metastases. Ann Surg Oncol 2013;20(8):2493–500.

123. Kishi Y, Abdalla EK, Chun YS, et al. Three hundred and one consecutive extended right hepatectomies: evaluation of outcome based on systematic liver volumetry. Ann Surg 2009;250(4):540–8.

124. Azoulay D, Castaing D, Krissat J, et al. Percutaneous portal vein embolization increases the feasibility and safety of major liver resection for hepatocellular carcinoma in injured liver. Ann Surg 2000;232(5):665–72.

125. Narita M, Oussoultzoglou E, Fuchshuber P, et al. What is a safe future liver remnant size in patients undergoing major hepatectomy for colorectal liver metastases and treated by intensive preoperative chemotherapy? Ann Surg Oncol 2012;19(8):2526–38.

126. Shirabe K, Shimada M, Gion T, et al. Postoperative liver failure after major hepatic resection for hepatocellular carcinoma in the modern era with special reference to remnant liver volume. J Am Coll Surg 1999;188(3):304–9.

127. Clavien PA, Petrowsky H, DeOliveira ML, et al. Strategies for safer liver surgery and partial liver transplantation. N Engl J Med 2007;356(15):1545–59.

128. Bruix J, Castells A, Bosch J, et al. Surgical resection of hepatocellular carcinoma in cirrhotic patients: prognostic value of preoperative portal pressure. Gastroenterology 1996;111(4):1018–22.

129. Franco D, Capussotti L, Smadja C, et al. Resection of hepatocellular carcinomas. Results in 72 European patients with cirrhosis. Gastroenterology 1990; 98(3):733–8.

130. Teh SH, Nagorney DM, Stevens SR, et al. Risk factors for mortality after surgery in patients with cirrhosis. Gastroenterology 2007;132(4):1261–9.

131. Schroeder RA, Marroquin CE, Bute BP, et al. Predictive indices of morbidity and mortality after liver resection. Ann Surg 2006;243(3):373–9.

132. Kamath PS, Wiesner RH, Malinchoc M, et al. A model to predict survival in patients with end-stage liver disease. Hepatology 2001;33(2):464–70.
133. Wiesner RH, McDiarmid SV, Kamath PS, et al. MELD and PELD: application of survival models to liver allocation. Liver Transpl 2001;7(7):567–80.
134. Teh SH, Christein J, Donohue J, et al. Hepatic resection of hepatocellular carcinoma in patients with cirrhosis: Model of End-Stage Liver Disease (MELD) score predicts perioperative mortality. J Gastrointest Surg 2005;9(9):1207–15 [discussion: 1215].
135. Cucchetti A, Ercolani G, Vivarelli M, et al. Impact of model for end-stage liver disease (MELD) score on prognosis after hepatectomy for hepatocellular carcinoma on cirrhosis. Liver Transpl 2006;12(6):966–71.
136. Pugh RN, Murray-Lyon IM, Dawson JL, et al. Transection of the oesophagus for bleeding oesophageal varices. Br J Surg 1973;60(8):646–9.
137. Maithel SK, Kneuertz PJ, Kooby DA, et al. Importance of low preoperative platelet count in selecting patients for resection of hepatocellular carcinoma: a multi-institutional analysis. J Am Coll Surg 2011;212(4):638–48 [discussion: 648–50].
138. Manizate F, Hiotis SP, Labow D, et al. Liver functional reserve estimation: state of the art and relevance for local treatments: the Western perspective. J Hepatobiliary Pancreat Sci 2010;17(4):385–8.
139. Cucchetti A, Ercolani G, Vivarelli M, et al. Is portal hypertension a contraindication to hepatic resection? Ann Surg 2009;250(6):922–8.
140. Jarnagin WR, Gonen M, Fong Y, et al. Improvement in perioperative outcome after hepatic resection: analysis of 1,803 consecutive cases over the past decade. Ann Surg 2002;236(4):397–406 [discussion: 406–7].
141. Poon RT, Fan ST, Lo CM, et al. Improving perioperative outcome expands the role of hepatectomy in management of benign and malignant hepatobiliary diseases: analysis of 1222 consecutive patients from a prospective database. Ann Surg 2004;240(4):698–708 [discussion: 708–10].
142. Kaneko K, Shirai Y, Wakai T, et al. Low preoperative platelet counts predict a high mortality after partial hepatectomy in patients with hepatocellular carcinoma. World J Gastroenterol 2005;11(37):5888–92.
143. Caesar J, Shaldon S, Chiandussi L, et al. The use of indocyanine green in the measurement of hepatic blood flow and as a test of hepatic function. Clin Sci 1961;21:43–57.
144. Imamura H, Seyama Y, Kokudo N, et al. One thousand fifty-six hepatectomies without mortality in 8 years. Arch Surg 2003;138(11):1198–206 [discussion: 1206].
145. Bennett JJ, Blumgart LH. Assessment of hepatic reserve prior to hepatic resection. J Hepatobiliary Pancreat Surg 2005;12(1):10–5.
146. Ijichi M, Makuuchi M, Imamura H, et al. Portal embolization relieves persistent jaundice after complete biliary drainage. Surgery 2001;130(1):116–8.
147. Uesaka K, Nimura Y, Nagino M. Changes in hepatic lobar function after right portal vein embolization. An appraisal by biliary indocyanine green excretion. Ann Surg 1996;223(1):77–83.
148. Hirai I, Kimura W, Fuse A, et al. Evaluation of preoperative portal embolization for safe hepatectomy, with special reference to assessment of nonembolized lobe function with 99mTc-GSA SPECT scintigraphy. Surgery 2003;133(5):495–506.
149. Abdalla EK, Hicks ME, Vauthey JN. Portal vein embolization: rationale, technique and future prospects. Br J Surg 2001;88(2):165–75.
150. Shindoh J, Tzeng CW, Aloia TA, et al. Portal vein embolization improves rate of resection of extensive colorectal liver metastases without worsening survival. Br J Surg 2013;100(13):1777–83.

151. Farges O, Belghiti J, Kianmanesh R, et al. Portal vein embolization before right hepatectomy: prospective clinical trial. Ann Surg 2003;237(2):208–17.

152. Shindoh J, Truty MJ, Aloia TA, et al. Kinetic growth rate after portal vein embolization predicts posthepatectomy outcomes: toward zero liver-related mortality in patients with colorectal liver metastases and small future liver remnant. J Am Coll Surg 2013;216(2):201–9.

153. Leung U, Simpson AL, Araujo RL, et al. Remnant growth rate after portal vein embolization is a good early predictor of post-hepatectomy liver failure. J Am Coll Surg 2014;219(4):620–30.

154. Di Stefano DR, de Baere T, Denys A, et al. Preoperative percutaneous portal vein embolization: evaluation of adverse events in 188 patients. Radiology 2005;234(2):625–30.

155. Hoekstra LT, van Lienden KP, Doets A, et al. Tumor progression after preoperative portal vein embolization. Ann Surg 2012;256(5):812–7 [discussion: 817–8].

156. Abdalla EK, Adam R, Bilchik AJ, et al. Improving resectability of hepatic colorectal metastases: expert consensus statement. Ann Surg Oncol 2006;13(10):1271–80.

157. Adam R, Laurent A, Azoulay D, et al. Two-stage hepatectomy: A planned strategy to treat irresectable liver tumors. Ann Surg 2000;232(6):777–85.

158. Lam VW, Laurence JM, Johnston E, et al. A systematic review of two-stage hepatectomy in patients with initially unresectable colorectal liver metastases. HPB (Oxford) 2013;15(7):483–91.

159. Wicherts DA, Miller R, de Haas RJ, et al. Long-term results of two-stage hepatectomy for irresectable colorectal cancer liver metastases. Ann Surg 2008;248(6):994–1005.

160. Schnitzbauer AA, Lang SA, Goessmann H, et al. Right portal vein ligation combined with in situ splitting induces rapid left lateral liver lobe hypertrophy enabling 2-staged extended right hepatic resection in small-for-size settings. Ann Surg 2012;255(3):405–14.

161. Alvarez FA, Ardiles V, Sanchez Claria R, et al. Associating liver partition and portal vein ligation for staged hepatectomy (ALPPS): tips and tricks. J Gastrointest Surg 2013;17(4):814–21.

162. Aloia TA, Vauthey JN. Associating liver partition and portal vein ligation for staged hepatectomy (ALPPS): what is gained and what is lost? Ann Surg 2012;256(3):e9 [author reply: e16–9].

163. Li J, Girotti P, Konigsrainer I, et al. ALPPS in right trisectionectomy: a safe procedure to avoid postoperative liver failure? J Gastrointest Surg 2013;17(5):956–61.

164. Vennarecci G, Laurenzi A, Levi Sandri GB, et al. The ALPPS procedure for hepatocellular carcinoma. Eur J Surg Oncol 2014;40(8):982–8.

165. Vennarecci G, Laurenzi A, Santoro R, et al. The ALPPS procedure: a surgical option for hepatocellular carcinoma with major vascular invasion. World J Surg 2014;38(6):1498–503.

166. Andriani OC. Long-term results with associating liver partition and portal vein ligation for staged hepatectomy (ALPPS). Ann Surg 2012;256(3):e5 [author reply: e16–9].

167. de Santibanes E, Clavien PA. Playing play-doh to prevent postoperative liver failure: the "ALPPS" approach. Ann Surg 2012;255(3):415–7.

168. Ratti F, Schadde E, Masetti M, et al. Strategies to increase the resectability of patients with colorectal liver metastases: a multi-center case-match analysis of alpps and conventional two-stage hepatectomy. Ann Surg Oncol 2015;22(6):1933–42.

Anatomy of Hepatic Resectional Surgery

Michael C. Lowe, MD[a], Michael I. D'Angelica, MD[a,b],*

KEYWORDS

- Liver anatomy • Hepatic resections • Parenchymal-sparing resections
- Intraoperative management

KEY POINTS

- Liver anatomy can be variable, and understanding of anatomic variations is crucial to performing hepatic resections, particularly parenchymal-sparing resections.
- Anatomic knowledge is a critical prerequisite for effective hepatic resection with minimal blood loss, parenchymal preservation, and optimal oncologic outcome.
- Each anatomic resection has pitfalls, about which the operating surgeon should be aware and comfortable managing intraoperatively.

LIVER ANATOMY
Historical Definitions

Historically, the liver was described as having 2 anatomic lobes, the larger right lobe and the smaller left lobe. These lobes are separated on the anterior surface of the liver by the falciform ligament, and on the inferior surface by the ligamentum teres as it enters the umbilical fissure. The liver is invested by peritoneum except on its posterior surface, where the peritoneum reflects to create the right and left triangular ligaments. The area between the folds of peritoneum that create the triangular ligaments is devoid of peritoneum and is referred to as the bare area. The retrohepatic inferior vena cava (IVC) lies within this bare area on the undersurface of the liver. The gastrohepatic ligament attaches to the ligamentum venosum, which separates the historically defined right and left lobes of the liver on its posterior surface (**Fig. 1**). This common early definition of liver anatomy was based on external landmarks and has no real relationship to functional anatomy. In fact, the liver does not have reliable external landmarks for most current functional definitions.

Conflicts of Interest/Funding Sources: None.
[a] Department of Surgery, Memorial Sloan Kettering Cancer Center, 1275 York Avenue, New York, NY 10065, USA; [b] Weill Cornell University School of Medicine, New York, NY 10065, USA
* Corresponding author.
E-mail address: dangelim@mskcc.org

Surg Clin N Am 96 (2016) 183–195
http://dx.doi.org/10.1016/j.suc.2015.11.003
0039-6109/16/$ – see front matter © 2016 Elsevier Inc. All rights reserved.

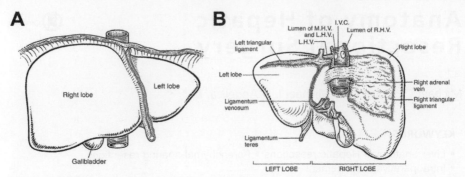

Fig. 1. The external anatomy of the liver as seen from the anterior (*A*) and posterior (*B*) surfaces. (*From* Blumgart LH, Hann LE. Surgical and radiologic anatomy of the liver, biliary tract, and pancreas. In: Jarnagin WR, Blumgart LH, eds. Blumgart's surgery of the liver, biliary tract and pancreas. 5th edition. Philadelphia: Elsevier; 2012; with permission.)

Vascular Anatomy

The hepatic veins drain the liver directly into the suprahepatic IVC. The larger right hepatic vein has a short 1 cm extrahepatic course, while the smaller middle and left hepatic veins usually join a common trunk 1 to 2 cm in length before entering the IVC separately from the right hepatic vein. Occasionally, the left and middle hepatic veins will drain separately into the IVC. The umbilical vein typically runs anterior to the umbilical fissure and most commonly drains into the left hepatic vein, but can join into the middle hepatic vein or join both the middle and left hepatic veins as a trifurcation. Although intrahepatic venous branching can be variable, there are common branches found in most cases. The right hepatic vein provides the dominant drainage of the posterior sector, and its branches typically drain from the right into the main trunk. The middle hepatic vein commonly drains a large right-sided branch which serves as the principal drainage of segment VIII. Segment IV typically derives its venous drainage from branches of the left hepatic and umbilical veins. There are variable and typically numerous retrohepatic venous branches that drain directly from the caudate lobe into the vena cava. Accessory hepatic veins are common and most frequently involve the right side of the liver as an inferior right hepatic vein draining directly into the vena cava independent of the right hepatic vein.

The hepatic artery and portal vein inflow to and biliary drainage of the liver have many anatomic variations. With conventional anatomy, the portal vein, common bile duct, and hepatic artery run in the porta hepatis. The portal vein sits posteriorly, while the bile duct runs anteriorly and to the right of the portal vein; the hepatic artery runs anteriorly and to the left of the portal vein.

The hepatic artery arises from the celiac axis and becomes the proper hepatic artery after giving off the gastroduodenal and right gastric arteries. It then branches into the right and left hepatic arteries. The left branch extends toward the base of the umbilical fissure and gives off branches to the caudate lobe and segments II-IV. Often the left hepatic artery branches into lateral and medial branches extrahepatically that feed segments II, II, and IV, respectively. The segment IV branch can also arise from the right hepatic artery and was historically referred to as the middle hepatic artery. The right hepatic artery usually passes posterior to the common hepatic duct, although it passes anteriorly in about 10% to 20% of cases. The right hepatic artery typically splits into an anterior and posterior branch, which can often be dissected in an extrahepatic location.

The most common variations in arterial anatomy are replaced or accessory right or left hepatic arteries arising from the superior mesenteric or left gastric arteries, respectively. A replaced branch has an aberrant origin and provides complete blood supply to a hemi-liver, whereas an accessory branch has an aberrant origin but only provides additional blood supply to a hemi-liver. Aberrant arterial anatomy occurs in approximately 40% of individuals, and almost any combination of arterial branches can be present. A replaced right hepatic artery runs laterally to the common bile duct and can easily be injured when dissecting the porta hepatis without prior knowledge of its aberrant location. A replaced left hepatic artery runs in the gastrohepatic ligament and can be injured when mobilizing the left lobe of the liver. The common hepatic artery can also originate from the superior mesenteric artery and run in the same plane as a replaced right hepatic artery. A summary of the most frequently occurring arterial anomalies can be found in **Fig. 2**.

The portal vein is created by the confluence of the splenic and superior mesenteric veins behind the neck of the pancreas. It ascends behind the common bile duct and the hepatic artery into the hilus of the liver, where it bifurcates into a larger right portal vein and smaller left portal vein. The left branch enters the umbilical fissure and supplies the left liver. The right branch, which has a much shorter extrahepatic course, divides into the right anterior and the right posterior sectoral branches. The most common variations of portal venous anatomy can be seen in **Fig. 3**. Although almost any variation is possible, the most common anatomic variation involves the branching of the right portal vein with either a lack of a main right portal vein or separate origins of the anterior and posterior sectoral branches.

Biliary drainage follows a remarkably similar anatomic pathway as the portal inflow. The right anterior and right posterior sectoral branches combine to form the right hepatic duct, which has a short extrahepatic course before joining the left hepatic duct at the biliary confluence to form the common hepatic duct. The left hepatic duct courses along the base of segment IV; it can be accessed by incising Glisson capsule at the base of the quadrate lobe, a maneuver referred to as lowering the hilar plate. Common anomalies in biliary anatomy include a trifurcation (12%) and ectopic drainage of right sectoral ducts into the common or left hepatic duct (20%). These and the remaining biliary anomalies can be seen in **Fig. 4**.

Functional Surgical Anatomy

Couinaud segments

Understanding the internal anatomy of the liver is essential to performing hepatic resections, and in particular, parenchymal-preserving resections. The functional anatomy of the liver described by Couinaud serves as the most useful for the surgeon and is quite different from the historically defined hepatic lobes based on external landmarks.[1] According to Couinaud descriptions, the 3 main hepatic veins separate the liver into 4 sectors, each of which is fed by a portal pedicle that includes a branch of the hepatic artery, portal vein, and bile duct. The right and left hemi-livers are divided by the main portal scissura, which contains the middle hepatic vein. This main portal scissura progresses from the gallbladder fossa anteriorly to the left of the IVC posteriorly, and these landmarks serve as external boundaries of the line between the functional right and left liver. Both the right and left hemi-livers are further divided into sectors by scissurae containing the right and left hepatic veins, respectively (**Fig. 5**).

The right portal scissura separates the right liver into the anterior and posterior sectors, which are further subdivided into segments. The right anterior sector is comprised of segments V inferiorly and VIII superiorly, and the right posterior sector

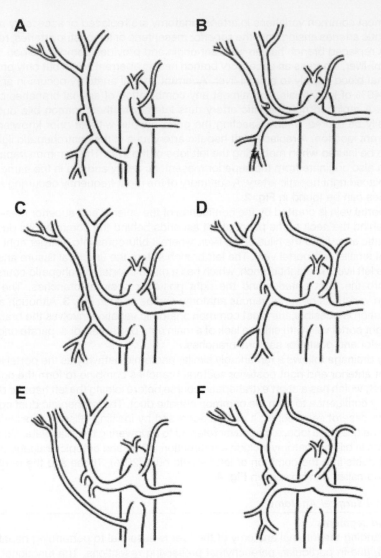

Fig. 2. Variations in hepatic arterial anatomy. These include a replaced common hepatic artery (*A*), a very short common hepatic artery origin from the celiac axis (*B*), a replaced (*C*) or accessory (*E*) right hepatic artery arising from the superior mesenteric artery, and a replaced (*D*) or accessory (*F*) left hepatic artery arising from the left gastric artery. (*From* Blumgart LH, Hann LE. Surgical and radiologic anatomy of the liver, biliary tract, and pancreas. In: Jarnagin WR, Blumgart LH, eds. Blumgart's surgery of the liver, biliary tract and pancreas. 5th edition. Philadelphia: Elsevier; 2012; with permission.)

is comprised of segments VI inferiorly and VII superiorly. The left portal scissura, which runs to the left of and posterior to the ligamentum teres along the course of the left hepatic vein, separates the left liver into the anterior and posterior sectors. Segments IV and III make up the anterior sector, and the posterior sector is comprised only of segment II (**Fig. 6**). Segment IV can further be divided into segment IVA superiorly and segment IVB inferiorly based on the branching of the left portal pedicle (see

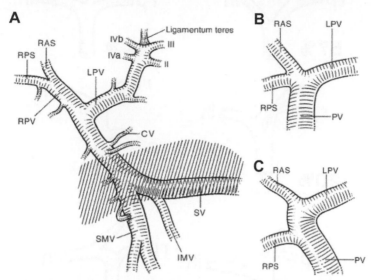

Fig. 3. Variations in portal venous anatomy. In normal anatomy the splenic vein (SV) and superior mesenteric vein combine to form the portal vein, which branches into the right portal vein (RPV) and left portal vein (LPV). The RPV further branches in right anterior sectoral (RAS) and right posterior sectoral (RPS) branches (*A*). The RAS, RPS, and LPV can all arise independently from the main portal vein (*B*). The RPS may arise early from the portal vein, which then bifurcates in the RAS and LPV (*C*). CV, coronary vein; IMV, inferior mesenteric vein; SMV, superior mesenteric vein. (*From* Blumgart LH, Hann LE. Surgical and radiologic anatomy of the liver, biliary tract, and pancreas. In: Jarnagin WR, Blumgart LH, eds. Blumgart's surgery of the liver, biliary tract and pancreas. 5th edition. Philadelphia: Elsevier; 2012; with permission.)

Fig. 5), although this branching is variable and does not often result in an easily defined segment IVA and B. The caudate lobe (segment I) is the portion of liver that lies between the IVC and the main portal pedicle and straddles the retrohepatic IVC (**Fig. 7**). It is supplied by vessels from both the right and left portal pedicles, and biliary drainage follows a similar pattern. The caudate lobe is the only portion of the liver that drains directly into the IVC.

Brisbane terminology

An alternative nomenclature was devised by the Scientific Committee of the International Hepato-Pancreato-Biliary Association (IHPBA) in Brisbane, Australia, in 2000.[2] This terminology was created in an attempt to clarify the confusion surrounding the terminology of liver anatomy and resections. The main difference between the Couinaud description and the Brisbane 2000 Terminology is the renaming of Couinaud sectors as sections. Furthermore, the left liver is not divided into 2 sectors based on the left hepatic vein. The left liver is defined as having a lateral section (segments II and III) and a medial section (segment IV). This new classification of the left liver is not based on the left portal scissura, but rather on the division of the left liver by the line between the falciform ligament and the umbilical fissure. The anatomic terms, Couinaud segments, and surgical resection terms for all anatomic resections are included in **Table 1**.

Variations in Anatomy

Ultimately, the true definition of segmental anatomy is dictated by the vascular/biliary pedicle supplying each segment. While the previously described anatomic

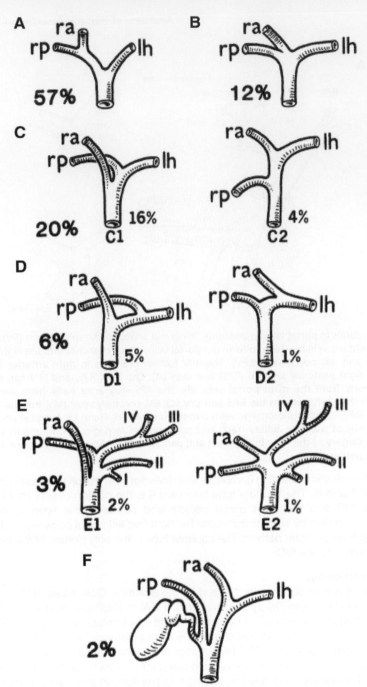

Fig. 4. Variations in biliary anatomy. With typical anatomy the right anterior and posterior sectoral branches combine to form the right hepatic duct, which combines with left hepatic duct to form the common hepatic duct (*A*). Variations include a triple confluence (*B*), ectopic drainage of the right sectoral duct into the common hepatic duct (*C*), ectopic drainage of either of the right sectoral branches into the left hepatic duct (*D*), absence of the confluence (*E*), and absence of the right hepatic duct and drainage of the right posterior duct into the cystic duct (*F*). (*From* Blumgart LH, Hann LE. Surgical and radiologic anatomy of the liver, biliary tract, and pancreas. In: Jarnagin WR, Blumgart LH, eds. Blumgart's surgery of the liver, biliary tract and pancreas. 5th edition. Philadelphia: Elsevier; 2012; with permission.)

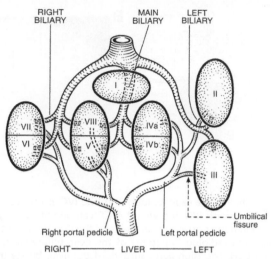

Fig. 5. The segmental anatomy of the liver, which is determined by the portal inflow and hepatic outflow. (*From* Blumgart LH, Hann LE. Surgical and radiologic anatomy of the liver, biliary tract, and pancreas. In: Jarnagin WR, Blumgart LH, eds. Blumgart's surgery of the liver, biliary tract and pancreas. 5th edition. Philadelphia: Elsevier; 2012; with permission.)

descriptions serve as a guide for resectional surgery, it is vital to recognize anatomic variations on preoperative imaging and confirm these findings using intraoperative ultrasound. There are an infinite number of anatomic variations in vascular branching patterns as well as segmental size and location that will not always follow the textbook definitions provided in this article. Every planned resection should be preceded by high-quality cross-sectional imaging with an assessment of vascular and segmental anatomy. Alterations in planned resections may be required if anatomic variations or additional malignant-appearing tumors are found. The ultimate goal is to accomplish an oncologically appropriate resection leaving a remnant with sufficient portal venous and hepatic arterial supply, biliary drainage, and unopposed venous outflow.

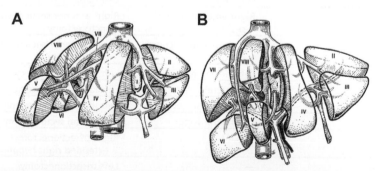

Fig. 6. The functional division of the liver as seen in the patient (*A*) and ex vivo (*B*). (*From* Blumgart LH, Hann LE. Surgical and radiologic anatomy of the liver, biliary tract, and pancreas. In: Jarnagin WR, Blumgart LH, eds. Blumgart's surgery of the liver, biliary tract and pancreas. 5th edition. Philadelphia: Elsevier; 2012; with permission.)

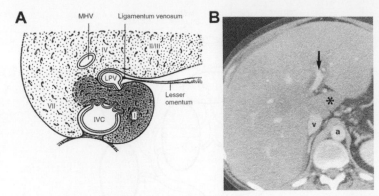

Fig. 7. (A) The relationship of the caudate lobe (I) to the IVC, portal vein (LPV), middle hepatic vein (MHV), and segments II/III and VII. (B) A CT scan demonstrating the caudate lobe (*asterisk*) situated between the portal vein (*arrow*) and the IVC (V). a, Aorta. (*From* Blumgart LH, Hann LE. Surgical and radiologic anatomy of the liver, biliary tract, and pancreas. In: Jarnagin WR, Blumgart LH, eds. Blumgart's surgery of the liver, biliary tract and pancreas. 5th edition. Philadelphia: Elsevier; 2012; with permission.)

USING ANATOMY TO GUIDE RESECTIONAL SURGERY
Minimizing Operative Morbidity

Parenchymal preservation without oncologic compromise
Historically, liver resection was associated with high morbidity and mortality related to blood loss and hepatic failure. With recent advancements in surgical technique and anesthesia, morbidity and mortality rates have dramatically decreased. A major part of the reason for this decrease is the increased use of parenchymal-preserving liver resection. In a recent single-institution analysis of 3876 patients undergoing 4152 liver resections for cancer from 1993 to 2012, the percentage of major hepatectomies

Table 1
Surgical resection terms and their related anatomic terms and Couinaud segments

Couinaud Segments	Anatomic Term	Surgical Resection Term
5–8	Right liver	Right hepatectomy
2–4	Left liver	Left hepatectomy
5, 8	Right anterior section/sector	Right anterior sectionectomy/sectorectomy
6, 7	Right posterior section/sector	Right posterior sectionectomy/sectorecomty
4	Left medial section	Left medial sectionectomy
2, 3	Left lateral section	Left lateral sectionectomy
4, 3	Left medial sector	Left medial sectorectomy
2	Left lateral sector	Left lateral sectorectomy
4–8	—	Right trisectionectomy/extended right hepatectomy
2–4, 5, 8	—	Left trisectionectomy/extended left hepatectomy
Any segment 1–8	Segment	Segmentectomy
Any 2 contguous segments	—	Bisegmentectomy

decreased from 66% to 36%. During this same period, the 90-day mortality decreased from 5% to 1.6%, and the perioperative morbidity decreased from 53% to 20%. Over this period of time, the mortality of major resections such as trisectionectomy (6%) and right hepatectomy (3%) did not change, strongly suggesting that the improvements in perioperative outcome were mostly related to the increase in the percentage of parenchymal-sparing resections.[3] The theoretic concern with parenchymal-sparing surgery is compromised oncologic outcome. To the contrary, numerous studies have shown that performing parenchymal-sparing resections does not result in inferior survival, particularly for colorectal liver metastases.[4–10] A meta-analysis of 7 non-randomized controlled studies found no significant difference in surgical margins, overall survival, and disease-free survival between patients undergoing anatomic and nonanatomic resections.[11]

Minimizing blood loss

Although specific techniques employed to minimize blood loss will be covered elsewhere, it is important to appreciate the importance of limiting hemorrhage, which historically has contributed to significant perioperative morbidity. This can be accomplished most successfully by maintaining a low central venous pressure (CVP) during parenchymal resection. This reduces hepatic venous distention, which significantly decreases backbleeding when the liver parenchymal is transected.[12] Maintaining low CVP during liver resection reduces intraoperative blood loss, in-hospital mortality, and postoperative morbidity.[13] Postoperative renal failure is possible after low CVP anesthesia, but this complication is rare if the patient is resuscitated to euvolemia immediately upon completion of the parenchymal transection. In a recent study of 2116 patients undergoing low CVP-assisted hepatectomy, less than 1% of patients developed clinically relevant acute kidney injury.[14]

Vascular occlusion also can contribute to control of intraoperative blood loss. Hepatic inflow arrest was first described by Pringle in the setting of trauma,[15] and this remains the standard method by which control of portal venous and hepatic arterial inflow is gained. Encircling the hepatoduodenal ligament allows for simultaneous occlusion of the portal vein and hepatic artery. Intermittent occlusion permits longer periods of occlusion, but the length of inflow occlusion should be limited as much as possible, particularly with an abnormal liver. More complex vascular exclusion techniques, such as hepatic vascular exclusion, will be covered elsewhere. Although inflow occlusion is not required for all cases, it is an important tool to be used if there is inflow bleeding during hepatic transection.

GENERAL ANATOMIC CONCEPTS AND PITFALLS IN SPECIFIC RESECTIONS
Right Hepatectomy

Descriptions of this operation are common, and there are numerous techniques to accomplish a safe and effective right hepatectomy. Most commonly, the right liver is mobilized completely off of the diaphragm and vena cava by dividing the often numerous retrohepatic venous branches. The right caval ligament, which runs laterally to the right hepatic vein and envelops the vena cava posteriorly circumferentially to join the left side of the caudate, must be encircled and divided to expose the right hepatic vein. Dissection along the vena cava to encircle the right hepatic vein can be accomplished after this ligament is divided. Inflow to the liver can be taken in a number of ways, including extrahepatic ligation of inflow vessels or ligation of the right inflow pedicle inside the liver. Pedicle ligation can be carried out through hepatotomies or by splitting the liver down to the pedicle in an anterior approach. If an extrahepatic ligation of vessels is carried out, it is advisable, if possible, to take the right hepatic bile duct intrahepatically in the main pedicle to minimize the chance of contralateral biliary injury. Regardless of the approach to the inflow vessels, knowledge of the inflow vessels and their anatomy and variation is critical. Once inflow is taken, the right hepatic vein is divided and most commonly divided extrahepatically. The line of transection is along the middle hepatic vein, which can be taken or preserved depending on the location of the tumor to be resected. Maintaining transection in this plane is important in order to prevent leaving ischemic liver tissue behind.

There are several anatomic variations that are relevant to the performance of this operation. A large inferior right hepatic vein can be present and serve as the primary venous drainage of segment VI. This needs to be divided as the liver is mobilized off of the vena cava. The right portal vein has a wide range of anatomic presentations ranging from a long segment prior to sectoral/segmental branching, to the complete lack of a true right portal vein with immediate branching into segmental/sectoral branches. Lastly, the right anterior portal vein and pedicle can originate off of the left inflow and necessitate intrahepatic control. The right portal vein almost always gives off a small posterior branch to the caudate process that can be a common source of bleeding during extrahepatic dissection. The right hepatic artery typically runs posterior to the common hepatic duct, but in about 10% to 20% of cases, it runs anterior to the duct. A replaced right hepatic artery is common and runs posteriorly in the porta between the portal vein and common bile duct. The most common biliary anomalies include a right sectoral branch draining into the left hepatic duct. Lastly, the left hepatic duct as it arises from the common hepatic duct can originate close to the right inflow, and injury to this duct during transection of right-sided inflow structures can be disastrous. Lowering of the hilar plate is helpful to both identify and protect the left hepatic duct. These abnormalities can all be detected on high-quality cross-sectional imaging and should be evaluated prior to operation.

Right Posterior Sectorectomy

This resection removes segments VI and VII of the liver, and the principle transection plane is the right portal scissura along the right hepatic vein. The right liver should be mobilized as is done for a right hepatectomy. Although not critical for every case, it is advisable to dissect and control the right hepatic vein. Knowledge of the posterior sectoral inflow anatomy is important. There often is not a common posterior sectoral trunk dividing into segment VI and VII branches. Often the segment VI and VII inflow pedicles branch almost immediately off of the right inflow pedicle. This requires taking these pedicles individually inside the liver. Although the posterior sectoral inflow vessels can be dissected extrahepatically, this is, in general, difficult and not necessary. The plane of the right hepatic vein can be visualized by intraoperative ultrasound and marked. The transection plane is somewhat horizontal toward the right edge of the vena cava. The transection plane is divided down to the inflow pedicles, which are divided intrahepatically to ensure that the dissection has not gone too far to the left into the anterior sectoral pedicles. Although preferable to preserve the right hepatic vein, this vessel can be taken, since the middle hepatic vein is the principal venous drainage for the anterior sector.

Right Anterior Sectorectomy

This resection is challenging in that it requires 2 long lines of transection to encompass segments V and VIII. The main anterior pedicle at its origin will almost always take all of the inflow to these segments, although occasionally segment V will have extra inflow pedicles from the posterior sectoral pedicle or the central inflow pedicles at the main branching points in the porta. The key to the operation is identification and ligation of the main anterior pedicle, which, is best accomplished intrahepatically if the tumor allows. The main anterior pedicle can be found by transecting along the middle hepatic vein, since it terminates in branches coursing to the left of and anterior to the anterior pedicle. Thus transection of the liver in the main portal scissura exposes the main right anterior pedicle after ligating and dividing these terminal middle hepatic vein branches. The middle hepatic vein can be taken in this operation, since segment IV can drain into the umbilical vein, which most commonly originates from the left hepatic vein. It is critical to preserve the right hepatic vein, since this is the venous drainage of the posterior sector. The posterior extent of dissection does not require division down to the vena cava, since the well-vascularized caudate lobe lies posteriorly and does not need to be taken as part of this operation.

Central Hepatectomy

This resection is similar to an anterior sectorectomy, except that the left extent of the resection takes some or all of segment IV and mandates resection of the middle hepatic vein. The inflow to segment IV can easily be taken intrahepatically while transecting the liver to the right of the umbilical fissure. The segment IV pedicles are almost always multiple and do not neatly divide into segment IVA and IVB branches. At the base of segment IV, the dissection must turn sharply to the right to avoid the main left inflow structures. Similar to an anterior sectorectomy, dissection then commences to the right, taking terminal middle hepatic vein branches to isolate the main right anterior inflow pedicle. Other technical issues are the same as an anterior sectorectomy.

Left Hepatectomy

The left liver is situated anterior to the caudate lobe and therefore does not require mobilization off of the vena cava. The inflow to the left liver is more accessible than the right-sided structures, and extrahepatic isolation and division are fairly straightforward. The left hepatic artery courses cephalad along the left side of the porta hepatis anteriorly and is relatively easy to encircle. Once encircled, it should be ensured that one has not come around the proper hepatic artery prior to branching; this can happen easily if the branching is more distal. Simple dissection or clamping with palpation of a right-sided pulse is sufficient. Often the left hepatic artery branches into medial (segment IV) and lateral (segments II and III) branches, but a common variation is that the segment IV branch (previously called the middle hepatic artery) comes off the right hepatic artery. Posteriorly, the left portal vein can be dissected. Confirmation of portal anatomy requires visualization of the portal bifurcation. The left portal vein gives off a small branch to the caudate lobe, which should be identified and preserved if possible. Just beyond the caudate branch, the ligamentum venosum inserts into the left portal vein and can be seen with careful dissection. This area of insertion usually is surrounded by fibrous tissue. The safest place to divide the left portal vein is between the caudate branch and the insertion of the ligamentum venosum. The left bile duct runs at the base of segment IV before branching into the left liver. Whenever possible, the left bile duct should be divided within the main left pedicle intrahepatically. Biliary anomalies are most relevant for left-sided resections, since right sectoral branches can be found draining into the left bile duct. If a tumor mandates division of the left bile duct extrahepatically, these biliary anomalies should be sought and defined with preoperative imaging and during dissection. The left hepatic vein typically courses anterior to the segment II pedicle and then runs posterior to the segment III pedicle.

A left hepatectomy can be performed either by taking or preserving the middle hepatic vein. Although the middle hepatic vein is typically the dominant venous drainage of the right anterior sector, there is almost always sufficient venous collateral to the right hepatic vein to provide adequate drainage. It is often difficult to isolate the left and middle hepatic vein individually in an extrahepatic location, but sometimes with careful dissection this can be done. In order to divide the left and middle hepatic veins at their common trunk extrahepatically, dissection between the right and middle hepatic veins superiorly at the suprahepatic vena cava demonstrates a wide tunnel. Posterior to the left liver, the ligamentum venosum is divided and retracted cephalad to expose a space anterior to the caudate lobe and between the hepatic parenchyma and the left/middle hepatic vein common trunk. This is often a tight space and requires meticulous dissection to avoid vascular injury or bleeding. Alternatively, either vein can be approached by splitting the liver back to its origin and dividing the veins after the parenchymal dissection has exposed their origin. As for a right hepatectomy, the plane of transection is in the main portal scissura in the plain of the middle hepatic vein.

Left Lateral Sectionectomy

A left lateral sectionectomy is a relatively straightforward resection that is most easily accomplished by taking inflow and outflow structures intrahepatically. The segment II and III pedicles are relatively constant in branching and location but can occasionally vary. Sometimes their origins are close, and they may even share a common trunk. Small branches other than the main segmental pedicles are commonly encountered. Although these inflow pedicles can be dissected in the umbilical fissure or encircled by making flanking hepatotomies, the simplest method to expose them is to split the liver in the plane just to the left of the umbilical fissure down to their origins. In this manner, each pedicle can be encircled and divided. The left hepatic vein typically joins the middle hepatic vein in a relatively intrahepatic position, and therefore isolating the left hepatic vein extrahepatically can be difficult and is usually not necessary. The left hepatic vein origin can be defined by splitting the liver to the point where the left hepatic vein joins the middle hepatic vein. The umbilical vein runs in the plane anterior to the umbilical fissure and most commonly joins the left hepatic vein, although sometimes it will come off the common channel or middle hepatic vein. The umbilical vein is in the plane of resection for a left lateral sectionectomy and can be preserved or taken; either way, its location should be noted as it can be a source of bleeding during transection.

Wedge/Atypical/Single Segment Resections

Detailed descriptions of every potential atypical or single segment resection are beyond the scope of this article. Nonetheless, careful review of anatomic variation and careful intrahepatic dissection with the help of intraoperative ultrasound should be able to identify any inflow or outflow structure in order to accomplish any of these resections in proper anatomic planes without devascularizing large amounts of hepatic parenchyma. Single-segment resections require careful isolation of the inflow pedicle or pedicles, and knowledge of common variations is necessary. For example, segment VIII typically has a single dominant pedicle that divides into a ventral and dorsal branch. This is a remarkably consistent anatomic finding. On the other hand, segment V typically does not have a dominant inflow pedicle and has numerous inflow branches, most commonly coming off the main right anterior pedicle. Segmental resections also mandate that parenchymal transection takes place in a scissura along the main hepatic veins. As operations for multiple bilobar tumors have become more common the use of wedge and atypical resections has become more common. From an anatomic perspective, the surgeon, with careful review of imaging and use of intraoperative ultrasound, must ensure that these resections do not divide major inflow and outflow vessels to other parts of the liver. As long as major vessels are preserved, these atypical resections outside of typical anatomic planes are safe and effective.

REFERENCES

1. Couinaud C. Anatomic principles of left and right regulated hepatectomy: technics. J Chir (Paris) 1954;70(12):933–66 [in French].
2. Strasberg SM. Nomenclature of hepatic anatomy and resections: a review of the Brisbane 2000 system. J Hepatobiliary Pancreat Surg 2005;12(5):351–5.
3. Kingham TP, Correa-Gallego C, D'Angelica MI, et al. Hepatic parenchymal preservation surgery: decreasing morbidity and mortality rates in 4,152 resections for malignancy. J Am Coll Surg 2015;220(4):471–9.
4. Gold JS, Are C, Kornprat P, et al. Increased use of parenchymal-sparing surgery for bilateral liver metastases from colorectal cancer is associated with improved mortality without change in oncologic outcome: trends in treatment over time in 440 patients. Ann Surg 2008;247(1):109–17.
5. Karanjia ND, Lordan JT, Quiney N, et al. A comparison of right and extended right hepatectomy with all other hepatic resections for colorectal liver metastases: a ten-year study. Eur J Surg Oncol 2009;35(1):65–70.
6. Kokudo N, Tada K, Seki M, et al. Anatomical major resection versus nonanatomical limited resection for liver metastases from colorectal carcinoma. Am J Surg 2001;181(2):153–9.
7. Lalmahomed ZS, Ayez N, van der Pool AE, et al. Anatomical versus nonanatomical resection of colorectal liver metastases: is there a difference in surgical and oncological outcome? World J Surg 2011;35(3):656–61.
8. Stewart GD, O'Súilleabháin CB, Madhavan KK, et al. The extent of resection influences outcome following hepatectomy for colorectal liver metastases. Eur J Surg Oncol 2004;30(4):370–6.
9. Tanaka K, Shimada H, Matsumoto C, et al. Impact of the degree of liver resection on survival for patients with multiple liver metastases from colorectal cancer. World J Surg 2008;32(9):2057–69.
10. von Heesen M, Schuld J, Sperling J, et al. Parenchyma-preserving hepatic resection for colorectal liver metastases. Langenbecks Arch Surg 2012; 397(3):383–95.
11. Sui CJ, Cao L, Li B, et al. Anatomical versus nonanatomical resection of colorectal liver metastases: a meta-analysis. Int J Colorectal Dis 2012;27(7):939–46.
12. Jones RM, Moulton CE, Hardy KJ. Central venous pressure and its effect on blood loss during liver resection. Br J Surg 1998;85(8):1058–60.
13. Chen H, Merchant NB, Didolkar MS. Hepatic resection using intermittent vascular inflow occlusion and low central venous pressure anesthesia improves morbidity and mortality. J Gastrointest Surg 2000;4(2):162–7.
14. Correa-Gallego C, Berman A, Denis SC, et al. Renal function after low central venous pressure-assisted liver resection: assessment of 2116 cases. HPB (Oxford) 2015;17(3):258–64.
15. Pringle JH. V. Notes on the arrest of hepatic hemorrhage due to trauma. Ann Surg 1908;48(4):541–9.

Preoperative Assessment and Optimization of the Future Liver Remnant

Pragatheeshwar Thirunavukarasu, MD, Thomas A. Aloia, MD*

KEYWORDS

- Liver cancer • Liver metastases • Liver surgery • Steatosis
- Chemotherapy-associated hepatotoxicity • Portal vein embolization

KEY POINTS

- Patients who undergo liver resection and have an inadequate future liver remnant (FLR) volume are at increased risk for postoperative morbidity and mortality.
- The absolute volume of FLR required to avoid postoperative liver insufficiency depends on patient, disease, and anatomic factors.
- Rapid expansion of the FLR can be achieved with portal venous embolization (PVE) of the contralateral liver segments.
- PVE is a safe and effective procedure, when performed at high-volume hepatobiliary centers.
- Following PVE, the kinetic growth rate is the most reliable predictor of freedom from postoperative liver insufficiency.

The principle that guides curative treatment of both primary and secondary hepatobiliary malignancies is complete resection of all tumors. Anatomy and tumor factors, including tumor size and location, often mandate resection of several liver segments to obtain adequate margins. Patients who undergo liver resection and have an inadequate future liver remnant (FLR) volume are at increased risk for postoperative morbidity and mortality.[1] In patients who are anticipated to have a marginal or inadequate FLR volume, rapid expansion of the FLR can be achieved with portal venous embolization (PVE) of the contralateral liver segments.

MEASUREMENT OF PREOPERATIVE LIVER VOLUME AND FUNCTION

When evaluating a candidate for liver resection, history and physical examination are essential. It is important to detect any stigmata of hepatic dysfunction, including

Disclosures: The authors have nothing to disclose.
HPB Surgery Section, Department of Surgical Oncology, UT-MD Anderson Cancer Center, 1400 Herman Pressler Drive, Unit 1484, Houston, TX 77030, USA
* Corresponding author.
E-mail address: taaloia@mdanderson.org

Surg Clin N Am 96 (2016) 197–205
http://dx.doi.org/10.1016/j.suc.2015.11.001
0039-6109/16/$ – see front matter © 2016 Elsevier Inc. All rights reserved.

jaundice, scleral icterus, hepatomegaly, or ascites. It is also important to inquire about the existence of viral hepatitis or other predispositions to liver disease, including alcohol use.

When planning for major liver resection, it is also vital to assess baseline liver volume and function. There are several methods for evaluating liver volumes and function with both imaging modalities and biochemical markers. With baseline liver volumetry, it is possible to calculate the FLR volume based on the planned resection in order to predict the need for preoperative liver augmentation as well as to predict procedure-related morbidity and mortality.

Although ultrasound was the first modality used to calculate liver volumes, it has largely been replaced by cross-sectional imaging techniques. The technique of computed tomography (CT) volumetry was described and validated in 1979 by comparing CT volumetry with actual explanted liver volumes.[2] This initial report established CT scan as a noninvasive, accurate, and reproducible means of assessing liver volumes. Subsequently, CT-based liver volumetry was shown to correlate with clinical outcomes.[3] The advent of helical, multidetector, thin-slice CT scanning has made the rapid acquisition of high-resolution images increasingly available. This technique allows the images to be obtained during a single breath-hold, minimizing artifact and increasing quality and accuracy.

Once images are obtained from the CT scan, either manual or automated techniques are used for calculating liver volumes. The manual process involves a radiologist electronically tracing the contours of the liver. Hepatic and portal vein branch anatomy is used to delineate segments.[4] Manual techniques, although time consuming, provide the most accurate estimate of liver volume.[5] Increased accuracy is achieved through the exclusion of nearby structures, including the gallbladder, vasculature, and major fissures. Automated algorithms, which work from source images alone, have also been described. These automated methods take significantly less time to calculate and have had adequate correlation when compared with manual calculations. Despite these findings, software for fully automated techniques remains expensive, and most centers continue to use manual calculations.

Individuals who have underlying liver parenchymal disease, such as cirrhosis or steatosis, may benefit from functional as well as anatomic volumetric assessment. Indocyanine green and technetium-99m galactosyl serum albumin have both been used to estimate FLR function. When combined with CT volumetry, the clearance of these substances can help stratify patients into groups who will need PVE versus those who do not. However, these functional tests are not available in most Western centers, explaining the dependence of these centers on volumetry alone. In these centers, hypertrophic response to PVE is used as the marker for functional capacity of the FLR.

INDICATIONS FOR FUNCTIONAL LIVER REMNANT AUGMENTATION

Many factors have to be considered when deciding whether a patient will require PVE before resection. The first step is characterizing the patient's liver with regard to underlying parenchymal disease. This step is necessary to define what an acceptable FLR volume following resection for that individual will be. Other patient-centered characteristics, such as height and body surface area (BSA), also need to be considered. Tall individuals with larger BSA will require higher FLR volume than shorter patients having the same magnitude of hepatectomy. Vauthey and colleagues[6] have shown that total liver volume (TLV) is best estimated when controlling for BSA in Western adults; they developed a BSA-based formula that remains the most accurate method of predicting TLV. In addition, the patient's age, nutritional status, comorbidities, and functional status can affect the degree of hypertrophy (DH) achieved after PVE. Finally, the surgical procedure itself must be characterized with regard to extent, complexity, and any simultaneously performed procedures. Once the patient factors have been considered and it is determined that resection will be undertaken, the next step in evaluation is volumetry. The mainstay of liver volume evaluation is CT volumetry, and once performed, the estimated TLV and FLR volume can be used to determine the need for PVE.

Considerable heterogeneity exists not only in TLV from person to person but also in individual liver segment volumes. CT volumetry across populations shows that the lateral left liver (segments II and III) contributes less than 20% of the TLV in more than 75% of patients.[1] Without preoperative liver augmentation, therefore, up to 20% of individuals undergoing right hepatectomy and most undergoing extended right hepatectomy would have inadequate FLR volume. In contrast, most patients undergoing extended left hepatectomy will not require PVE because the right posterior sector (segments VI and VII) typically comprises 33% of the liver.

Although considerable debate exists over the hypertrophic efficacy of PVE versus portal venous ligation (PVL), it is now clear that that PVE performed with microspheres is superior to PVL. PVL failures are likely secondary to intrahepatic porto-porto shunting that is eliminated by PVE, but remains a deterrent to hypertrophy in patients treated with PVL.

Noncirrhotic liver has a greater regenerative capacity than a cirrhotic liver, tolerates injury better, and ultimately functions more efficiently. Individuals with normal liver function and no parenchymal disease can survive resection of up to 80% of the liver provided vascular inflow, vascular outflow, and biliary drainage are maintained. Cirrhotic patients can tolerate far less parenchymal loss and are unlikely to survive resection of more than 60% of the liver.[7] Even with considerably smaller parenchymal resections, patients with cirrhosis remain at elevated risk of perioperative morbidity, including fluid retention, ascites, and wound breakdown. When any individual undergoes liver resection and the FLR volume is inadequate, the sequela is postresection hepatic failure that frequently leads to multisystem organ failure and death.

In patients with normal livers, the indications for PVE have evolved with the greater accuracy of CT volumetry and the use of standardized liver volumes. It has been shown that the likelihood of postoperative complications is predicted more accurately by FLR volume than resected liver volume.[8] Extended resections can be achieved with very low risk of death from liver failure; however, standardized FLR volume less than 20% of TLV is associated with a greatly increased risk of complications.

A considerable number of patients will have undergone neoadjuvant chemotherapy before liver resection. In these patients, the chemotherapeutic agents that they have been exposed to must be known before any operative planning. Both irinotecan-based and oxaliplatin flouropyrimidine chemotherapy regimens can induce liver injury.[9] In particular, the use of irinotecan in patients with metabolic syndrome is associated with steatohepatitis, impaired liver regeneration, and death after major hepatectomy. For patients who received preoperative chemotherapy, there is likely to be benefit to PVE when the FLR volume is estimated to be less than 30% of TLV (**Fig. 1**).

The impact of steatosis and steatohepatitis on decision-making for PVE is complex. To date, there have been no large clinical trials that address selection of patients with steatosis and steatohepatitis and, consequently, there is no uniform formula that can be used to adjust FLR expectations before resection. In patients with mild to moderate steatosis and normal liver function tests, proceeding according to established volumetric guidelines is usually safe. In patients with severe steatosis or any evidence of

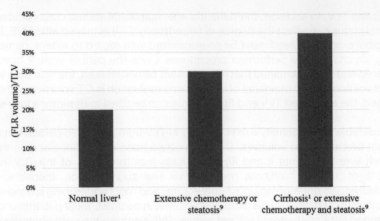

Fig. 1. Minimum FLR volume cutoff values typically used to inform the risk of postoperative liver insufficiency. TLV, total liver volume. (*Data from* Abdalla EK, Denys A, Chevalier P, et al. Total and segmental liver volume variations: implications for liver surgery. Surgery 2004;135:404–10; and Vauthey JN, Pawlik TM, Ribero D, et al. Chemotherapy regimen predicts steatohepatitis and an increase in 90-day mortality after surgery for hepatic colorectal metastases. J Clin Oncol 2006;24:2065–72.)

steatohepatitis, surgical planning should be undertaken cautiously and higher FLR volumes should be targeted.

In patients with chronic liver disease, preoperative assessment is essential. Extended hepatectomy is rarely an option for cirrhotic patients; however, major hepatectomy can often be performed safely in carefully selected patients who have preserved liver function, Child-Turcotte-Pugh class A status, and low model for end-stage liver disease score.[10] In these patients, PVE is indicated when the FLR volume is less than 40% of the TLV.[11] Patients with cirrhosis who undergo PVE before right hepatectomy have been shown to have fewer complications and shorter intensive care unit and hospital length of stay than those who do not.[12] In patients with hepatocellular carcinoma and cirrhosis, it is possible to perform resection following sequential chemoembolization and PVE. This strategy has been shown to atrophy the embolized liver and cause a greater DH in the FLR.[13] Patients who have severe portal hypertension are not candidates for liver resection and are therefore not candidates for PVE. The absolute contraindications to performing PVE are portal hypertension (gradient >~14 mm Hg) and extensive tumor thrombus in the targeted branch of the portal vein. Severe portal hypertension usually precludes hepatic resection, and therefore, PVE would only serve to create additional morbidity. Relative contraindications include uncorrectable coagulopathy, undrained biliary obstruction of the FLR, and renal insufficiency.

PORTAL VENOUS EMBOLIZATION TECHNIQUES

There are 2 major steps in PVE: obtaining access to the portal venous system and embolization of target vessels. It is important to note that the selection of vascular access to the portal venous system can dictate what embolic materials can be safely used. Several factors may dictate the selection of approach and embolic materials, including patient-specific clinical and technical considerations, operator experience and preference, and the type and extent of planned resection.

Percutaneous transhepatic portal vein embolization (PTPE) can be performed by either the ipsilateral or the contralateral approach. The ipsilateral approach involves puncture of a peripheral right portal vein branch and use of a 180° reverse curved catheter in order to embolize the right portal branches, whereas the contralateral approach involves the puncture of a left portal vein branch to gain access to the right portal circulation to facilitate embolization. These procedures can be performed safely as an outpatient procedure under sedation or general anesthesia, although some centers elect to admit patients for observation. Unless a simultaneous biliary procedure is performed, there is no need for periprocedural antibiotics. With either the ipsilateral or the contralateral approach, it is important to leave at least 1 cm of the proximal main portal vein free of embolic material in order to facilitate surgical control at the time of resection.

For the ipsilateral technique, portal venous access is obtained within the portion of the liver that is planned for resection; this has the advantage of leaving the FLR untouched and less susceptible to vascular injury/thrombosis from the percutaneous puncture. When embolization of the right portal vein needs to be extended to segment IV, it is recommended that segment IV embolization be performed first.[14] This sequencing is preferred due to the difficulty in exchanging catheters through a previously embolized segment of portal vein and the risk of dislodging embolic materials.

The contralateral approach has the advantage of antegrade cannulation of the right portal branches without the sharp angulation that is often encountered during ipsilateral embolization. This approach allows the embolic material to be delivered in a prograde fashion and also allows portograms to be obtained without the risk of dislodging embolic materials. When embolizing the right portal vein, the portal vein of segment III is usually punctured because it is the most anterior and allows access to segment IV branches when needed. Puncture through the recess of Rex should be avoided because of thick and fibrotic tissues in the periportal area. The operator should also be aware of a frequent variant of liver anatomy wherein the right anterior portal vein enters the left main portal vein.

Although most centers favor PTPE because of its simplicity, a transileocolic portal vein embolization (TIPE) has been described.[15] This approach requires the patient to be placed under general anesthesia and a laparotomy performed with a pararectus skin incision in the right lower quadrant. After confirming that there is no peritoneal dissemination or tumor extension that would jeopardize a subsequent liver resection, a portion of the ileum is extracted from the abdomen. A branch of the ileocolic vein is selected, cannulated, and used to facilitate portography and embolization.

There are several embolic agents available for use in PVE. There are no large randomized trials that compare embolic agents and most information is derived from small retrospective cohorts and expert opinion. The guiding principles behind selection of embolic materials were introduced by Madoff and colleagues[16] as an agent that causes permanent PVE without recanalization, is well tolerated by the patient, and is easy to use. In the authors' experience at a high-volume center, PVE with embolic microspheres produces the most complete distal (small vessel) embolization, which induces greater subsequent FLR hypertrophy.

POSTPROCEDURAL COMPLICATIONS

PVE is a technique that is used to improve the morbidity and mortality after liver resection. It is important to weigh the risk reduction at the time of resection versus immediate morbidity from the embolization itself. Although it is considered relatively safe, PVE does have the potential for complications or failure.

The Cardiovascular and Interventional Radiological Society of Europe guidelines indicate that PVE should be performed with a minor complication rate of less than 20% to 25% and major complication rate of less than 5%. In addition, it is important that even major complications not preclude major hepatectomy.[17] Complications, like the procedure itself, can be divided into 2 groups: those occurring secondary to vascular access and those secondary to embolization.

Complications related to access include mechanical injuries that occur along the puncture route and include arterial, venous, biliary, and pleural injuries. Arterial injuries are typically the most morbid and usually occur from injury of hepatic or intercostal arteries. These injuries manifest as subcapsular or intrahepatic hematomas, pseudoaneurysm, or hemothorax. When investigating an occult injury, signs such as hypotension and tachycardia may manifest, but often there are more subtle indicators including right upper quadrant pain, shoulder pain, dyspnea, or confusion. Upon suspecting an arterial injury, immediate resuscitative measures to treat hemorrhagic shock should be undertaken. Only after the patient is hemodynamically stable, a contrast CT scan of the chest and abdomen, including arterial and portal venous phase, should be obtained. Arterial injuries are generally considered major complications because they almost always require reintervention in order to control bleeding. Subcapsular hematoma, even when not associated with a pseudoaneurysm, requires close clinical follow-up, because the hematoma can limit or prevent hypertrophy of the FLR. Pseudoaneurysm typically requires transarterial embolization, but this must be used with care because it can compromise the remaining blood supply to the FLR.

Venous injuries are typically limited to the contralateral approach because it requires puncture of the contralateral portal vein. These injuries can lead to slow-growing subcapsular hematomas that do not present as acutely as arterial injuries. These hematomas, if unrecognized, can also cause compression of the FLR and impair hypertrophy.

Biliary injuries are typically less serious than vascular injuries. It is not uncommon for the bile duct to be inadvertently punctured; despite this, biliary injuries rarely become symptomatic or severe. Bile leak and hemobilia are the most common manifestations. Bile leak typically requires treatment with biliary drainage. Hemobilia may indicate an iatrogenic arteriobiliary fistula that will require embolization if it is persistent or severe. In patients with biliary obstruction, cholangitis after PVE can occur because of inadvertent biliary puncture and presents with classic symptoms. This complication can be avoided by draining the biliary tree before PVE, particularly in patients with cholangiocarcinoma and central biliary obstruction.

Pneumothorax and hemothorax are rare injuries usually resulting from pleural injury during a right transhepatic approach. Acute onset of chest pain, dyspnea, tachypnea, tachycardia, cyanosis, and/or absent breath sounds should raise clinical concerns for pleural injury resulting in pneumothorax or hemothorax. Any suspicion of these conditions warrants immediate chest radiograph to diagnose and guide therapy. Pneumothorax should be treated following conventional algorithms. Injury to an intercostal artery may cause hemothorax that can ultimately require chest tube placement and embolization of the offending intercostal branch to restore hemodynamic stability.

TIPE eliminates some of the risk associated with direct parenchymal or pleural injury. However, this comes at the cost of the injuries typically associated with laparotomy, including bleeding, ileus, enterotomy related to bowel manipulation or freeing of adhesions, wound complications, and more. TIPE must also be performed under general anesthesia and carries the inherent risks of this technique.

Embolization-related complications include nontarget embolization, portal vein thrombosis, hepatic infarction, portal hypertension, postembolization syndrome, and delayed recanalization. Postembolization syndrome is the most common and can include a constellation of minor symptoms, including right upper quadrant abdominal pain, fever, nausea, and vomiting. Transient liver dysfunction can also occur with elevated liver enzymes, but typically these return to baseline within 7 to 10 days.

Nontarget embolization within the FLR is one of the most feared complications of PVE; this can occur from nontarget administration of embolization materials or traumatic catheter manipulation in an embolized section of the portal vein. Certain techniques are thought to minimize nontarget embolization, including careful monitoring of flow stasis, using particulate embolic agents for distal vein occlusion and coils for proximal vein occlusion.

Central or main portal vein thrombosis is another potentially devastating complication related to embolization. Portal vein thrombosis that develops in the FLR may inhibit hypertrophy or even cause atrophy and could render the patient unsuitable for liver resection. Thrombus extension from the targeted to the nontargeted portal vein is rare but does occur. If thrombosis is acute and mild, it may be adequately treated with systemic anticoagulation to prevent further clot propagation. Extensive or symptomatic thrombosis may require catheter-directed thrombolysis with or without mechanical thrombectomy.

ASSESSMENT OF HYPERTROPHY AFTER PORTAL VEIN EMBOLIZATION

After PVE, it is important to quantify the amount of induced hypertrophy. Simply performing PVE in an individual with inadequate preprocedure FLR does not guarantee adequate hypertrophy for resection particularly in patients with underlying parenchymal disease. Repeat CT volumetry is performed in order to determine the adequacy of hypertrophy 2 to 8 weeks after PVE. The DH following PVE is a direct measure of FLR function and, most importantly, it predicts the ability of the FLR to regenerate after resection, avoiding liver failure.

A simple method for determining the eligibility of a patient for liver resection is using the same criteria used to select patients for PVE. For patients with normal livers, prolonged chemotherapy and cirrhosis adequacy is typically judged at 20%, 30%, and 40%, respectively.[1] However, these values serve as guidelines with final decision-making for resectability individualized to the patient and their burden of underlying disease and chemotherapy-related injury. Using only these figures as guides will still result in postresection acute liver failure in ~15% of patients.

After using these guidelines for several years, the authors' group noted that there were patients who hypertrophied rapidly but did not meet the absolute cutoff values (ie, postchemotherapy FLR volume 24% to 29%). These patients tended to do well after major hepatectomy. In contrast, other patients hypertrophied slowly but did achieve these guideline values (ie, cirrhotic FLR volume 38% to 41%). This subset did very poorly after liver resection. Based on these observations, the authors proposed that DH is a more accurate method of determining postoperative liver function.[18] DH is determined at the time of post-PVE CT volumetry by calculating the percentage-point difference between the FLR volume before and after the PVE. Review of patients who demonstrated at least a 5% point increase in FLR volume found a decrease to only 5% of patients experiencing postresection acute liver failure.

Subsequently, the authors refined these calculations, identifying the FLR kinetic growth rate (KGR) as the most accurate way for the clinician to predict the future growth of the FLR and readiness to proceed with liver resection. The KGR is calculated with the following formula: KGR = DH (%) ÷ time elapsed since PVE (weeks). Among patients with a KGR greater than 2.0 percentage points per week, less than 5% will require additional waiting time before proceeding to resection. In addition, the authors found that KGR greater than 2.0 percentage points per week was the strongest predictor of successful resection without hepatic insufficiency[19] and has been associated with 0% liver failure at the authors' institution over the past 4 years.

Several studies have looked at the effects of chemotherapy on FLR hypertrophy itself. Although it is intuitive that hypertrophy may be inhibited by the hepatotoxic effects of chemotherapy, these studies have determined that no difference in post-PVE growth was seen in patients who underwent neoadjuvant chemotherapy.[20]

SUMMARY

Because of its inherent regenerative capacity, the liver presents an interesting target for preoperative evaluation and intervention. Patients who have low FLR before surgery have increased postoperative morbidity and mortality, but rapid expansion of FLR volume is possible with minimal morbidity by using preoperative PVE. Indeed, the ability to hypertrophy after PVE is the best predictor of FLR function after major hepatectomy. Once adequate hypertrophy is achieved, patients who would otherwise be inoperable due to the burden of their disease can safely undergo curative liver resection.

REFERENCES

1. Abdalla EK, Denys A, Chevalier P, et al. Total and segmental liver volume variations: implications for liver surgery. Surgery 2004;135:404–10.
2. Heymsfield SB, Fulenwider T, Nordlinger B, et al. Accurate measurement of liver, kidney, and spleen volume and mass by computerized axial tomography. Ann Intern Med 1979;90:185–7.
3. Shirabe K, Shimada M, Gion T, et al. Postoperative liver failure after major hepatic resection for hepatocellular carcinoma in the modern era with special reference to remnant liver volume. J Am Coll Surg 1999;188:304–9.
4. Couinaud C. Liver anatomy: portal (and suprahepatic) or biliary segmentation. Dig Surg 1999;16:459–67.
5. Nakayama Y, Li Q, Katsuragawa S, et al. Automated hepatic volumetry for living related liver transplantation at multisection CT. Radiology 2006;240:743–8.
6. Vauthey JN, Abdalla EK, Doherty DA, et al. Body surface area and body weight predict total liver volume in Western adults. Liver Transpl 2002;8:233–40.
7. Abdalla EK, Barnett CC, Doherty D, et al. Extended hepatectomy in patients with hepatobiliary malignancies with and without preoperative portal vein embolization. Arch Surg 2002;137:675–80 [discussion: 680–1].
8. Shoup M, Gonen M, D'Angelica M, et al. Volumetric analysis predicts hepatic dysfunction in patients undergoing major liver resection. J Gastrointest Surg 2003;7:325–30.
9. Vauthey JN, Pawlik TM, Ribero D, et al. Chemotherapy regimen predicts steatohepatitis and an increase in 90-day mortality after surgery for hepatic colorectal metastases. J Clin Oncol 2006;24:2065–72.
10. Teh SH, Christein J, Donohue J, et al. Hepatic resection of hepatocellular carcinoma in patients with cirrhosis: Model of End-Stage Liver Disease (MELD) score predicts perioperative mortality. J Gastrointest Surg 2005;9:1207–15 [discussion: 1215].
11. Kubota K, Makuuchi M, Kusaka K, et al. Measurement of liver volume and hepatic functional reserve as a guide to decision-making in resectional surgery for hepatic tumors. Hepatology 1997;26:1176–81.

12. Farges O, Belghiti J, Kianmanesh R, et al. Portal vein embolization before right hepatectomy: prospective clinical trial. Ann Surg 2003;237:208–17.
13. Ogata S, Belghiti J, Farges O, et al. Sequential arterial and portal vein embolizations before right hepatectomy in patients with cirrhosis and hepatocellular carcinoma. Br J Surg 2006;93:1091–8.
14. Madoff DC, Hicks ME, Vauthey JN, et al. Transhepatic portal vein embolization: anatomy, indications, and technical considerations. Radiographics 2002;22: 1063–76.
15. Makuuchi M, Thai BL, Takayasu K, et al. Preoperative portal embolization to increase safety of major hepatectomy for hilar bile duct carcinoma: a preliminary report. Surgery 1990;107:521–7.
16. Madoff DC, Hicks ME, Abdalla EK, et al. Portal vein embolization with polyvinyl alcohol particles and coils in preparation for major liver resection for hepatobiliary malignancy: safety and effectiveness–study in 26 patients. Radiology 2003;227: 251–60.
17. Denys A, Bize P, Demartines N, et al. Quality improvement for portal vein embolization. Cardiovasc Intervent Radiol 2010;33:452–6.
18. Ribero D, Abdalla EK, Madoff DC, et al. Portal vein embolization before major hepatectomy and its effects on regeneration, resectability and outcome. Br J Surg 2007;94:1386–94.
19. Shindoh J, Truty MJ, Aloia TA, et al. Kinetic growth rate after portal vein embolization predicts posthepatectomy outcomes: toward zero liver-related mortality in patients with colorectal liver metastases and small future liver remnant. J Am Coll Surg 2013;216:201–9.
20. Tanaka K, Kumamoto T, Matsuyama R, et al. Influence of chemotherapy on liver regeneration induced by portal vein embolization or first hepatectomy of a staged procedure for colorectal liver metastases. J Gastrointest Surg 2010;14:359–68.

Chemotherapy-Associated Hepatotoxicities

Michael A. White, MD[a], Yuman Fong, MD[b],*, Gagandeep Singh, MD[c]

KEYWORDS

- Liver injury • Chemotherapy • Hepatectomy • Steatosis • Steatohepatitis
- Sinusoidal obstruction syndrome

KEY POINTS

- Steatosis is most commonly associated with irinotecan and 5-fluorouracil, whereas sinusoidal obstruction syndrome is more frequently noted with oxaliplatin. Steatohepatitis has only been linked to irinotecan.
- Most investigators agree that presence of steatosis has little impact on surgical outcomes, whereas steatohepatitis leads to increased mortality.
- Sinusoidal obstruction syndrome can predispose patients to increased blood loss, earlier disease recurrence, and decreased overall survival.
- Duration of preoperative chemotherapy and time interval after completion of chemotherapy before surgery can be optimized to reduce liver toxicities.

OVERVIEW

The number of chemotherapy options and combination regimens for a multitude of malignancies has vastly increased in the last few decades. An unfortunate consequence of using increasingly effective systemic cytotoxic therapies before hepatectomy is their off-target effects that result in concurrent damage to normal tissues. The mechanisms and readouts for level of host tissue damage are increasingly understood. Hepatic toxicities are notable, as they can not only impact a patient's overall health and recovery from surgery but also impair the regenerative capacity that is the basis of potentially curative resections of the liver, a common site for metastatic disease to present. Surgeons in particular must account for chemotherapy-associated liver injuries when considering liver resection for metastasectomy in planning safe surgery.

Disclosures: The authors have no relevant financial disclosures to report.
a Complex Surgical Oncology, Division of Surgical Oncology, Department of Surgery, City of Hope National Medical Center, 1500 East Duarte Road, Duarte, CA 91010, USA; b Department of Surgery, City of Hope National Medical Center, 1500 East Duarte Road, Duarte, CA 91010, USA; c Hepatobiliary and Pancreatic Surgery, Division of Surgical Oncology, Department of Surgery, City of Hope National Medical Center, 1500 East Duarte Road, Duarte, CA 91010, USA
* Corresponding author.
E-mail address: yfong@coh.org

Surg Clin N Am 96 (2016) 207–217
http://dx.doi.org/10.1016/j.suc.2015.11.005
0039-6109/16/$ – see front matter © 2016 Elsevier Inc. All rights reserved.

surgical.theclinics.com

CATEGORIES OF HEPATOTOXICITY

Two major categories of hepatic tissue damage commonly occur as a consequence of chemotherapy. The first is similar to nonalcoholic fatty liver disease and often referred to as *CASH*, for chemotherapy-associated steatohepatitis.[1] This form of nonalcoholic fatty liver disease can be further divided into steatosis and steatohepatitis. Nonalcoholic fatty liver disease is classified as a greater than 5% infiltration of hepatocytes by triglycerides in patients without significant alcohol consumption.[2] In steatosis, lipid accumulates to abundance in hepatocytes, whereas steatohepatitis indicates concurrent inflammatory changes and ballooning degeneration of the hepatocytes.[2] These fatty liver diseases lead to the classic fatty or yellow liver that can be noted on gross examination owing to a yellowed (or frequently pink) hue of the liver parenchyma (**Fig. 1**A). A scoring system for these fatty liver changes has been developed by Kleiner and colleagues and termed the Nonalcoholic Fatty Liver Disease Activity Score (**Table 1**).[3] This scoring system includes 14 histologic categories. Three of those—degree of steatosis, lobular inflammation, and hepatocellular ballooning—are given quantitative scores with a range from 0 to 8. The sum of these unweighted scores is used to classify histologic findings as steatosis versus steatohepatitis with good reproducibility among evaluators. Scores greater than 5 are consistent with steatohepatitis, whereas scores less than 3 are considered not steatohepatitis.[3] Patients with steatohepatitis are at risk for progressive disease culminating in fibrosis and possible cirrhosis and have a 10-fold increased risk of death from liver disease.[2]

The second category results from injury to the sinusoids causing venous congestion and blue liver, a term coined because of its macroscopic appearance (**Fig. 1**B). Endothelial cells in the sinusoids become damaged leading to initiation of the coagulation cascade within the subendothelial space of Disse and ultimately sinusoidal obstruction as fibrotic changes occur to the central venules.[4] Sinusoidal injury can also be scored based on a system devised by Rubbia-Brandt and colleagues[5] with grades 0 to 3 (**Table 2**). The range of sinusoidal injury can go from mild changes such as sinusoidal dilation progressing on the extreme end to veno-occlusive changes with regenerative nodular hyperplasia.[5] Severe chemotherapy-associated veno-occlusive disease can have the behavior and radiologic appearance of the Budd-Chiari syndrome.[5]

SCOPE OF THE PROBLEM

Although primary liver cancers are common worldwide, metastatic disease to the liver is far more abundant in the United States. The most common primary site for

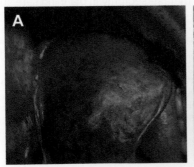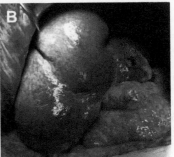

Fig. 1. (*A*) Blue liver consistent with sinusoidal obstruction syndrome. (*B*) Yellow liver with steatosis and some nodularity consistent with fibrotic changes.

Table 1 Nonalcoholic fatty liver disease activity scoring system	
	Scoring Criteria
Steatosis	0: <5% Fatty infiltration 1: 5%–33% 2: 33%–66% 3: >66%
Lobular inflammation	0: None 1: <2 Foci/200x field 2: 2–4 Foci/200x field 3: > 4 Foci/200x field
Hepatocyte ballooning	0: None 1: Minimal ballooning 2: Prominent ballooning

Scores from 0 to 2 are not consistent with steatohepatitis. Scores from 5 to 8 correlate with a diagnosis of steatohepatitis.
Data from Kleiner DE, Brunt EM, Van Natta M, et al. Design and validation of a histologic scoring system for nonalcoholic fatty liver disease. Hepatology 2005;41(6):1319.

metastatic lesions to the liver is from colorectal cancers. More than 136,000 new cases of colon and rectal cancer were diagnosed in the United States last year, making it the second most common cancer in men and third most common in women.[6] Approximately 25% of these patients present at initial diagnosis with synchronous liver metastases, and up to 60% of colorectal cancer patients will have metastatic disease to the liver during the course of their disease.[7] The treatment and prognosis for these patients has significantly improved in the last 20 years in large part because of improvements in systemic therapy and a better understanding of the surgical management of liver metastases. We have learned that with colorectal cancer patients that have liver-only metastases, long-term survival and often cure can be achieved if complete surgical resection is possible.[8] These patients will frequently get chemotherapy either in the preoperative setting or adjuvantly. Use of neoadjuvant chemotherapy can convert disease initially deemed unresectable to resectable disease 10% to 15% of the time.[9] These patients are also found to have similar survival outcomes to those who were upfront surgical candidates.[10] As a result of these advancements in the treatment regimen for patients with hepatic metastases from colorectal cancer, a large number of patients receive systemic chemotherapy that can be potentially damaging to the liver.

Table 2 Sinusoidal obstruction syndrome grading system	
Grade 0	No sinusoidal dilation identified
Grade 1	(Mild) Sinusoidal dilation of up to 1/3 of the lobular surface
Grade 2	(Moderate) Sinusoidal dilation of up to 2/3 of the lobular surface
Grade 3	(Severe) Sinusoidal dilation throughout

Grading system for sinusoidal obstruction syndrome of the liver.
Adapted from Rubbia-Brandt L, Audard V, Sartoretti P, et al. Severe hepatic sinusoidal obstruction associated with oxaliplatin-based chemotherapy in patients with metastatic colorectal cancer. Ann Oncol 2004;15(3):461.

Paramount to the advancement of our treatment of colorectal cancers has been the development of 3 primary cytotoxic chemotherapy agents, 5-Fluorouracil (5-FU), oxaliplatin, and irinotecan. Use of these agents has now been linked to predictable hepatotoxicities including steatosis, steatohepatitis, and sinusoidal obstructive syndrome. Irinotecan and 5-FU are more associated with steatosis.[11] Steatohepatitis has only been linked to irinotecan,[12] whereas oxaliplatin regimens can result in sinusoidal injuries leading to sinusoidal obstruction syndrome.[11–13]

In addition, patients with elevated body mass index, type 2 diabetes mellitus, or metabolic syndrome have an increased risk for steatosis irrespective of chemotherapy. Up to one-third of the population is thought to likely have some degree of nonalcoholic fatty liver disease caused by the worldwide obesity epidemic.[2] Although mild steatosis is thought to be relatively benign, it is thought that patients with baseline nonalcoholic fatty liver disease are at higher risk for chemotherapy-associated liver injuries than those without.

MECHANISMS

The basic underlying principle for hepatotoxicities from cytotoxic chemotherapies is related to the development of reactive oxygen species leading to cellular damage and apoptosis pathways. It is thought that livers with preexisting nonalcoholic steatosis changes are most susceptible to further damage from use of chemotherapy. 5-FU and Irinotecan specifically are thought to affect mitochondrial membranes allowing for an increase in reactive oxygen species and setting off a cascade of events leading to lipid peroxidation, fibrosis, and cell death.[14,15] Sinusoidal injury is also thought to result from reactive oxygen species. Once these endothelial cells are injured, the coagulation cascade is activated and can lead to sinusoidal obstruction.[5]

IDENTIFICATION OF LIVER INJURY

Although definitive diagnosis of any of these chemotherapy-associated hepatotoxicities requires histologic examination of tissue, it is often helpful to be able to predict or identify these patients, especially in a preoperative setting.

Nonalcoholic fatty liver disease is usually asymptomatic; thus, clinical suspicion (such as identifying overweight, diabetic, and chemotherapy-treated patients) is necessary to diagnose this disease. Laboratory abnormalities are insensitive but an increase in alanine aminotransferase greater than aspartate aminotransferase is frequently present in nonalcoholic fatty liver disease.[2] With elevation of liver transaminases, other causes of liver injury including but not limited to alcohol use, hepatitis, and autoimmune hepatitis should be ruled out.[2] Steatohepatitis can progress to fibrosis and ultimately cirrhosis of the liver. In these cases, thrombocytopenia that is not corrected after cessation of chemotherapy is often noted.[1] In sinusoidal obstruction syndrome, rather than elevated transaminases, a picture of cholestasis with elevations in alkaline phosphatase or γ-glutamyl transpeptidase is seen[13] (**Table 3**).

Ultrasound scan, computed tomography (CT) and MRI are all commonly used imaging modalities to help identify liver injuries. Ultrasound scan is inexpensive but user dependent and not as sensitive for early steatosis.[2] CT imaging, which is often obtained to look for metastatic disease, can identify steatosis with low attenuation of liver tissue on nonenhanced images with Hounsfield unit values of less than 40 compared with a normal range of 50 to 57.[1,2] Another metric that is often used is an attenuation ratio of liver to spleen greater than 1.1 that is predictive of more than 30% steatosis.[2] Findings of splenomegaly are suggestive of more advanced liver disease such as cirrhosis[1] (**Fig. 2**). MRI, the most expensive, is thought to be the most accurate at

Table 3
Characteristics of chemotherapy-associated liver injury categories

	Steatosis	Steatohepatitis	Sinusoidal Obstruction
Mechanism	Reactive oxygen species causing cellular damage and apoptosis. Mitochondrial membrane damage, lipid peroxidation, fibrosis, cellular death.	Reactive oxygen species causing cellular damage and apoptosis. Mitochondrial membrane damage, lipid peroxidation, fibrosis, cellular death.	Reactive oxygen species causing damage to endothelial cells, extravasation of red blood cells into perisinusoidal spaces, venous outflow obstruction and subsequent dilation of sinusoids.
Laboratory abnormalities	Increased ALT > AST	Increased ALT > AST	Increased Alk Phos or gGT
Gross appearance	Yellow, fatty	Yellow, fatty	Blue, congested
Pathology	Greater that 5% triglyceride infiltration into hepatocytes	Steatosis changes plus lobular inflammation, hepatocellular ballooning, fibrosis	Sinusoidal dilation, fibrotic changes to central venules, perisinusoidal fibrosis, possible regenerative nodular hyperplasia

Abbreviations: Alk Phos, Alkaline phosphatase; ALT, alanine aminotransferase; AST, aspartate aminotransferase; gGT, Gamma-glutamyl transpeptidase.

predicting steatosis and is proposed by some as a method for identifying sinusoidal injury.[2] A study by Cho and colleagues[16] in 2008 compared noncontrast CT, contrast-enhanced CT, and MRI for detection of steatosis and compared these findings with histologic analysis of tissues. In their study, sensitivity and specificity for each modality (noncontrast CT, contrast-enhanced CT, MRI) were 33% and 100%, 50% and 83%, and 88% and 63%, respectively. They concluded that significant steatosis could be identified on noncontrast CT, but a CT read as normal could not exclude the diagnosis. MRI was good for exclusion of steatosis but had poor ability to identify nonalcoholic fatty liver changes.[16]

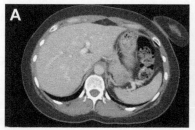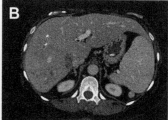

Fig. 2. (*A*) CT scan axial image of normal liver without evidence of chemotherapy-associated hepatotoxicities. (*B*) CT scan axial image of a fatty liver consistent with steatosis. Note the low attenuation of the liver relative to the spleen and associated splenomegaly suggesting possible fibrosis or cirrhotic changes.

The current gold standard would include laparoscopic evaluation of the liver to assess macroscopic changes and tissue biopsy for pathologic review of uninvolved liver parenchyma. Despite this finding, because of the invasive nature of laparoscopy and biopsy, they are often not performed before the definitive operation.

IMPACT OF CHEMOTHERAPY-ASSOCIATED HEPATOTOXICITIES

In general, many surgeons believe chemotherapy-associated liver injuries are deleterious to surgical outcomes related to liver resections. The literature has not demonstrated a true consensus on this common perception. Numerous studies looked at the impact of chemotherapy-induced liver injury, and key studies are discussed in this review.

A study by Vigano and colleagues[17] in 2013 looked at 323 patients over a span of 13 years who were undergoing liver resection for metastatic colorectal cancers. All patients were treated preoperatively with either oxaliplatin or irinotecan-based chemotherapy regimens. Grade 2 or 3 sinusoidal obstruction was noted in 38.4% (all grades 64.1%) of patients and grade 2 or 3 steatosis in 22.6%. Steatohepatitis was seen in 9.3% of the patients. They noted that patients who had moderate or severe sinusoidal obstruction had less of a pathologic response of the tumor to chemotherapy. Although tumor response to chemotherapy was prognostically significant, chemotherapy-associated liver injuries did not have a negative impact on long-term survival. Steatosis was actually noted to have a protective survival impact that has also been shown in other studies.[17,18]

Reddy and colleagues[19] performed a retrospective study looking at hepatic steatosis and compared the likelihood of progression to advanced hepatic fibrosis in patients previously treated with chemotherapy versus those who had never received chemotherapy. They found on multivariable analysis that chemotherapy treatment, especially 5-FU and irinotecan, was a negative predictor for having a low probability of finding advanced fibrosis in patients with steatosis. They suggest that chemotherapy-treated patients with steatosis at least 6 months after their last treatment should be closely evaluated for development of progressive fibrosis of the liver.[19]

Additional studies looked at perioperative morbidity and mortality as it relates to chemotherapy-associated liver injury (**Table 4**). In a 2006 study by Vauthey and colleagues,[12] 406 patients who underwent hepatectomy for colorectal cancer metastases were reviewed retrospectively. More than 60% of the patients had received preoperative chemotherapy (n = 248), and common agents included 5-FU, oxaliplatin, and irinotecan. Approximately 9% of patients had steatosis, 8% had steatohepatitis, and 5% had sinusoidal changes. Consistent with many other studies, oxaliplatin was associated with sinusoidal obstruction, whereas irinotecan was independently associated with steatohepatitis. They noted that patients with steatohepatitis had a significantly increased risk of 90-day mortality at 14.7% compared with 1.6% in those without.[12]

Pawlik and colleagues[11] similarly looked at 212 patients retrospectively in 2007 that had hepatic resections for metastatic colorectal cancer. They similarly found an association of sinusoidal injury with oxaliplatin use, and steatosis of nearly 30% was associated with irinotecan use. In their study, only 3 patients were identified to have steatohepatitis, 2 of whom had received irinotecan. They found no statistical difference in perioperative morbidity rates or 60-day mortality when comparing patients who received preoperative chemotherapy with those who did not.

A recent European study by Parkin and colleagues[20] identified 4329 patients through the LiverMetSurvey that had first-time liver resections after neoadjuvant

Table 4
Perioperative morbidity and mortality related to chemotherapy-associated liver injury

Study, Year	Number of Patients Treated with Chemotherapy	Agents Used (% Patients)	Hepatotoxicities (% of Total)	Chemotherapy Agent and Toxicity (Odds Ratio or % of Treated Patients)	Conclusions
Vauthey et al,[12] 2006	248	5-FU alone (15.5%) 5-FU + irinotecan (23.1%) 5-FU + oxaliplatin (19.5%)	Steatosis (8.9%) Steatohepatitis (8.4%) Sinusoidal dilation (5.4%)	Oxaliplatin–sinusoidal dilation (OR, 8.3; $P<.001$) Irinotecan–steatohepatitis (OR, 5.4; $P<.001$)	Steatohepatitis– increased 90-d mortality (OR, 10.5; $P = .001$)
Pawlik et al,[11] 2007	153	5-FU alone (31.6%) 5-FU + irinotecan (25.9%) 5-FU + oxaliplatin (14.6%)	Steatosis (19.6%) Steatohepatitis (2.0%) Sinusoidal dilation (4.6%)	Irinotecan–steatosis (27.3%) Oxaliplatin–sinusoidal dilation (9.7%)	Unchanged perioperative complication rate and 60-d mortality between chemotherapy and no chemotherapy groups
Parkin et al,[20] 2014	4329	5-FU (76%) Irinotecan (29.2%) Oxaliplatin (55.6%) Capecitabine (15%) Bevacizumab (23.4%) Cetuximab (7.1%)	NR	NR	No difference in 5-y OS or CSS in patients with steatosis vs those without
Wolf et al,[21] 2013	250	Oxaliplatin (66.4%) Irinotecan (43.6%) Bevacizumab (29.2%)	Steatosis (38%) Steatohepatitis (6%) Sinusoidal dilation (10%)	Irinotecan–steatosis (46%; $P<.01$), steatohepatitis (8%; $P = .01$)	No association between early postoperative mortality, steatohepatitis or preoperative chemotherapy
Tamandl et al,[13] 2011	161	FOLFOX/XELOX (52.2%) FOLFOX/XELOX + Bevacizumab (30%) FOLFIRI or FOLFOX conversion to FOLFIRI (16.1%)	Sinusoidal dilation grade 2–3 (27%)	FOLFOX or XELOX–sinusoidal dilation grade 2–3 (18.1%; $P = .011$)	Sinusoidal obstruction syndrome decreases recurrence-free survival and overall survival. No increase in perioperative morbidity.

Abbreviations: CSS, cancer specific survival; FOLFIRI, Folinic acid (leucovorin), 5-Fluorouracil, irinotecan; FOLFOX, Folinic acid (leucovorin), 5-Fluorouracil, oxaliplatin; NR, not reported; OR, odds ratio; OS, overall survival; XELOX, capecitabine, oxaliplatin.
Data from Refs.[11–13,20,21]

chemotherapy. This study compared 90-day mortality, 5-year overall survival, and 5-year cancer specific survival based on 3 liver histology groups that included normal liver, steatosis and other. They found no statistically significant difference in any of their survival endpoints across the 3 groups, suggesting that steatosis should not compromise oncologic outcomes or perioperative mortality in this patient population.

In 2013, Wolf and colleagues[21] reviewed 384 patients who had pathologic tissue available for review after resection of metastatic colorectal metastases to the liver. In this retrospective study, 65% of patients had preoperative chemotherapy for a median of 24 weeks. They found chemotherapy to be protective against major perioperative morbidity and mortality.

In contrast, Tamandl and colleagues[13] were able to identify a worsened outcome in patients with sinusoidal obstruction after preoperative chemotherapy before hepatic metastasectomy for colorectal cancer. In their study, 18% of patients receiving oxaliplatin-based chemotherapy regimens subsequently had grade 2 or 3 sinusoidal obstruction. They were able to show in their study that these patients had earlier recurrence of their disease and decreased overall survival; however, there was no increase in perioperative morbidity.

MANAGEMENT OF CHEMOTHERAPY-ASSOCIATED HEPATOTOXICITIES

With a greater understanding of the specific agents that cause chemotherapy-associated liver injuries, efforts have been made to minimize the extent of damage that is induced. Many chemotherapy-associated liver injuries are noted to be reversible, especially in earlier stages if surgery is delayed after completion of chemotherapy.[4,22] Duration of therapy is thought to correlate with the extent of liver damage and have an impact on perioperative outcomes. Aloia and colleagues[23] demonstrated that patients receiving more than 12 cycles of preoperative chemotherapy were more likely to require reoperation (11% vs 0%) and to have a longer hospital length of stay (15 days vs 11). As a result of this and other studies, some suggest stopping chemotherapy in the preoperative setting once metastatic lesions are resectable rather than treating to maximal response. Others suggest 4 months as the optimal duration of treatment to obtain the greatest tumor response balanced with minimizing liver toxicity.[12]

Other investigators looked at the interval between the last dose of chemotherapy and date of surgery as a way to minimize operative complications that could be related to treatment-induced liver injuries. Numerous studies show a reduction in chemotherapy-associated liver injuries with longer time intervals after chemotherapy; however, this also must be balanced against the risk of regrowth of the tumor during that treatment-free period. Many surgeons consider 4 to 6 weeks the appropriate interval, and these authors recommend waiting 5 weeks from the last chemotherapy treatment before taking a patient to surgery for hepatic resection.[24,25]

A proper assessment of the estimated functional liver remnant is important before taking a patient for large-volume liver resections. In patients with suspected chemotherapy-induced liver injuries, most surgeons agree that a future liver remnant of at least 30% is necessary to minimize risk for postoperative hepatic failure.[26] This is compared with 20% to 25% in patients with healthy liver tissue. Methods to optimize the future liver remnant including portal vein embolization are beyond the scope of this report and are discussed elsewhere.

Combined ablation and resection is a technique that can be used to spare liver parenchyma in patients with extensive liver disease that would previously be considered unresectable. This technique was evaluated in a multicenter study to look at complication rates and survival outcomes.[27] Combined ablation and resection was performed on 288 patients across 4 centers, most with synchronous and bilateral colorectal liver metastases. Median hepatic recurrence-free survival in these patients was 14 months. Complications occurred in 35% of patients and were an independent risk factor for overall survival. Five-year overall survival rate was 45% in patients without and 25.6% for those with complications. The 30-day mortality rate was low at 1%.

Lastly, some investigators noted that use of bevacizumab may have a protective effect against sinusoidal injuries to the liver if used in the preoperative setting. Although the percentage of patients with grade 2 or 3 sinusoidal injuries was reduced, the surgical complication rate was not significantly changed.[28,29]

SUMMARY

Hepatotoxic side effects from chemotherapy remain a major hurdle for the treatment of numerous malignancies. These effects have become better characterized over the last decade and include a spectrum of nonalcoholic fatty liver disease including steatosis and steatohepatitis (chemotherapy-associated steatohepatitis) and sinusoidal injuries. The incidence of these liver injuries is predictable based on chemotherapy regimen, and their presence can complicate attempts for curative surgical resection of liver metastases. Oxaliplatin-based chemotherapy regimens are more commonly associated with sinusoidal obstructive liver injury, whereas irinotecan and 5-FU are more frequently associated with steatosis. Steatohepatitis has only been linked to irinotecan. Increased awareness and understanding of these chemotherapy-induced side effects has allowed medical oncologists and liver surgeons to develop treatment plans that help minimize risk for severe liver injury and to appropriately plan preoperatively to avoid serious complications. Further work remains to be done to increase our knowledge of the mechanisms for these injuries, to identify those patients at highest risk, and to help prevent these side effects entirely in the future.

REFERENCES

1. Fong Y, Bentrem DJ. CASH (chemotherapy-associated steatohepatitis) costs. Ann Surg 2006;243(1):8–9.
2. Dyson JK, McPherson S, Anstee QM. Non-alcoholic fatty liver disease: non-invasive investigation and risk stratification. J Clin Pathol 2013;66(12):1033–45.
3. Kleiner DE, Brunt EM, Van Natta M, et al. Design and validation of a histological scoring system for nonalcoholic fatty liver disease. Hepatology 2005;41(6): 1313–21.
4. Maor Y, Malnick S. Liver injury induced by anticancer chemotherapy and radiation therapy. Int J Hepatol 2013;2013:815105.
5. Rubbia-Brandt L, Audard V, Sartoretti P, et al. Severe hepatic sinusoidal obstruction associated with oxaliplatin-based chemotherapy in patients with metastatic colorectal cancer. Ann Oncol 2004;15(3):460–6.
6. DeSantis CE, Lin CC, Mariotto AB, et al. Cancer treatment and survivorship statistics, 2014. Cancer J Clinicians 2014;64(4):252–71.
7. Donadon M, Ribero D, Morris-Stiff G, et al. New paradigm in the management of liver-only metastases from colorectal cancer. Gastrointest Cancer Res 2007;1(1): 20–7.
8. Figueras J, Torras J, Valls C, et al. Surgical resection of colorectal liver metastases in patients with expanded indications: a single-center experience with 501 patients. Dis Colon Rectum 2007;50(4):478–88.

9. Adam R, Miller R, Pitombo M, et al. Two-stage hepatectomy approach for initially unresectable colorectal hepatic metastases. Surg Oncol Clin North America 2007;16(3):525–36, viii.

10. Fong Y. Chemotherapy and resection for colorectal metastases. Lancet Oncol 2013;14(12):1148–9.

11. Pawlik TM, Olino K, Gleisner AL, et al. Preoperative chemotherapy for colorectal liver metastases: impact on hepatic histology and postoperative outcome. J Gastrointest Surg 2007;11(7):860–8.

12. Vauthey JN, Pawlik TM, Ribero D, et al. Chemotherapy regimen predicts steatohepatitis and an increase in 90-day mortality after surgery for hepatic colorectal metastases. J Clin Oncol 2006;24(13):2065–72.

13. Tamandl D, Klinger M, Eipeldauer S, et al. Sinusoidal obstruction syndrome impairs long-term outcome of colorectal liver metastases treated with resection after neoadjuvant chemotherapy. Ann Surg Oncol 2011;18(2):421–30.

14. Laurent A, Nicco C, Tran Van Nhieu J, et al. Pivotal role of superoxide anion and beneficial effect of antioxidant molecules in murine steatohepatitis. Hepatology 2004;39(5):1277–85.

15. Pessayre D, Berson A, Fromenty B, et al. Mitochondria in steatohepatitis. Semin Liver Dis 2001;21(1):57–69.

16. Cho CS, Curran S, Schwartz LH, et al. Preoperative radiographic assessment of hepatic steatosis with histologic correlation. J Am Coll Surgeons 2008;206(3): 480–8.

17. Vigano L, Capussotti L, De Rosa G, et al. Liver resection for colorectal metastases after chemotherapy: impact of chemotherapy-related liver injuries, pathological tumor response, and micrometastases on long-term survival. Ann Surg 2013; 258(5):731–40 [discussion: 41–2].

18. Parkin E, O'Reilly DA, Adam R, et al. The effect of hepatic steatosis on survival following resection of colorectal liver metastases in patients without preoperative chemotherapy. HPB 2013;15(6):463–72.

19. Reddy SK, Reilly C, Zhan M, et al. Long-term influence of chemotherapy on steatosis-associated advanced hepatic fibrosis. Med Oncol 2014;31(6):971.

20. Parkin E, O'Reilly DA, Adam R, et al. Equivalent survival in patients with and without steatosis undergoing resection for colorectal liver metastases following pre-operative chemotherapy. Eur J Surg Oncol 2014;40(11):1436–44.

21. Wolf PS, Park JO, Bao F, et al. Preoperative chemotherapy and the risk of hepatotoxicity and morbidity after liver resection for metastatic colorectal cancer: a single institution experience. J Am Coll Surgeons 2013;216(1):41–9.

22. Nakano H, Oussoultzoglou E, Rosso E, et al. Sinusoidal injury increases morbidity after major hepatectomy in patients with colorectal liver metastases receiving preoperative chemotherapy. Ann Surg 2008;247(1):118–24.

23. Aloia T, Sebagh M, Plasse M, et al. Liver histology and surgical outcomes after preoperative chemotherapy with fluorouracil plus oxaliplatin in colorectal cancer liver metastases. J Clin Oncol 2006;24(31):4983–90.

24. Kopetz S, Vauthey JN. Perioperative chemotherapy for resectable hepatic metastases. Lancet 2008;371(9617):963–5.

25. Welsh FK, Tilney HS, Tekkis PP, et al. Safe liver resection following chemotherapy for colorectal metastases is a matter of timing. Br J Cancer 2007;96(7):1037–42.

26. Ferrero A, Vigano L, Polastri R, et al. Postoperative liver dysfunction and future remnant liver: where is the limit? Results of a prospective study. World J Surg 2007;31(8):1643–51.

27. Evrard S, Poston G, Kissmeyer-Nielsen P, et al. Combined ablation and resection (CARe) as an effective parenchymal sparing treatment for extensive colorectal liver metastases. PLoS One 2014;9(12):e114404.
28. Rubbia-Brandt L, Lauwers GY, Wang H, et al. Sinusoidal obstruction syndrome and nodular regenerative hyperplasia are frequent oxaliplatin-associated liver lesions and partially prevented by bevacizumab in patients with hepatic colorectal metastasis. Histopathology 2010;56(4):430–9.
29. van der Pool AE, Marsman HA, Verheij J, et al. Effect of bevacizumab added preoperatively to oxaliplatin on liver injury and complications after resection of colorectal liver metastases. J Surg Oncol 2012;106(7):892–7.

Hemostasis and Hepatic Surgery

Gareth Eeson, MD, MSc, Paul J. Karanicolas, MD, PhD*

KEYWORDS

- Liver resection • Blood loss • Blood transfusion • Hemostasis • Vascular occlusion
- Parenchymal transection • Topical hemostatic agents • Low central venous pressure

KEY POINTS

- Operative blood loss and allogeneic transfusions are independently associated with worse perioperative and long-term outcomes following hepatectomy.
- Restrictive transfusion protocols are safe and effective at minimizing exposure to allogeneic blood in surgical patients.
- Maintenance of low intraoperative central venous pressure is associated with decreased operative blood loss.
- Vascular inflow occlusion is well tolerated and can decrease blood loss during hepatectomy.
- Topical hemostatic agents may decrease intraoperative blood loss from the remnant surface.

INTRODUCTION

The liver hosts the most complex vascular anatomy of any human organ. Liver resection was once deemed an impossible feat largely because of its propensity for hemorrhage, but is now the mainstay for the treatment of primary and secondary tumors of the liver.

Significant progress in anatomic approaches, surgical technique, diagnostic imaging, and perioperative care has led to vast improvements in outcomes of patients undergoing hepatic resection. In the 1970s, operative mortality from hepatic resection occurred in approximately 20 to 30% of patients.[1] Contemporary series now report rates of major morbidity and mortality in high-volume centers to be less than 40% and 5%, respectively.[2,3] Despite these improvements, bleeding continues to be a major source of morbidity for patients and remains a pervasive challenge to hepatic surgeons. Intraoperative blood loss averages between 200 and 2000 mL for major

The authors have no financial conflicts of interest to disclose relevant to this article.

Division of General Surgery, Sunnybrook Health Sciences Centre, University of Toronto, 2075 Bayview Avenue, Room T2016, Toronto, ON M4N 3M5, Canada

* Corresponding author.

E-mail address: paul.karanicolas@sunnybrook.ca

Surg Clin N Am 96 (2016) 219–228
http://dx.doi.org/10.1016/j.suc.2015.12.001
0039-6109/16/$ – see front matter © 2016 Elsevier Inc. All rights reserved.

hepatic resection, and perioperative blood transfusions are used in 20% to 50% of patients.[2,4,5] Operative blood loss and exposure to allogeneic blood are independently associated with worse perioperative and long-term outcomes in patients undergoing hepatic resection.[2,3,6,7] These observations highlight the paramount importance of minimizing blood loss and blood transfusion in hepatic surgery. This review discusses strategies to minimize blood loss and the utilization of blood transfusion pertaining to oncologic hepatic surgery.

ALLOGENEIC RED BLOOD CELL TRANSFUSION IN HEPATIC RESECTION

The development of modern blood banking has contributed significantly to the improvements in outcomes in hepatic surgery and greatly expanded what is technically feasible for hepatic surgeons. Allogeneic blood transfusion is necessary in cases of severe hemorrhage to maintain hemodynamic stability and end-organ perfusion. However, blood transfusions carry risks of infectious disease transmission, transfusion reaction, and immune suppression and contribute notable economic costs. Furthermore, immunosuppression attributable to allogeneic transfusion has been strongly linked to increases in postoperative infectious complications and cancer recurrence.[3,6,8,9]

The evolution of surgical techniques has led to a reduction in blood loss and transfusion requirements, but paradigm shifts in transfusion strategies have further contributed to these trends. Randomized controlled trials have demonstrated that restrictive transfusion strategies are at least equivalent if not superior for patients who are critically ill, undergoing major elective surgery, or suffering from acute hemorrhage.[10–12] Specific transfusion triggers in surgical patients remain somewhat elusive, although consensus guidelines generally suggest consideration of transfusion in asymptomatic, hemodynamically stable patients with a hemoglobin lower than 6 to 8 g/dL.[13,14] Our institutional practice is to transfuse for a hemoglobin less than 7 g/dL in the asymptomatic nonbleeding patient. Considerable reductions in unnecessary blood transfusion are achievable through implementation of institutional transfusion policies.[15]

NONOPERATIVE TECHNIQUES TO MINIMIZE BLOOD LOSS DURING HEPATIC RESECTION

Improvements in outcomes of hepatectomy are not solely attributable to refinements in surgical techniques. Anesthetic and perioperative care have made substantial contributions to the progress of hepatic surgery.

Low Central Venous Pressure Anesthesia

The strategy of maintaining a low central venous pressure (CVP) during liver resection is based on the premise that blood loss during hepatectomy is derived largely from backflow from the vena cava and hepatic veins. As such, blood loss is exacerbated by normovolemic or hypervolemic states that result from aggressive fluid resuscitation. Decreased blood loss, transfusion requirements, and perioperative morbidity have been demonstrated with the use of low CVP anesthesia.[16–19] With the strategy of low CVP anesthesia, the procedure is divided into the (1) pretransection phase and the (2) posttransection phase.[16] During the pretransection phase, a low CVP (<5 mm Hg) is accomplished primarily through volume restriction. Intravenous fluids are limited (<1 mL/kg per hour) and marginal urine output (25 mL/h) is accepted. Trendelenburg positioning (15°) is used to increase venous return to the heart while decreasing CVP in the inferior vena cava.

A number of pharmacologic adjuncts may assist achieving a low CVP, including loop diuretics, intravenous nitroglycerin, and morphine, although with judicious fluid management these are rarely required. Hypoventilation has been suggested to aid in CVP reduction by lowering intrathoracic pressures, but the results of a randomized controlled trial failed to demonstrate any difference in bleeding, despite modest reductions in CVP.[20] Clamping of the infrahepatic inferior vena cava has also been proposed as a measure to decrease CVP and has been shown to significantly reduce blood loss in randomized controlled trials.[21,22] One of these trials demonstrated a statistically significant increase in symptomatic pulmonary embolism, tempering enthusiasm for this technique.[21]

The development of hypotension may necessitate the administration of vasopressors (eg, dopamine) or small corrective fluid boluses to target a systolic pressure of greater than 90 mm Hg. Other safety concerns include air embolus and organ hypoperfusion (eg, renal insufficiency) due to prolonged hypotension, yet these have not been substantiated.[16,19]

The posttransection phase commences once the specimen has been removed and hemostasis is achieved. This phase is characterized by restoration of euvolemia with fluid resuscitation and normalization of blood pressure and urine output. This strategy has clearly been associated with decreased operative blood loss and is accompanied by a good safety profile when performed by a capable hepatobiliary team.

Autotransfusion Strategies

Three main strategies of autotransfusion have been described: (1) preoperative autologous blood donation (PABD), (2) acute normovolemic hemodilution (ANH), and (3) intraoperative cell salvage (ICS).

Preoperative autologous blood donation requires patients to donate blood in advance of surgery that can then be transfused in the perioperative period. Several limitations have restricted the use of this technique, including high processing costs and the time interval necessary for the patient to reconstitute blood stores between donation and surgery. In patients undergoing hepatic resection, PABD does not appear to reduce the need for allogeneic blood or improve perioperative outcomes.[23,24] Furthermore, the economics of PABD programs are unjustifiable when one considers that 50% to 60% of donated units are discarded.[25]

ANH involves the removal of whole blood from patients immediately before surgery and autotransfusion during the posttransection phase. The premise of ANH is that shed blood contains a lower red cell mass due to the hemodilution and can reduce the need for allogeneic transfusion. Euvolemia is restored with crystalloid or colloid resuscitation to target a hemoglobin of 8 g/dL or a hematocrit approximately 24%. The whole blood is stored at room temperature in the operating theater and is retransfused intraoperatively if a transfusion trigger is encountered (typically <7 g/dL) or at the termination of surgery. The removed volume of whole blood can be calculated by using the following formula:

$$V_L = EBV \times (H_0 - H_F/H_{AV}),$$

Where V_L is allowable blood loss; EBV, estimated blood volume; H_0, initial Hgb; H_F, minimal allowable Hgb; and H_{AV}, average of initial and minimal allowable Hgb.

A meta-analysis including 4 randomized trials of ANH demonstrated a significant reduction in requirements for allogeneic transfusion (relative risk [RR] 0.41; 95% confidence interval 0.25–0.66).[19] ANH avoids the high processing costs of PABD, risks of clerical error, and degradation associated with blood storage. Conversely, the technique is quite labor-intensive and can lead to transient hypotension. The benefit of

ANH is most pronounced in patients with operative blood loss that exceeds 800 mL and its use should be considered in patients deemed to be at risk of major blood loss.[26]

Intraoperative cell salvage with autotransfusion is routinely used in high blood loss procedures with demonstrable reductions in need for allogeneic transfusions.[27] Shed blood is collected intraoperatively and filtered before being autotransfused. Due to the theoretic concerns of dissemination of malignant cells, ICS has not been widely used during oncologic surgery. A recent systematic review, however, failed to identify any evidence that ICS increases the risk of tumor recurrence, suggesting that ICS in oncologic surgery should be more carefully considered.[28]

Pharmacologic Strategies to Minimize Bleeding

Several pharmacologic agents are available to reduce bleeding and transfusion requirements in surgery. The main drug classes include (1) antifibrinolytics and (2) procoagulants.

Antifibrinolytic agents inhibit plasmin directly (eg, aprotinin) or block the conversion of plasminogen to plasmin (eg, tranexamic acid and epsilon aminocaproic acid). These agents have been extensively studied in high blood loss procedures, including liver transplantation, where they have demonstrated reduction in blood loss and transfusion requirements with acceptable safety profiles. Additionally, concerns regarding the risk of thromboembolic complications have not been demonstrated in large prospective trials.[29] Fewer trials have evaluated the effect of antifibrinolytics on hemostasis in elective hepatic resection, but both tranexamic acid and aprotinin appear to reduce blood loss and transfusion requirements in small randomized studies.[30,31] The ongoing HeLiX trial (Hemorrhage During Liver Resection: traneXamic Acid; ClinicalTrials.gov ID: NCT02261415) is currently investigating the effect of tranexamic acid in the setting of a multicentered randomized placebo-controlled clinical trial.

Impairments in coagulation due to underlying liver disease (eg, cirrhosis) or due to extensive hepatectomy have encouraged the study of procoagulant agents in controlling perioperative bleeding. The most noteworthy agents include recombinant factor VIIa, antithrombin III, and desmopressin, all of which have been investigated in randomized controlled trials with disappointing results.[5] Although the safety of procoagulants has been surprisingly favorable, none of these drugs has demonstrated clinical benefits with regard to bleeding endpoints in patients undergoing hepatic resection and are therefore not recommended.

OPERATIVE STRATEGIES TO MINIMIZE BLOOD LOSS
Vascular Occlusion Techniques

Occlusion of the inflow vessels by encircling and compressing the portal pedicle was first reported by Pringle[32] for the arrest of hemorrhage in the setting of liver trauma. The hemodynamic effects of pedicular clamping are minimal, and periods of warm ischemia up to 60 minutes are well tolerated in patients with healthy liver parenchyma. Various modifications have been proposed to minimize blood loss during parenchymal transection and mitigate the risks of ischemia-reperfusion injury to the liver remnant. Belghiti and colleagues[33] established the safety and improved tolerance of intermittent pedicular clamping achieved with 15-minute to 20-minute clamping alternating with 5-minute reperfusion periods. With intermittent clamping, total warm ischemic times can be safely extended up to 120 minutes.[33] Selective inflow occlusion strategies have been proposed to reduce the risk of ischemia to the remnant parenchyma, including hemihepatic inflow occlusion or total portal vein occlusion. These techniques require more advanced portal dissection, and the available trials have failed to demonstrate any clinical benefit over total inflow occlusion.[34]

Despite the intuitive appeal of inflow occlusion, the evidentiary basis is conflicting and based on a few small prospective controlled studies. Three small trials have reported modest improvements in blood loss and transfusion rates in patients randomized to intermittent Pringle maneuver.[35–37] This is in contrast to 2 more recent trials that have demonstrated no difference in blood loss or transfusion rates with vascular inflow occlusion.[38,39] No available trials have been adequately powered to address the impact of pedicle clamping on major morbidity or mortality. As such, published meta-analyses report conflicting findings with regard to the benefits of vascular inflow occlusion.[34,40] Overall, vascular inflow occlusion is well tolerated in patients, appears to reduce blood loss during transection, and should be used liberally to reduce bleeding and need for transfusion in patients undergoing hepatic resection.

A notable shortcoming of inflow occlusion alone is that major bleeding during liver resection can result from backflow through the hepatic veins. Various techniques have been proposed to control vascular outflow, which in conjunction with inflow control are referred to as hepatic vascular exclusion (HVE). These strategies are particularly suited for tumors abutting or involving the hepatic veins or vena cava or in patients with elevated CVP (eg, right-sided heart failure). Although the liver is excluded from the systemic circulation, the blood flow within the vena cava is also interrupted, which can result in significant hemodynamic sequelae. The available trials that have compared total HVE with inflow occlusion alone revealed no difference in blood loss, transfusion rates, liver failure, or mortality.[34] Operative times, length of stay, and intraoperative hemodynamic changes, however, were significantly greater in patients receiving HVE. In an effort to avoid the physiologic effects of caval interruption, selective HVE has been used whereby the hepatic veins are encircled extraparenchymally, leaving the caval inflow intact. Despite better physiologic tolerance, selective HVE is technically demanding and potentially hazardous, and is of no value in tumors that encroach on the hepatocaval junction. For routine hepatic resection, HVE is not recommended given its technical requirements, hemodynamic effects, and comparable clinical outcomes.

Parenchymal Transection

Transection of the liver parenchyma is responsible for most blood loss attributable to hepatectomy. Transection requires the careful exposure of vascular and biliary structures followed by division and sealing. The traditional technique against which newer techniques are compared is the clamp-crush technique (a refinement of the finger-fracture technique). This technique involves the controlled crushing of parenchyma, leaving behind exposed blood vessels and biliary channels that are subsequently clipped, ligated, cauterized, or otherwise sealed. Numerous devices have been devised to improve on the performance characteristics of liver transection, including blood loss, biliary leak, and transection time. Several small randomized trials have been conducted with this objective in mind, but none have clearly demonstrated superiority of any technique.[41,42] In practice, this is reflected by the enormous variation in the utilization of these devices among hepatobiliary surgeons (**Table 1**).[43]

Other commonly used techniques for dissection of vasculobiliary structures include the ultrasonic dissector and water-jet dissector. Ultrasonic dissection offers excellent quality of visualization of blood and biliary vessels. Division of the parenchyma is achieved using an oscillating tip that causes fragmentation of hepatocytes, sparing collagen-rich blood vessels and biliary structures. The hand piece is coupled with a saline irrigator and aspiration system that removes cellular debris from the surgical

Table 1
Comparison of parenchymal transection techniques

	Technique	Characteristics
Dissection	Clamp-crush technique	• Simple, reliable method
		• No specialized equipment required
		• Permits good exposure of vascular and biliary structures
	Ultrasonic dissection	• Excellent visualization of vascular and biliary structures
		• No vessel-sealing or coagulation functionality
		• Time consuming
	Water-jet dissection	• Precise, tissue-selective dissection of vascular and biliary structures
		• No zone of tissue injury
		• No vessel-sealing or coagulation function
Vessel ligation	Clip/ties	• Simple method
		• Time consuming
	Bipolar electrothermal vessel sealer	• Coagulates, seals and divides tissue
		• Decreased transection time demonstrated in some studies[51]
		• Meta-analysis suggested decrease in blood loss, biliary leak and hospital stay compared with CC[47]
	Radiofrequency dissecting sealer	• Coagulates and seals zone of tissue
		• Maintains low tissue temperatures
		• No difference in blood loss or tumor recurrence compared with CC[44]
		• Higher infective and bleeding complications when compared with CC[42]
	Stapler transection	• Faster transection with comparable blood loss compared with CC[52]
		• Concerns that staples inadequately seal small biliary channels
		• Highly costly

CC refers to traditional clamp-crush method with clips/ties alone for vessel ligation.
Data from Refs.[42,44,47,51,52]

plane. Water-jet dissection uses a high-velocity laminar water jet to allow precise dissection of hepatic parenchyma with preservation of fibrous structures in the absence of a surrounding zone of cellular injury. The water jet is favored by many surgeons for its utility in the exposure of major pedicles and hepatic veins. The limited available trials do not show any technique to be clearly superior and the choice currently remains a matter of surgeon preference.[44–46]

Ligation of intraparenchymal vasculobiliary structures can be achieved with a similar variety of techniques. Bipolar electrothermal vessel sealers are attractive, as they are able to seal and divide vessels up to 7 mm in diameter. Despite theoretic concerns of improper sealing of biliary channels, no trials have demonstrated an increase in postoperative bile leaks.[47] Radiofrequency dissecting sealer devices have also been suggested to offer improved hemostasis by creating a region of ablation that is subsequently transected. Of potential concern, radiofrequency-assisted techniques generate a zone of coagulation on each side of the planned transection plane, resulting in additional tissue loss. Although very few well-conducted trials have evaluated radiofrequency devices in hepatic resection, the available data suggest that it offers

Table 2 Summary of topical hemostatic agents		
Topical Hemostatic Agent	**Active Component**	**Selected Examples**
Matrix agents	Collagen Cellulose Gelatin Microporous polysaccharide spheres	Avitene, Instat Surgicel Gelfoam, Surgifoam Arista
Coagulation factor-based agents	Fibrin sealant (fibrinogen and thrombin) Topical thrombin	Tisseel Evithrom
Combination agents	Gelatin/Thrombin Collagen/Fibrinogen/Thrombin	Floseal, Surgiflo TachoSil

modest reductions in blood loss but is associated with increased postoperative abscess formation and possibly more frequent bile leaks.[48–50]

Management of the Remnant Surface

Hemorrhage from the raw liver surface can lead to significant blood loss in the post-transection and postoperative phases. Meticulous inspection of the cut surface of the liver remnant allows identification of small blood and biliary vessels that can be controlled with ligation, clips, or other sealing techniques. Topical hemostatic agents are adjuncts commonly used to facilitate the development of a stable coagulum to seal the cut surface of the remnant. Available agents can be broadly classified as (1) hemostatic matrix agents, (2) coagulation factor-based agents, and (3) combination agents (**Table 2**). Matrix agents provide a scaffold for endogenous coagulation to occur and contain no active coagulation factors. These matrices are typically composed of oxidized cellulose, microfibrillar collagen, microporous polysaccharide spheres, or gelatin. The coagulation factor–based agents are the most common topical hemostatic agents currently in use by liver surgeons.[53] These compounds typically contain fibrinogen or thrombin along with various compositions of coagulation cofactors (eg, calcium, factor XII, aprotinin) and serve to reenact the endogenous coagulation cascade. Fibrinogen is converted to fibrin by thrombin as a final stage of the coagulation cascade, permitting the formation of clot. Topical thrombin is also available and is similarly applied to activate endogenous fibrinogen. Many of the commercially available agents are combination agents that contain both active hemostatic components and a coagulation matrix.

Fibrin sealants reduce time to hemostasis and increase rates of complete intraoperative hemostasis.[54] There is no definitive evidence that any topical hemostatic agent decreases clinically significant outcomes, such as blood loss, transfusion, and perioperative morbidity in liver resection, although few studies are adequately powered for these endpoints.[40,53] Furthermore, little evidence exists to suggest whether combination agents are more efficacious than matrix agents alone.[55–57] The interpretation of the available evidence is complex due to the quality of studies and diversity of topical hemostatic agents. The data appear to suggest that intraoperative blood loss can be improved with topical hemostatic agents, yet the superiority of any one agent has not been demonstrated and the substantial costs of many of these agents have not been justified.

SUMMARY

Although outcomes following hepatectomy have improved substantially over time, blood loss continues to pose a challenge to liver surgeons. Perioperative blood loss and allogeneic transfusion are clearly associated with inferior short-term and long-term outcomes in patients. With modern approaches and techniques, blood loss can be minimized and allogeneic transfusion can be avoided in the vast majority of patients undergoing major hepatic resection. The techniques described herein and their appropriate application should be familiar to the hepatic surgeon to ensure best outcomes in patients undergoing hepatic resection.

REFERENCES

1. Foster JH. Survival after liver resection for cancer. Cancer 1970;26(3):493–502.
2. Jarnagin WR, Gonen M, Fong Y, et al. Improvement in perioperative outcome after hepatic resection: analysis of 1,803 consecutive cases over the past decade. Ann Surg 2002;236(4):397–406.
3. Hallet J, Tsang M, Cheng ESW, et al. The impact of perioperative red blood cell transfusions on long-term outcomes after hepatectomy for colorectal liver metastases. Ann Surg Oncol 2015;22(12):4038–45.
4. Bui LL, Smith AJ, Bercovici M, et al. Minimising blood loss and transfusion requirements in hepatic resection. HPB (Oxford) 2002;4(1):5–10.
5. Gurusamy KS, Li J, Sharma D, et al. Pharmacological interventions to decrease blood loss and blood transfusion requirements for liver resection. Cochrane Database Syst Rev 2009;(4):CD008085.
6. Kooby DA, Stockman J, Ben-Porat L, et al. Influence of transfusions on perioperative and long-term outcome in patients following hepatic resection for colorectal metastases. Ann Surg 2003;237(6):860–9.
7. Ejaz A, Spolverato G, Kim Y, et al. Variation in triggers and use of perioperative blood transfusion in major gastrointestinal surgery. Br J Surg 2014;101(11):1424–33.
8. Amato A, Pescatori M. Perioperative blood transfusions for the recurrence of colorectal cancer. Cochrane Database Syst Rev 2006;(1):CD005033.
9. Rohde JM, Dimcheff DE, Blumberg N, et al. Health care–associated infection after red blood cell transfusion. JAMA 2014;311(13):1317–26.
10. Hébert PC, Wells G, Blajchman MA, et al. A multicenter, randomized, controlled clinical trial of transfusion requirements in critical care. Transfusion requirements in critical care investigators, Canadian critical care trials group. N Engl J Med 1999;340(6):409–17.
11. Villanueva C, Colomo A, Bosch A, et al. Transfusion strategies for acute upper gastrointestinal bleeding. N Engl J Med 2013;368(1):11–21.
12. Carson JL, Terrin ML, Noveck H, et al. Liberal or restrictive transfusion in high-risk patients after hip surgery. N Engl J Med 2011;365(26):2453–62.
13. Carson JL, Grossman BJ, Kleinman S, et al. Red blood cell transfusion: a clinical practice guideline from the AABB*. Ann Intern Med 2012;157(1):49–58.
14. American Society of Anesthesiologists Task Force on Perioperative Blood Management. Practice guidelines for perioperative blood management: an updated report by the American Society of Anesthesiologists task force on perioperative blood management*. Anesthesiology 2015;122(2):241–75.
15. Wehry J, Cannon R, Scoggins CR, et al. Restrictive blood transfusion protocol in liver resection patients reduces blood transfusions with no increase in patient morbidity. Am J Surg 2015;209(2):280–8. Elsevier Inc.
16. Melendez JA, Arslan V, Fischer ME, et al. Perioperative outcomes of major hepatic resections under low central venous pressure anesthesia: blood loss, blood transfusion, and the risk of postoperative renal dysfunction. J Am Coll Surg 1998;187(6):620–5.

17. Wang W-D, Liang L-J, Huang X-Q, et al. Low central venous pressure reduces blood loss in hepatectomy. World J Gastroenterol 2006;12(6):935–9.
18. Smyrniotis V, Kostopanagiotou G, Theodoraki K, et al. The role of central venous pressure and type of vascular control in blood loss during major liver resections. Am J Surg 2004;187(3):398–402.
19. Gurusamy KS, Li J, Vaughan J, et al. Cardiopulmonary interventions to decrease blood loss and blood transfusion requirements for liver resection. Cochrane Database Syst Rev 2012;(5):CD007338.
20. Hasegawa K, Takayama T, Orii R, et al. Effect of hypoventilation on bleeding during hepatic resection: a randomized controlled trial. Arch Surg 2002;137(3): 311–5.
21. Rahbari NN, Koch M, Zimmermann JB, et al. Infrahepatic inferior vena cava clamping for reduction of central venous pressure and blood loss during hepatic resection: a randomized controlled trial. Ann Surg 2011;253(6):1102–10.
22. Zhu P, Lau W-Y, Chen Y-F, et al. Randomized clinical trial comparing infrahepatic inferior vena cava clamping with low central venous pressure in complex liver resections involving the Pringle manoeuvre. Br J Surg 2012;99(6):781–8.
23. Hashimoto T, Kokudo N, Orii R, et al. Intraoperative blood salvage during liver resection. Ann Surg 2007;245(5):686–91.
24. Park JO, Gonen M, D'Angelica MI, et al. Autologous versus allogeneic transfusions: no difference in perioperative outcome after partial hepatectomy. J Gastrointest Surg 2007;11(10):1286–93.
25. Sima CS, Jarnagin WR, Fong Y, et al. Predicting the risk of perioperative transfusion for patients undergoing elective hepatectomy. Ann Surg 2009;250(6):914–21.
26. Jarnagin WR, Gonen M, Maithel SK, et al. A prospective randomized trial of acute normovolemic hemodilution compared to standard intraoperative management in patients undergoing major hepatic resection. Ann Surg 2008;248(3):360–9.
27. Carless PA, Henry DA, Moxey AJ, et al. Cell salvage for minimising perioperative allogeneic blood transfusion. Cochrane Database Syst Rev 2010;4:CD001888.
28. Waters JH, Yazer M, Chen Y-F, et al. Blood salvage and cancer surgery: a meta-analysis of available studies. Transfusion 2012;52(10):2167–73.
29. Henry DA, Carless PA, Moxey AJ, et al. Anti-fibrinolytic use for minimising perioperative allogeneic blood transfusion. Cochrane Database Syst Rev 2011;3:CD001886.
30. Wu CC, Ho WM, Cheng SB, et al. Perioperative parenteral tranexamic acid in liver tumor resection. Ann Surg 2006;243(2):173–80.
31. Lentschener C, Benhamou D, Mercier FJ, et al. Aprotinin reduces blood loss in patients undergoing elective liver resection. Anesth Analg 1997;84(4):875–81.
32. Pringle JH. V. Notes on the arrest of hepatic hemorrhage due to trauma. Ann Surg 1908;48(4):541–9.
33. Belghiti J, Noun R, Malafosse R, et al. Continuous versus intermittent portal triad clamping for liver resection: a controlled study. Ann Surg 1999;229(3):369–75.
34. Gurusamy KS, Sheth H, Kumar Y, et al. Methods of vascular occlusion for elective liver resections. Cochrane Database Syst Rev 2009;(1):CD007632.
35. Man K, Fan ST, Ng IO, et al. Prospective evaluation of Pringle maneuver in hepatectomy for liver tumors by a randomized study. Ann Surg 1997;226(6):704–11.
36. Man K, Lo CM, Liu CL, et al. Effects of the intermittent Pringle manoeuvre on hepatic gene expression and ultrastructure in a randomized clinical study. Br J Surg 2003;90(2):183–9.
37. Chouker A. Effects of Pringle manoeuvre and ischaemic preconditioning on haemodynamic stability in patients undergoing elective hepatectomy: a randomized trial. Br J Anaesth 2004;93(2):204–11.

38. Capussotti L, Muratore A, Ferrero A, et al. Randomized clinical trial of liver resection with and without hepatic pedicle clamping. Br J Surg 2006;93(6):685–9.
39. Lee KF, Cheung YS, Wong J, et al. Randomized clinical trial of open hepatectomy with or without intermittent Pringle manoeuvre. Br J Surg 2012;99(9):1203–9.
40. Sanjay P, Ong I, Bartlett A, et al. Meta-analysis of intermittent Pringle manoeuvre versus no Pringle manoeuvre in elective liver surgery. ANZ J Surg 2013;83(10): 719–23.
41. Pamecha V, Gurusamy KS, Sharma D, et al. Techniques for liver parenchymal transection: a meta-analysis of randomized controlled trials. HPB (Oxford) 2009;11(4):275–81.
42. Gurusamy KS, Pamecha V, Sharma D, et al. Techniques for liver parenchymal transection in liver resection. Cochrane Database Syst Rev 2009;(1):CD006880.
43. Truong JL, Cyr DP, Lam-McCulloch J, et al. Consensus and controversy in hepatic surgery: a survey of Canadian surgeons. J Surg Oncol 2014;110(8):947–51.
44. Lesurtel M, Selzner M, Petrowsky H, et al. How should transection of the liver be performed? Ann Surg 2005;242(6):814–23.
45. Rau HG, Wichmann MW, Schinkel S, et al. Surgical techniques in hepatic resections: ultrasonic aspirator versus Jet-Cutter. A prospective randomized clinical trial. Zentralbl Chir 2001;126(8):586–90 [in German].
46. Takayama T, Makuuchi M, Kubota K, et al. Randomized comparison of ultrasonic vs clamp transection of the liver. Arch Surg 2001;136(8):922–8.
47. Alexiou VG, Tsitsias T, Mavros MN, et al. Technology-assisted versus clamp-crush liver resection: a systematic review and meta-analysis. Surg Innov 2013;20(4): 414–28.
48. Xiao WK, Chen D, Hu AB, et al. Radiofrequency-assisted versus clamp-crush liver resection: a systematic review and meta-analysis. J Surg Res 2014;187(2): 471–83.
49. Lupo L, Gallerani A, Panzera P, et al. Randomized clinical trial of radiofrequency-assisted versus clamp-crushing liver resection. Br J Surg 2007;94(3):287–91.
50. Arita J, Hasegawa K, Kokudo N, et al. Randomized clinical trial of the effect of a saline-linked radiofrequency coagulator on blood loss during hepatic resection. Br J Surg 2005;92(8):954–9.
51. Saiura A, Yamamoto J, Koga R, et al. Usefulness of LigaSure for liver resection: analysis by randomized clinical trial. Am J Surg 2006;192(1):41–5.
52. Rahbari NN, Elbers H, Koch M, et al. Randomized clinical trial of stapler versus clamp-crushing transection in elective liver resection. Br J Surg 2014;101(3):200–7.
53. Boonstra EA, Molenaar IQ, Porte RJ, et al. Topical haemostatic agents in liver surgery: do we need them? HPB (Oxford) 2009;11(4):306–10.
54. Sanjay P, Watt DG, Wigmore SJ. Systematic review and meta-analysis of haemostatic and biliostatic efficacy of fibrin sealants in elective liver surgery. J Gastrointest Surg 2012;17(4):829–36.
55. Öllinger R, Mihaljevic AL, Schuhmacher C, et al. A multicentre, randomized clinical trial comparing the Veriset™ haemostatic patch with fibrin sealant for the management of bleeding during hepatic surgery. HPB (Oxford) 2012;15(7):548–58.
56. Chapman WC, Clavien PA, Fung J, et al. Effective control of hepatic bleeding with a novel collagen-based composite combined with autologous plasma: results of a randomized controlled trial. Arch Surg 2000;135(10):1200–4.
57. Moench C, Mihaljevic AL, Hermanutz V, et al. Randomized controlled multicenter trial on the effectiveness of the collagen hemostat Sangustop® compared with a carrier-bound fibrin sealant during liver resection (ESSCALIVER study, NCT00918619). Langenbecks Arch Surg 2014;399(6):725–33.

Technical Aspects of Gallbladder Cancer Surgery

Motaz Qadan, MD, PhD, T. Peter Kingham, MD*

KEYWORDS

- Gallbladder cancer • Incidental • Nonincidental • Laparoscopic • Robotic
- Segment IVB/V • Biliary tract cancer

KEY POINTS

- Gallbladder cancer is a rare disease that may be diagnosed incidentally following cholecystectomy or nonincidentally, often with more advanced disease.
- The principal aim of surgical resection is attainment of negative margins.
- Jaundice is considered an ominous sign in the presentation of gallbladder cancer.
- Minimally invasive resection techniques are well described in the surgical treatment of gallbladder cancer.
- The roles of adjuvant and neoadjuvant therapies in the treatment of gallbladder cancer remain poorly elucidated.

INTRODUCTION

Gallbladder cancer is a rare disease, although it is the most common disease of the biliary tract. Its incidence has increased over the last 20 years. This increase may be a result of the increasing prevalence of laparoscopic cholecystectomy, which is responsible for incidentally discovered gallbladder cancer.[1] Despite the increasing incidence of gallbladder cancer, laparoscopic cholecystectomy has permitted earlier detection and improved survival of what was once considered a disease associated with a dismal prognosis.[2]

In this review, an updated description of gallbladder cancer is divided into 2 sections based on presentation: disease that presents incidentally following laparoscopic cholecystectomy and malignancy that is suspected preoperatively. Elements pertaining to technical aspects of surgical resection provide the critical focus of this review

The authors have no conflicts of interests, financial or otherwise, to disclose.
Department of Surgery, Memorial Sloan Kettering Cancer Center, 1275 York Avenue, New York, NY 10065, USA
* Corresponding author.
E-mail address: kinghamt@mskcc.org

and are discussed in the context of evidence-based literature on gallbladder cancer today.

EPIDEMIOLOGY

The estimated incidence of gallbladder cancer is approximately 2 per 100,000 of the population in the United States.[3] As of 2015, there are an estimated 10,910 cases in the United States annually, including other biliary tumors, compared with only approximately 9250 cases in 2008.[3,4] The incidence seems to be significantly higher in women (3:1) and more commonly occurs in patients older than 40 years.[5] Incidence of gallbladder cancer is based on the central etiologic factor of cholelithiasis, with variations in geography and race mirroring the incidence of gallstone disease. For example, the incidence of gallbladder cancer in Norway, where cholelithiasis rates are low, ranges from 0.2 to 0.4 per 100,000 people. Conversely, the incidence of gallbladder cancer ranges from 9.3 to 25.3 per 100,000 among Chilean Mapuche Indian women, in whom gallstone disease is more prevalent.[6] Furthermore, mortality rates seem to also be higher in Andean populations within South America.[7] Finally, even within the United States, the incidence among Native Americans in the state of New Mexico is approximately 14.5 per 100,000, a rate that is dramatically higher than the national average.[8]

CAUSE AND PATHOGENESIS

Cholelithiasis is considered a primary etiologic factor in gallbladder cancer, which results in chronic mucosal inflammation, dysplasia, and subsequent malignant transformation, with the development of porcelain features clinically.[7] Only approximately 0.3% to 3.0% of patients with long-standing cholelithiasis will develop gallbladder cancer, highlighting the rarity of gallbladder cancer.[9] Interestingly, in a case-control study that compared gallstones in patients with and without gallbladder cancer, there were significantly more stones and heavier stones in patients who developed gallbladder cancer.[10] Despite this, the mechanistic association between gallstones and frank malignancy is not fully established. In a study by Jain and colleagues,[11] the investigators examined 350 gallbladder specimens from patients with gallstones and found mucosal hyperplasia in 32.0%, metaplasia in 47.8%, dysplasia in 15.7%, and carcinoma in situ in 0.6% of specimens. The investigators were able to show loss of genetic heterozygosity in 2.1% to 47.8% of preneoplastic lesions at 8 different loci for several tumor suppressor genes associated with gallbladder cancer but showed no loss of heterozygosity in normal gallbladders, thereby suggesting a possible mechanistic association between gallstones and gallbladder cancer beyond inflammation and neoplasia.

In keeping with other gastrointestinal malignancies, progression from adenoma to carcinoma has also been stipulated in gallbladder cancer, particularly in sessile adenomata greater than 1 cm in size.[12] Although adenomatous polyps exist in only about 1% of gallbladder specimens, up to 7% of lesions harbor malignancy.[13,14] Cancer was more likely to exist in isolated, broad-based polyps, with increasing size. A size cutoff of 1 cm is often considered relevant.

Although porcelain gallbladder does not automatically imply malignancy, gallbladder cancer may occur in approximately 1 in 13 patients with a porcelain appearance.[15] These data are still debated, as demonstrated by a recent case series evaluating the risk of gallbladder cancer in patients with a porcelain gallbladder. This series found 13 patients with porcelain gallbladder identified among 1200 cholecystectomy patients. None of the 13 patients had evidence of carcinoma.[16]

Systematic reviews including 60,665 cholecystectomies reported 0.2% of patients had porcelain gallbladders. Only 15% of those patients (ie, 0.03% of the total cohort) were diagnosed with gallbladder carcinomas. The issue of cholecystectomy for porcelain gallbladder remains unsettled; but given the possibility of an elevated relative risk of cancer in porcelain gallbladder compared with nonporcelain gallbladder and the potential for cure in patients treated with early cholecystectomy, it is reasonable to consider cholecystectomy.[17]

TNM STAGING SYSTEM

The American Joint Commission for Cancer (AJCC) gallbladder cancer TNM staging system is described in **Table 1**. Most cases of gallbladder cancer are adenocarcinomas, although variants, including papillary, mucinous, squamous, and adenosquamous subtypes, are well described. Importantly, and while describing the T-stage (depth of tumor invasion), emphasis should be placed on where the gallbladder cancer is in the gallbladder, given that the gallbladder hepatic interface lacks serosa and consists only of the perimuscular connective tissue that is continuous with hepatic connective tissue (cystic plate). This has implications in the surgical management of resectable disease as described later. Nodal drainage patterns are shown in **Fig. 1**.

INCIDENTAL GALLBLADDER CARCINOMA

Incidental gallbladder cancer following cholecystectomy is found in approximately 0.2% to 1.1% of all laparoscopic cholecystectomies.[18] When discovered intraoperatively, the procedure should be aborted and patients should be transferred to a

Table 1
AJCC seventh edition TNM staging system for gallbladder cancer

Primary Tumor	
T_X	Primary tumor cannot be assessed
T0	No evidence of primary tumor
T_{is}	Carcinoma in situ
T1a	Tumor invades lamina propria
T1b	Tumor invades muscular layer
T2	Tumor invades perimuscular connective tissue without extension into serosa
T3	Tumor perforates serosa (visceral peritoneum) and/or directly invades liver or an adjacent organ
T4	Tumor invades main portal vein or hepatic artery or invades 2 or more organs
Regional Lymph Nodes	
N_X	Regional nodes cannot be assessed
N0	No regional lymph node metastasis
N1	Metastases to nodes along the cystic duct, common bile duct, hepatic artery, and/or portal vein
N2	Metastases to para-aortic, para-caval, superior mesenteric artery, and/or celiac artery lymph nodes
Distant Metastasis	
M0	No distant metastasis
M1	Distant metastasis

From AJCC: gallbladder. In: Edge SB, Byrd DR, Compton CC, et al, editors. AJCC cancer staging manual. 7th edition. New York: Springer; 2010. p. 211–7.

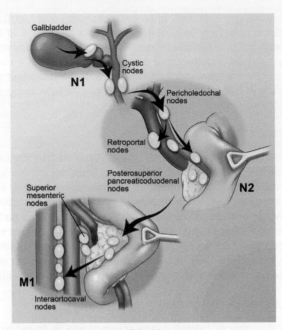

Fig. 1. Lymph node drainage basins in gallbladder cancer.

hepatobiliary center. Outcomes of patients with an incidental finding of gallbladder cancer have a better prognosis than nonincidentally discovered disease, provided patients are staged and managed appropriately with R0 resection.[19] Critically, however, the presence of any residual disease following attempted resection dramatically reduces disease-free interval and disease-specific survival, with survival comparable with stage 4 gallbladder cancer. In a report by Butte and colleagues,[20] disease-free survival in patients with residual disease was 11.2 months, compared with 93.4 months in patients without residual disease.

Preoperative Work-up

Following referral of cases with incidentally discovered gallbladder cancer within the gallbladder specimen after cholecystectomy, high-resolution imaging is uniformly utilized to evaluate for residual disease, nodal metastases, and identification of distant metastatic disease. Given associated postoperative changes, the role of ultrasound imaging is limited. However, review of precholecystectomy ultrasound findings in order to determine the location of the tumor is often helpful, in addition to discussing intraoperative findings with the referring surgeon of record.

Although computed tomography (CT) or magnetic resonance imaging (MRI) provide critical information in restaging patients following laparoscopic cholecystectomy, the role of fluorodeoxyglucose-positron emission tomography (FDG-PET) in this setting is not established. FDG-PET scans have shown a 78% sensitivity and 80% specificity in detecting residual disease.[21] In addition, FDG-PET helped detect metastatic disease in 29% to 55% of patients who had undergone cholecystectomy.[22] A complementary role with CT in detecting extrahepatic metastases has been demonstrated.[23] Significant false positivity associated with nonspecific FDG-avidity in the postcholecystectomy gallbladder fossa has also been elucidated in these studies. A recent report from the authors' institution correlated CT and MRI findings with FDG-PET scans in patients with gallbladder cancer.[24] Of 100 total patients included in the study, there were 63 patients with incidental gallbladder cancer. Three of the 100 patients had additional disease on FDG-PET, which prevented unnecessary operation; 2 patients had suspicious CT findings refuted by FDG-PET that permitted operation; 12 patients had equivocal CT findings confirmed by FDG-PET; and 3 patients had additional invasive procedures performed owing to FDG-PET avidity in other sites. The findings confirmed a modest impact on management of patients with gallbladder cancer, particularly in patients with suspicious nodal disease and those without a prior cholecystectomy (nonincidental gallbladder cancer). FDG-PET caused a change in management, however, in only 13% of patients with incidental gallbladder cancer, compared with 31% in patients with in situ gallbladder cancer ($P = .035$).

Surgical Restaging of Incidental Postcholecystectomy Gallbladder Cancer

Selection for reoperation is based on surgical staging, as evaluated by the AJCC staging system discussed earlier. In general, M1 disease is considered unresectable, with no role for surgical intervention. Approximately one-quarter of patients with gallbladder cancer have metastatic disease.[25] Because there is a limited role for palliative surgical intervention in this disease process, unnecessary laparotomy should be avoided; starting with staging laparoscopy provides a logical approach in the treatment of incidentally discovered postcholecystectomy gallbladder cancer. In a review performed at the authors' institution, Butte and colleagues[26] evaluated the role of staging laparoscopy in patients with incidental gallbladder carcinoma. In 136 consecutive patients, staging laparoscopy was carried out in 46 patients, of whom 10 had disseminated disease. Only 2 of these patients, however, had disease detected during laparoscopy, before conversion to laparotomy (yield 4.3% and accuracy 20.0%). Although disseminated disease was a relatively infrequent event, the likelihood of disseminated disease correlated with an increasing T-stage, positive margin at initial cholecystectomy, and increasing tumor grade. Given the low risks associated with the procedure, high yield, and significant benefit associated with avoidance of unnecessary laparotomy in this population, the authors perform staging laparoscopy in all patients undergoing resection of incidental gallbladder cancer.

Timing of Radical Reresection

There are now data that show delaying reresection of patients with incidental gallbladder cancer may improve patient selection. Ausania and colleagues[27] reported results using a treatment algorithm with intentional delayed staging of incidental T2 and T3 gallbladder cancer following cholecystectomy by 3 months. This delay permitted careful evaluation for residual disease and extrahepatic spread as well as observation of the biological behavior of the tumor. Importantly, the investigators were able to show that this strategy permitted the avoidance of unnecessary laparotomy in patients who, arguably, may not have benefited from surgical resection. This delay was done without adversely affecting survival in patients who remained candidates for resection. Median overall survival among the 24 patients who underwent radical resection was 54.8 months. There were 24 patients who were found to be unresectable on preoperative imaging and 1 found to be unresectable at operation, in whom median survival was 9.7 months.

Surgical Treatment of Early (T1 and T2) Incidental Gallbladder Cancer

Because T1a gallbladder cancer only extends into the lamina propria, a simple cholecystectomy is often considered sufficient for the treatment of these tumors. With negative margins, the cure rate after simple cholecystectomy has ranged from 85% to 100%.[28] Therefore, no additional resection is warranted in this group of patients.

With T1b tumors, survival data did not similarly support the concept that simple cholecystectomy would suffice. For example, in a report by Principe and colleagues, the investigators reported a 1-year survival rate of 50% only following margin negative simple cholecystectomy, despite a lack of invasion of the tumor into the perimuscular connective tissue.[29] The reduced survival rate and importance of radical resection in this setting arises because of a residual disease incidence of up to 10% and lymph node metastatic incidence of 10% to 20% described in the literature, with potential locoregional recurrence rates of up to 20% to 50%.[1,30] Radical resection, including reresection of the hepatic bed (segments IVB and V) and portal nodal lymphadenectomy, is recommended for T1b tumors detected incidentally after cholecystectomy.

With T2 tumors, early studies showed 5-year survival rates of 20% to 40% after cholecystectomy, compared with 70% to 80% in patients who underwent radical resection.[1,28,30–32] Although residual disease rates are, once again, increased with increasing T-stage, nodal involvement is thought to occur in approximately one-third of cases, although other studies have reported involvement in more than 60% of cases.[33] Radical resection, including reresection of the hepatic bed in an operation that includes segments IVB and V, with portal nodal lymphadenectomy, is recommended for T2 tumors detected incidentally after cholecystectomy. Reresection additionally provides accurate staging information, which allows patients to be referred for appropriate adjuvant therapy.

Of recent interest in the treatment and selection of patients for resection with T2 disease is tumor location. In a recent multi-institutional study by Shindoh and colleagues,[34] the investigators examined 437 patients with gallbladder cancer who were analyzed with tumor location defined as hepatic side or peritoneal side, given the anatomic discrepancy described earlier between the 2 locations. The investigators showed that in patients with tumors on the hepatic side, patients had higher rates of vascular invasion, neural invasion, and nodal metastases when compared with tumors located on the peritoneal side (51% vs 19%, 33% vs 8%, and 40% vs 17%, respectively). Five-year survival rates were 64.7% versus 42.6% ($P = .0006$) for peritoneal and hepatic tumors, respectively, with tumor location serving as a predictor of liver and distant nodal recurrence despite radical resection. Additional studies have confirmed the importance of tumor location in T2 disease and even recommended reservation of radical resection for T2 cancers located on the hepatic side.[35]

Surgical Treatment of Advanced (T3 and T4) Incidental Gallbladder Cancer

Treatment of T3 incidental gallbladder cancers is similar to T2 cancers and includes a radical resection of the gallbladder fossa with portal nodal lymphadenectomy. Outcomes following radical resection of T3 disease, although historically poor, now range widely from 21% to 63% in some studies, with an operative mortality less than 5%.[36,37] The incidence of residual disease and lymph node metastases is higher again, estimated at 36% and 46%, respectively.[25] With advanced disease stage, the need for more extensive hepatic and bile duct resections are often indicated in the attainment of negative surgical margins.[38]

In the case of T4 disease, the role of extensive vascular reconstructions in the treatment of gallbladder cancer has not been shown to provide a durable survival benefit. The perioperative morbidity and mortality associated with extensive reconstructions generally outweigh any survival benefit, and extensive resection and vascular reconstruction is generally not recommended. The role of neoadjuvant therapy in the treatment of advanced gallbladder cancers (T3 and T4) is discussed later.

Surgical Treatment of the Extrahepatic Bile Duct

Routine resection of the extrahepatic bile duct has not been uniformly associated with improved outcomes.[39] Rather, resection of the common bile duct has been shown to increase perioperative morbidity, with little additional benefit when performed empirically.[31,40] Unless there is a positive cystic duct margin to warrant additional re-excision, bile duct resection can be avoided. In cases when there is concern, intraoperative frozen section of the cystic duct stump margin can help determine the need for extended duct resection. If detected, a positive duct margin warrants bile duct excision in order to ensure negative margins. In this setting, bile duct resection may be performed following adequate exposure with a Kocher maneuver and division of the duct at the level of the duodenum. Reconstruction is then carried out with a Roux-en-Y hepaticojejunostomy. In the case of jaundice arising from malignant infiltration of the bile duct, the prognosis is often poor, so a biliary stent and neoadjuvant chemotherapy is warranted.[41] Finally, resection of the extrahepatic bile duct has not been associated with a more effective portal nodal lymphadenectomy.

Surgical Treatment of the Hepatic Margin and Extended Liver Resections

In terms of radical reresection, recommendations for liver resection have varied from limited 2-cm wedge resections of the gallbladder fossa to routine extended right hepatectomy. In reality, the size of the wedge liver resection will depend on the pathologic depth of the tumor and stage of disease, ranging from limited segment IVB and V wedge resections to formal anatomic resections (**Fig. 2**). With the aid of intraoperative ultrasound, vascular anatomy should be delineated to guide the resection margin, ensuring full tumor clearance and identifying branches of the middle hepatic vein to allow for a controlled transection. Pedicles to segment 4b can be dissected in the umbilical fissure and divided before parenchymal transection begins. The main right anterior sectoral branches must be carefully preserved, although the pedicle to segment V is often also divided. In larger tumors, dividing the entire right anterior pedicle may be necessary. Pringle occlusion of the hepatic vascular inflow is helpful during parenchymal transection.

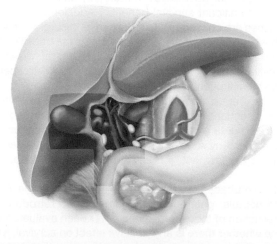

Fig. 2. Radical cholecystectomy, including cholecystectomy, segment IVB and V resection, and portal lymphadenectomy.

With respect to extended hepatic resections, if the tumor invades hepatic inflow vascular structures, particularly the right portal vein with larger tumors, a right hepatectomy may be required in order to ensure adequate tumor clearance and an R0 resection. The importance of meticulous preoperative planning must not be underestimated in this setting. If clearly visualized, right inflow involvement may be used as justification for administration of neoadjuvant chemotherapy. This treatment provides an opportunity for response to therapy to be determined, with potential avoidance of an unnecessary extensive operation. In cases whereby extended hepatectomy is necessary, bile duct resection is often also necessary because of the size of the tumor. In a study by D'Angelica and colleagues,[40] empirical resections of liver (15 of 36 patients) and bile duct (32 of 68 patients) did not predict outcome after resection for gallbladder cancer. Instead, there was an increased rate of perioperative morbidity among patients who underwent major hepatectomy and common bile duct excision, with outcomes correlating only with tumor biology and disease stage. These data are used to justify the authors' approach of using extensive resection only as needed to clear disease.

Finally, in well-selected patients, the resection of other organs, including the stomach, colon, and duodenum, in the absence of distant metastatic disease, may be resected to ensure an R0 resection. Combined pancreaticoduodenectomy with hepatectomy can be performed after treating with chemotherapy.[42]

Surgical Treatment of Lymph Nodes

Lymph node dissections have historically ranged from excision of the cystic duct lymph node to a complete portal lymphadenectomy with pancreaticoduodenectomy in the Japanese literature.[43,44] In the authors' experience, the addition of hepatic and pancreatic resections contributes to additional morbidity without significant improvement in long-term survival and is not recommended.[5]

The presence of N1 nodal disease is not considered an absolute contraindication to surgical resection. Long-term survival with the presence of nodal metastatic disease, however, remains rare.[5] Given these poor outcomes, the authors usually treat patients with positive lymph nodes with neoadjuvant chemotherapy. More extensive nodal involvement that extends outside the hepatoduodenal ligament (N2) is considered unresectable, given the major postoperative morbidity and mortality associated with resection without any significant survival benefit.[45] Additional celiac and para-aortic lymph node metastases are considered M1 disease, and surgical resection is contraindicated. The highest peripancreatic lymph node marks the transition between the N1 and N2 fields and has been found to be prognostic of disease-specific and recurrence-free survival in biliary tract adenocarcinoma in a retrospective study performed at the authors' institution.[46]

At laparotomy, every effort should be made to carefully examine lymph nodes outside the radical resection field. Therefore, the exploration should begin with a Kocher maneuver to evaluate aortocaval and retropancreatic nodes, with careful examination of celiac nodes. Any suspicious nodes should be evaluated intraoperatively with frozen pathologic assessment; if positive, the procedure should be aborted at that time.

A standard portal lymphadenectomy for gallbladder cancer beyond T1a includes nodes in the porta hepatis, gastrohepatic ligament, and retroduodenal space (N1 nodes). Although resection of those nodes has never been evaluated in a prospective setting to determine whether there is any positive effect on survival, lymph node evaluation in this setting provides accurate staging and prognostic information at the very least. Indeed, the detection of lymph node disease, particularly in early stage gallbladder cancer, may influence the decision to administer adjuvant systemic therapy, which is discussed later.

Surgical Resection of Previous Port Sites

In a recent study from the authors' institution, patients who underwent port-site resection (69 patients) were compared with patients who underwent operation without port-site removal (44 patients).[47] Thirteen patients were noted to have port-site metastases, which occurred in patients with T2 and T3 cancer tumors, and correlated significantly with the development of peritoneal metastases. Survival was reduced from 42 months to 17 months when port-site disease was detected. However, port-site resection was not associated with overall survival or recurrence-free survival when R0-resected patients were compared and adjusted for T and N stage. Instead, port-site metastases were considered a harbinger of generalized peritoneal recurrence that would not be prevented with resection of these sites.[38] Fuks and colleagues[48] confirmed this finding in a separate study.[48] As a result of these combined findings, the authors do not routinely resect previous port-sites during radical resection.

Gallbladder Perforation During Cases of Incidental Gallbladder Cancer

In a recent German retrospective study by Goetze and Paolucci,[49] the investigators examined the rate of intraoperative perforation combined with the use of retrieval bags and showed that the rate of overall gallbladder cancer recurrence in perforated patients was significantly higher at 38.4%, compared with 27.2% in nonperforated patients. Once perforated, however, the use of retrieval bags did not reduce the recurrence rate, as evidenced by no significant difference in recurrence between cases with and without use of retrieval bags (32.5% vs 27.0%, respectively). Similarly, a recent study by Lee and colleagues[50] showed that bile spillage compared with no spillage was associated with a profound decline on disease-free survival (71.4% vs 20.9%, respectively) and overall survival (72.6% vs 25.8%, respectively). Although the diagnosis of incidental gallbladder cancer is only available following operation, the authors advocate for resection of the cystic plate in cases where clinical suspicion for malignancy arises during routine cholecystectomy, in order to significantly reduce the incidence of detrimental gallbladder perforation.

NONINCIDENTAL GALLBLADDER CARCINOMA

Early diagnosis of gallbladder cancer is uncommon in patients presenting with nonincidental gallbladder cancer. Interestingly, outcomes are significantly worse compared with incidentally discovered disease, even when matched for disease stage.[1,25] Given the frequently advanced stage on diagnosis, presenting signs and symptoms are wide ranging and include local signs and symptoms, such as jaundice, abdominal pain, abnormal stools, vomiting, and presence of a palpable mass, as well as nonspecific symptoms, such as weight loss, lethargy, and loss of appetite.

In addition, patients may present with generalized phenomena that are related to underlying malignancy, such as venous thromboembolism, including migratory thrombophlebitis (Trousseau sign), or with signs and symptoms that may be secondary to metastatic disease at presentation, such as shortness of breath in the case of pulmonary metastases or pathologic bone pain and/or fracture in osseous metastases.

Jaundice as a Presenting Sign

In cases of nonincidentally diagnosed gallbladder cancer, patients may present with jaundice as their initial presenting sign, which suggests malignant invasion of the biliary tree. In a study by Hawkins and colleagues[41] from the authors' institution, the investigators retrospectively reviewed the significance of jaundice in patients with gallbladder cancer. The investigators identified 82 jaundiced patients among 240 patients with gallbladder cancer who were more likely to have advanced stage disease. A mere total of 6 patients were resected with curative intent, and only 4 underwent resection with negative margins. The median disease-specific survival among jaundiced patients was 6 months, compared with 16 months in nonjaundiced patients. There were no disease-free survivors at 2 years among jaundiced patients, compared with 21% in nonjaundiced patients.

Conversely, in a later study by Varma and colleagues,[51] resection with negative margins was possible among 50% of patients with gallbladder cancer who presented with jaundice. The investigators showed that, although disease was significantly advanced among jaundiced patients, jaundice per se was not associated with disease unresectability in their patient cohort.

Although the authors do not recommend preclusion of resectability based on presentation with jaundice, meticulous evaluation of resectability is warranted, given that only 4 of 82 patients were resected with negative margins among patients reviewed at the authors' institution. Jaundice is considered to be an ominous sign in the authors' opinion and usually provides grounds for consideration of neoadjuvant therapy in the initial setting, in addition to endoscopic or percutaneous decompression of the biliary tree.

Preoperative Work-up

In cases of preoperative diagnosis of malignancy, disease is often locally advanced as described earlier. Radiologic staging is often carried out using CT or MRI to evaluate the extent of tumor invasion and depth, nodal metastases, and distant disease, with an ability to accurately delineate anatomic anomalies and detect vascular involvement, invasion into the biliary tree, hepatic parenchymal invasion, and nodal metastases. It is estimated that 75% of cases are already considered unsuitable for resection in nonincidentally diagnosed patients. FDG-PET, which is associated with lower false-positive rates than in incidentally diagnosed postcholecystectomy disease, has been used with more than 80% sensitivity and specificity in differentiating between malignant and nonmalignant disease in this setting.[52]

Preoperative Tissue Diagnosis

Although in incidental gallbladder cancer a diagnosis is already available, by definition, pathologic diagnosis in nonincidental disease is considered unnecessary for patients who are potentially resectable. Gallbladder cancer is characterized by an ability to seed the peritoneum, biopsy tracts, and surgical wounds; therefore, unnecessary biopsy may increase the risk of tumor dissemination.[53,54] In unresectable patients, percutaneous biopsy offers a reliable diagnosis with a documented sensitivity of approximately 88%.[55] Attempts to provide a pathologic diagnosis by removing the gallbladder are ill advised, given the significant risk of tumor spillage.

Extent of Surgical Resection of Nonincidental Gallbladder Cancer

In cases of nonincidental gallbladder cancer, many of the principles discussed following incidental diagnosis of gallbladder cancer apply, with the principal objective being attainment of negative surgical margins, including wedge, anatomic, or more extensive hepatic resections, with portal lymphadenectomy and extrahepatic bile duct resection only in the attainment of negative duct margins.[38] Simple cholecystectomy is almost never the treatment of choice in cases of nonincidental gallbladder cancer, given that T1a tumors, by definition, are unlikely to present or be detected radiologically in nonincidental disease.

MINIMALLY INVASIVE RESECTION OF GALLBLADDER CANCER

Traditionally, laparoscopic surgery has not been routinely recommended in the surgical management of suspected gallbladder cancer in the nonincidental setting. Several studies have pointed toward an increased incidence of port-site recurrence due to the manipulation of instruments through ports but also due to the chimney effect associated with carbon dioxide insufflation within the abdominal cavity.[7,56–59] However, more recent studies have failed to demonstrate any detrimental effect from purely laparoscopic approaches in the management of gallbladder cancer, with recent studies suggesting equivalent outcomes between laparoscopic and open approaches (**Table 2**).[60–65] Robotic-assisted procedures have also been described and are carried out at the authors' institution.[66]

When performing minimally invasive radical cholecystectomy, the authors begin by placing patients in a low lithotomy position, with the surgeon standing between the patients' legs. Robotic port placement is shown in **Fig. 3**. The procedure commences with staging intraoperative ultrasound. Use of laparoscopic energy devices is required, and the authors recommend use of a laparoscopic bipolar device for hemostasis during parenchymal transection (**Fig. 4**). Given inevitable blood loss during hepatic transection, the authors perform portal lymphadenectomy before parenchymal transection in order to ensure optimal visualization during portal triad dissection. Performing a Kocher maneuver is essential for adequate lymph node dissection. Retrieval bags should be used when extracting all specimens through port sites. Principles of resection, including lymphadenectomy, cystic duct margin analysis, and extrahepatic bile duct resections, are similar to open radical cholecystectomy.

SYSTEMIC THERAPY

Despite conflicting data on the use of adjuvant regimens in the treatment of gallbladder cancer, there are only limited level I data to support use, with most data being based on empirical therapies, phase II studies, or retrospective analyses. Phase III trials are emerging and now include gemcitabine-based therapies, which have shown improved efficacy over 5-fluorouracil (5-FU) regimens. In a recent 3-arm trial by

Table 2
Laparoscopic radical cholecystectomy series to date

	Cho et al,[63] 2010	Gumbs et al,[65] 2013	Agarwal et al,[64] 2015
Study period	2004–2007	2005–2011	2011–2013
Patient number	18	15	24
Inclusion of primary gallbladder cancer	Primary T1–T2	Primary T1–T3	Primary T1–3
Inclusion of incidental gallbladder cancer	No	Yes	Yes
Aortocaval node sampling	No	No	Yes
Extent of liver resection	2-mm wedge	Segment IVB/V	Segment IVB/V
Lymph node yield	8 (4–21)	4 (1–11)	10 (4–31)

Data from Refs.[63–65]

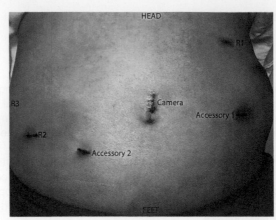

Fig. 3. Robotic port configuration in minimally invasive radical cholecystectomy. One or 2 accessory ports are used depending on the body habitus of patients.

Sharma and colleagues,[67] gemcitabine was compared with best supportive care and 5-FU in patients with unresectable disease. Gemcitabine was shown to improve median overall survival compared with both best supportive care and 5-FU, which exhibited similar survival (9.5 months versus 4.6 months, versus 4.5 months, respectively). In an earlier landmark Japanese phase III multi-institutional trial that included 140 patients with gallbladder cancer, patients were randomized to undergo resection followed by adjuvant mitomycin and 5-FU vs resection alone.[68] The study showed actuarial 5-year survivals of 20.3% vs 11.6% in favor of adjuvant therapy in patients with gallbladder cancer. Additional prospective trials have shown benefit from combining gemcitabine-based regimens with platinum agents, such as oxaliplatin and cisplatin, providing the rationale for current therapies in practice today.[69,70]

In a review of the published literature examining the role of radiation therapy in the treatment of gallbladder cancer, Houry and colleagues[71] demonstrated a slight improvement in survival in patients who received some form of radiation treatment. Most recently, a phase II trial combining gemcitabine, capecitabine, and radiation therapy in patients with extrahepatic biliary tract and gallbladder cancers showed promising efficacy and limited toxicity from use of this regimen, thereby allowing for future phase III trials incorporating gemcitabine-based radiation regimens to be investigated.[72]

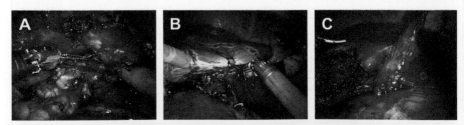

Fig. 4. (*A*) Intraoperative image of portal lymphadenectomy during robotic radical cholecystectomy. (*B*) Intraoperative image of preparation for segment IVB and V wedge resection during robotic radical cholecystectomy. (*C*) Intraoperative image of the completed radical cholecystectomy.

As described earlier, neoadjuvant chemotherapy is thought to provide an opportunity for response to therapy to be determined, during which time patients with biologically aggressive tumors who, arguably, may not benefit from extensive operations may declare themselves. Data investigating the regimens and outcomes related to neoadjuvant therapies are limited and have produced disappointing results in general. In a recent study from the MD Anderson Cancer Center, the investigators performed a retrospective review of their gallbladder cancers that were resected with wide 1-cm negative margins and had received either neoadjuvant or adjuvant therapy.[73] Five-year survival was 50.6%. A total of 17.8% of patients received neoadjuvant therapy; 48.7% received adjuvant chemotherapy; and 15.8% received adjuvant chemoradiation. Adjuvant therapy showed no improvement in survival, and neoadjuvant treatment had only served to significantly delay time to operation in their study, with immediate resection increasing survival from 42.3 months to 53.5 months. The investigators concluded the neither neoadjuvant treatment nor adjuvant therapies affected outcomes in patients who were resected with clear negative margins. Small case series have suggested possible efficacy associated with gemcitabine-platinum based combinations used in the neoadjuvant setting in the treatment of gallbladder and biliary tract cancers.[74–77]

LONG-TERM OUTCOMES

Many patients with gallbladder cancer will recur, with increased recurrence rates in nonincidental gallbladder cancer compared with incidental disease.[1] In a report published from the authors' institution by Jarnagin and colleagues,[78] 97 patients who underwent curative-intent resection were analyzed for long-term survival and outcomes. Overall, the median time to recurrence was 11.5 months, with 66% experiencing a recurrence at 24 months from their index procedure. Isolated locoregional recurrence occurred in only 15% of patients, compared with 85% presenting with distant disease that most commonly recurred in the peritoneum and was unrelated to initial disease stage on multivariate analysis. The systemic nature of gallbladder cancer was apparent. Positive resection margin was the only factor associated with distant recurrence on multivariate analysis, highlighting the importance of the aforementioned surgical principles in the definitive treatment of gallbladder cancer.

REFERENCES

1. Hueman MT, Vollmer CM Jr, Pawlik TM. Evolving treatment strategies for gallbladder cancer. Ann Surg Oncol 2009;16:2101–15.
2. Steinert R, Nestler G, Sagynaliev E, et al. Laparoscopic cholecystectomy and gallbladder cancer. J Surg Oncol 2006;93:682–9.
3. Randi G, Franceschi S, La VC. Gallbladder cancer worldwide: geographical distribution and risk factors. Int J Cancer 2006;118:1591–602.
4. Jemal A, Thun MJ, Ries LA, et al. Annual report to the nation on the status of cancer, 1975-2005, featuring trends in lung cancer, tobacco use, and tobacco control. J Natl Cancer Inst 2008;100:1672–94.
5. Miller G, Jarnagin WR. Gallbladder carcinoma. Eur J Surg Oncol 2008;34: 306–12.
6. Randi G, Malvezzi M, Levi F, et al. Epidemiology of biliary tract cancers: an update. Ann Oncol 2009;20:146–59.
7. Lazcano-Ponce EC, Miquel JF, Munoz N, et al. Epidemiology and molecular pathology of gallbladder cancer. CA Cancer J Clin 2001;51:349–64.

8. Barakat J, Dunkelberg JC, Ma TY. Changing patterns of gallbladder carcinoma in New Mexico. Cancer 2006;106:434–40.
9. Bartlett DL. Gallbladder cancer. Semin Surg Oncol 2000;19:145–55.
10. Roa I, Ibacache G, Roa J, et al. Gallstones and gallbladder cancer-volume and weight of gallstones are associated with gallbladder cancer: a case-control study. J Surg Oncol 2006;93:624–8.
11. Jain K, Mohapatra T, Das P, et al. Sequential occurrence of preneoplastic lesions and accumulation of loss of heterozygosity in patients with gallbladder stones suggest causal association with gallbladder cancer. Ann Surg 2014; 260:1073–80.
12. Fong Y, Malhotra S. Gallbladder cancer: recent advances and current guidelines for surgical therapy. Adv Surg 2001;35:1–20.
13. Yeh CN, Jan YY, Chao TC, et al. Laparoscopic cholecystectomy for polypoid lesions of the gallbladder: a clinicopathologic study. Surg Laparosc Endosc Percutan Tech 2001;11:176–81.
14. Tazuma S, Kajiyama G. Carcinogenesis of malignant lesions of the gall bladder. The impact of chronic inflammation and gallstones. Langenbecks Arch Surg 2001;386:224–9.
15. Kwon AH, Inui H, Matsui Y, et al. Laparoscopic cholecystectomy in patients with porcelain gallbladder based on the preoperative ultrasound findings. Hepatogastroenterology 2004;51:950–3.
16. Khan ZS, Livingston EH, Huerta S. Reassessing the need for prophylactic surgery in patients with porcelain gallbladder: case series and systematic review of the literature. Arch Surg 2011;146:1143–7.
17. Brown KM, Geller DA. Porcelain gallbladder and risk of gallbladder cancer. Arch Surg 2011;146:1148.
18. Pitt SC, Jin LX, Hall BL, et al. Incidental gallbladder cancer at cholecystectomy: when should the surgeon be suspicious? Ann Surg 2014;260:128–33.
19. Smith GC, Parks RW, Madhavan KK, et al. A 10-year experience in the management of gallbladder cancer. HPB (Oxford) 2003;5:159–66.
20. Butte JM, Kingham TP, Gonen M, et al. Residual disease predicts outcomes after definitive resection for incidental gallbladder cancer. J Am Coll Surg 2014;219: 416–29.
21. Anderson CD, Rice MH, Pinson CW, et al. Fluorodeoxyglucose PET imaging in the evaluation of gallbladder carcinoma and cholangiocarcinoma. J Gastrointest Surg 2004;8:90–7.
22. Corvera CU, Blumgart LH, Akhurst T, et al. 18F-fluorodeoxyglucose positron emission tomography influences management decisions in patients with biliary cancer. J Am Coll Surg 2008;206:57–65.
23. Shukla PJ, Barreto SG, Arya S, et al. Does PET-CT scan have a role prior to radical re-resection for incidental gallbladder cancer? HPB (Oxford) 2008;10:439–45.
24. Leung U, Pandit-Taskar N, Corvera CU, et al. Impact of pre-operative positron emission tomography in gallbladder cancer. HPB (Oxford) 2014;16:1023–30.
25. Pawlik TM, Gleisner AL, Vigano L, et al. Incidence of finding residual disease for incidental gallbladder carcinoma: implications for re-resection. J Gastrointest Surg 2007;11:1478–86.
26. Butte JM, Gonen M, Allen PJ, et al. The role of laparoscopic staging in patients with incidental gallbladder cancer. HPB (Oxford) 2011;13:463–72.
27. Ausania F, Tsirlis T, White SA, et al. Incidental pT2-T3 gallbladder cancer after a cholecystectomy: outcome of staging at 3 months prior to a radical resection. HPB (Oxford) 2013;15:633–7.

28. Shirai Y, Yoshida K, Tsukada K, et al. Radical surgery for gallbladder carcinoma. Long-term results. Ann Surg 1992;216:565–8.
29. Principe A, Del GM, Ercolani G, et al. Radical surgery for gallbladder carcinoma: possibilities of survival. Hepatogastroenterology 2006;53:660–4.
30. de Aretxabala X, Roa I, Burgos L, et al. Gallbladder cancer in Chile. A report on 54 potentially resectable tumors. Cancer 1992;69:60–5.
31. Bartlett DL, Fong Y, Fortner JG, et al. Long-term results after resection for gallbladder cancer. Implications for staging and management. Ann Surg 1996;224: 639–46.
32. Oertli D, Herzog U, Tondelli P. Primary carcinoma of the gallbladder: operative experience during a 16 year period. Eur J Surg 1993;159:415–20.
33. Shimada H, Endo I, Fujii Y, et al. Appraisal of surgical resection of gallbladder cancer with special reference to lymph node dissection. Langenbecks Arch Surg 2000;385:509–14.
34. Shindoh J, de Aretxabala X, Aloia TA, et al. Tumor location is a strong predictor of tumor progression and survival in T2 gallbladder cancer: an international multicenter study. Ann Surg 2015;261:733–9.
35. Lee H, Choi DW, Park JY, et al. Surgical strategy for T2 gallbladder cancer according to tumor location. Ann Surg Oncol 2015;22:2779–86.
36. Dixon E, Vollmer CM Jr, Sahajpal A, et al. An aggressive surgical approach leads to improved survival in patients with gallbladder cancer: a 12-year study at a North American center. Ann Surg 2005;241:385–94.
37. Fong Y, Jarnagin W, Blumgart LH. Gallbladder cancer: comparison of patients presenting initially for definitive operation with those presenting after prior noncurative intervention. Ann Surg 2000;232:557–69.
38. Shoup M, Fong Y. Surgical indications and extent of resection in gallbladder cancer. Surg Oncol Clin N Am 2002;11:985–94.
39. Fuks D, Regimbeau JM, Le Treut YP, et al. Incidental gallbladder cancer by the AFC-GBC-2009 Study Group. World J Surg 2011;35:1887–97.
40. D'Angelica M, Dalal KM, DeMatteo RP, et al. Analysis of the extent of resection for adenocarcinoma of the gallbladder. Ann Surg Oncol 2009;16:806–16.
41. Hawkins WG, DeMatteo RP, Jarnagin WR, et al. Jaundice predicts advanced disease and early mortality in patients with gallbladder cancer. Ann Surg Oncol 2004;11:310–5.
42. Wakai T, Shirai Y, Tsuchiya Y, et al. Combined major hepatectomy and pancreaticoduodenectomy for locally advanced biliary carcinoma: long-term results. World J Surg 2008;32:1067–74.
43. Matsumoto Y, Fujii H, Aoyama H, et al. Surgical treatment of primary carcinoma of the gallbladder based on the histologic analysis of 48 surgical specimens. Am J Surg 1992;163:239–45.
44. Sasaki R, Takahashi M, Funato O, et al. Hepatopancreatoduodenectomy with wide lymph node dissection for locally advanced carcinoma of the gallbladder-long-term results. Hepatogastroenterology 2002;49:912–5.
45. Niu GC, Shen CM, Cui W, et al. Surgical treatment of advanced gallbladder cancer. Am J Clin Oncol 2015;38:5–10.
46. Kelly KJ, Dukleska K, Kuk D, et al. Prognostic significance of the highest peripancreatic lymph node in biliary tract adenocarcinoma. Ann Surg Oncol 2014; 21:979–85.
47. Maker AV, Butte JM, Oxenberg J, et al. Is port site resection necessary in the surgical management of gallbladder cancer? Ann Surg Oncol 2012;19: 409–17.

48. Fuks D, Regimbeau JM, Pessaux P, et al. Is port-site resection necessary in the surgical management of gallbladder cancer? J Visc Surg 2013;150:277–84.
49. Goetze TO, Paolucci V. Use of retrieval bags in incidental gallbladder cancer cases. World J Surg 2009;33:2161–5.
50. Lee HY, Kim YH, Jung GJ, et al. Prognostic factors for gallbladder cancer in the laparoscopy era. J Korean Surg Soc 2012;83:227–36.
51. Varma V, Gupta S, Soin AS, et al. Does the presence of jaundice and/or a lump in a patient with gall bladder cancer mean that the lesion is not resectable? Dig Surg 2009;26:306–11.
52. Rodriguez-Fernandez A, Gomez-Rio M, Llamas-Elvira JM, et al. Positron-emission tomography with fluorine-18-fluoro-2-deoxy-D-glucose for gallbladder cancer diagnosis. Am J Surg 2004;188:171–5.
53. Merz BJ, Dodge GG, Abellera RM, et al. Implant metastasis of gallbladder carcinoma in situ in a cholecystectomy scar: a case report. Surgery 1993;114:120–4.
54. Fong Y, Brennan MF, Turnbull A, et al. Gallbladder cancer discovered during laparoscopic surgery. Potential for iatrogenic tumor dissemination. Arch Surg 1993;128:1054–6.
55. Akosa AB, Barker F, Desa L, et al. Cytologic diagnosis in the management of gallbladder carcinoma. Acta Cytol 1995;39:494–8.
56. Bouvy ND, Marquet RL, Jeekel H, et al. Impact of gas(less) laparoscopy and laparotomy on peritoneal tumor growth and abdominal wall metastases. Ann Surg 1996;224:694–700.
57. Lundberg O, Kristoffersson A. Open versus laparoscopic cholecystectomy for gallbladder carcinoma. J Hepatobiliary Pancreat Surg 2001;8:525–9.
58. Ricardo AE, Feig BW, Ellis LM, et al. Gallbladder cancer and trocar site recurrences. Am J Surg 1997;174:619–22.
59. Steinert R, Lippert H, Reymond MA. Tumor cell dissemination during laparoscopy: prevention and therapeutic opportunities. Dig Surg 2002;19:464–72.
60. Yoon YS, Han HS, Cho JY, et al. Is laparoscopy contraindicated for gallbladder cancer? A 10-year prospective cohort study. J Am Coll Surg 2015;221(4):847–53.
61. Gumbs AA, Hoffman JP. Laparoscopic radical cholecystectomy and Roux-en-Y choledochojejunostomy for gallbladder cancer. Surg Endosc 2010;24:1766–8.
62. Gumbs AA, Hoffman JP. Laparoscopic completion radical cholecystectomy for T2 gallbladder cancer. Surg Endosc 2010;24:3221–3.
63. Cho JY, Han HS, Yoon YS, et al. Laparoscopic approach for suspected early-stage gallbladder carcinoma. Arch Surg 2010;145:128–33.
64. Agarwal AK, Javed A, Kalayarasan R, et al. Minimally invasive versus the conventional open surgical approach of a radical cholecystectomy for gallbladder cancer: a retrospective comparative study. HPB (Oxford) 2015;17:536–41.
65. Gumbs AA, Jarufe N, Gayet B. Minimally invasive approaches to extrapancreatic cholangiocarcinoma. Surg Endosc 2013;27:406–14.
66. Shen BY, Zhan Q, Deng XX, et al. Radical resection of gallbladder cancer: could it be robotic? Surg Endosc 2012;26:3245–50.
67. Sharma A, Dwary AD, Mohanti BK, et al. Best supportive care compared with chemotherapy for unresectable gall bladder cancer: a randomized controlled study. J Clin Oncol 2010;28:4581–6.
68. Takada T, Amano H, Yasuda H, et al. Is postoperative adjuvant chemotherapy useful for gallbladder carcinoma? A phase III multicenter prospective randomized controlled trial in patients with resected pancreaticobiliary carcinoma. Cancer 2002;95:1685–95.

69. Sharma A, Mohanti B, Raina V, et al. A phase II study of gemcitabine and oxaliplatin (Oxigem) in unresectable gall bladder cancer. Cancer Chemother Pharmacol 2010;65:497–502.
70. Valle J, Wasan H, Palmer DH, et al. Cisplatin plus gemcitabine versus gemcitabine for biliary tract cancer. N Engl J Med 2010;362:1273–81.
71. Houry S, Barrier A, Huguier M. Irradiation therapy for gallbladder carcinoma: recent advances. J Hepatobiliary Pancreat Surg 2001;8:518–24.
72. Ben-Josef E, Guthrie KA, El-Khoueiry AB, et al. SWOG S0809: a phase II intergroup trial of adjuvant capecitabine and gemcitabine followed by radiotherapy and concurrent capecitabine in extrahepatic cholangiocarcinoma and gallbladder carcinoma. J Clin Oncol 2015;33:2617–22.
73. Glazer ES, Liu P, Abdalla EK, et al. Neither neoadjuvant nor adjuvant therapy increases survival after biliary tract cancer resection with wide negative margins. J Gastrointest Surg 2012;16:1666–71.
74. Sirohi B, Rastogi S, Singh A, et al. Use of gemcitabine-platinum in Indian patients with advanced gall bladder cancer. Future Oncol 2015;11:1191–200.
75. Selvakumar VP, Zaidi S, Pande P, et al. Resection after neoadjuvant chemotherapy in advanced carcinoma of the gallbladder: a retrospective study. Indian J Surg Oncol 2015;6:16–9.
76. Walker EJ, Simko JP, Nakakura EK, et al. A patient with cholangiocarcinoma demonstrating pathologic complete response to chemotherapy: exploring the role of neoadjuvant therapy in biliary tract cancer. J Gastrointest Oncol 2014;5: E88–95.
77. Kato A, Shimizu H, Ohtsuka M, et al. Surgical resection after downsizing chemotherapy for initially unresectable locally advanced biliary tract cancer: a retrospective single-center study. Ann Surg Oncol 2013;20:318–24.
78. Jarnagin WR, Ruo L, Little SA, et al. Patterns of initial disease recurrence after resection of gallbladder carcinoma and hilar cholangiocarcinoma: implications for adjuvant therapeutic strategies. Cancer 2003;98:1689–700.

Resection of Perihilar Cholangiocarcinoma

Hermien Hartog, MD, PhD[a], Jan N.M. Ijzermans, MD, PhD[a],
Thomas M. van Gulik, MD, PhD[b], Bas Groot Koerkamp, MD, PhD[a],*

KEYWORDS

- Perihilar cholangiocarcinoma • Hepatectomy • Caudate lobectomy
- Staging laparoscopy • Vascular reconstruction

KEY POINTS

- Staging laparoscopy avoids unnecessary laparotomy in 1 out of 4 patients with perihilar cholangiocarcinoma (PHC) scheduled for potential resection.
- Key anatomic features essential to recognize for resection of PHC:
  - Proximity of the biliary confluence to the right hepatic artery, except in cases of aberrant right hepatic artery.
  - The relation of the umbilical fissure and the confluence of the segment II and III bile ducts.
  - The relation of the right posterior bile duct and the right portal vein branches.
- Arterial involvement, lobar atrophy, and proximal biliary involvement together determine the feasibility of a complete resection and the optimal extent of resection.
- Portal venous resection may be required for a complete resection. Experts disagree whether arterial reconstructions should be considered in selected patients.
- Concomitant caudate lobectomy is the standard of care for resections of PHC based on level 2 evidence of increasing R0 resection rates.

INTRODUCTION

Perihilar cholangiocarcinoma (PHC) is located at the confluence of the left and right hepatic ducts. It is distinguished from distal cholangiocarcinoma by arising proximal to the cystic duct confluence.[1] Intrahepatic cholangiocarcinoma typically involves large liver tumors arising proximal to the second-order bile ducts.[1] The location of

[a] Division of HPB and Transplant Surgery, Department of Surgery, Erasmus MC, Postbus 2040, 3000 CA Rotterdam, The Netherlands; [b] Department of Surgery, Academic Medical Center, Meibergdreef 9, 1105 AZ Amsterdam, The Netherlands
* Corresponding author. Department of Surgery, Erasmus MC, Postbus 2040, Rotterdam 3000 CA, The Netherlands.
E-mail address: b.grootkoerkamp@erasmusmc.nl

Surg Clin N Am 96 (2016) 247–267
http://dx.doi.org/10.1016/j.suc.2015.12.008
0039-6109/16/$ – see front matter © 2016 Elsevier Inc. All rights reserved.

PHC at the biliary confluence near the bifurcation of the portal vein and the right hepatic artery explains why surgical resection is challenging.

The incidence of PHC is about 1 to 2 patients per 100,000 in Western countries. Patients typically present at an advanced stage with jaundice, weight loss, and abdominal discomfort.[2–4] Up to 65% of patients have unresectable or metastatic disease at time of presentation or surgical exploration and are ineligible for surgical resection.[3,5] Surgery for PHC is complex low-volume surgery, and therefore mainly performed in tertiary referral centers. The role of surgery for palliation is limited. Palliative treatment involves endoscopic and percutaneous biliary drainage and systemic chemotherapy.[6–8]

Most patients with resectable PHC require a major liver resection, which may entail complex biliary and vascular reconstruction. Over the past decades, the safety of major liver resections has increased because of improvements in perioperative management, resulting in a postoperative mortality of 1% to 3% in Eastern series.[9] However, 90-day postoperative mortality after resection of PHC was about 10% in 2 large nationwide Western series.[10,11] The main challenge in the preoperative management for patients with PHC is biliary drainage. A major liver resection may result in liver failure without prior biliary drainage of the future liver remnant (FLR). However, biliary drainage itself may cause cholangitis and liver failure.

This article gives an overview of current standards in surgical treatment of PHC and a description of signature strategies to PHC. Updates of twenty-first century management and outcomes have been published by all major groups and are summarized in this article (Appendix 1, **Table 1**).

PREOPERATIVE STAGING AND MANAGEMENT
Classification

Several tumor-staging systems have been developed to classify PHC for resectability and prognosis. The Bismuth-Corlette system[12] describes the extent of involvement of the biliary tree, but is insufficient to determine resectability and poorly predicts survival (**Fig. 1**B). The Blumgart/Memorial Sloan Kettering Cancer Center (MSKCC) system added portal vein involvement and lobar atrophy to the biliary extent of the tumor.[5] This addition led to a 3-stage system that is associated with both resectability and survival (see **Fig. 1**B–D).[13]

The seventh edition of the American Joint Committee on Cancer (AJCC)/Union for International Cancer Control staging system requires histopathologic data that become available only after surgical resection.[1] The recently proposed Mayo staging system is based on imaging features, performance status, and cancer antigen 19.9 level.[14] The AJCC and the Mayo staging are not useful to determine resectability in the preoperative setting.

Preoperative Staging

Staging of PHC typically starts with an abdominal and chest computed tomography (CT) scan to rule out stage IV disease. Both distant metastases and lymph node involvement beyond the hepatoduodenal ligament (ie, N2 nodes) are considered stage IV disease.[1] Suspicious lymph nodes beyond the hepatoduodenal ligament (ie, celiac or periaortic) may be assessed by endoscopic ultrasonography and fine-needle aspiration. Biliary extent of the tumor (Bismuth classification), portal vein and hepatic artery involvement, and anatomic variants are also addressed by multiphase contrast-enhanced liver CT. Magnetic resonance cholangiopancreatography is recommended if surgical decision making requires more detail of the biliary extent of the tumor. With high suspicion of malignancy on imaging, pathologic confirmation of PHC before surgery is not imperative. A negative brush or biopsy does not rule out cancer. Series of resection for PHC typically find a benign cause in about 10%.[15–17]

Anatomy

Several anatomic relations may determine resectability and the extent of liver resection (see **Fig. 1A**):

- The biliary confluence is located eccentrically to the right side of the hepatoduodenal ligament. The right portal vein and right hepatic artery are at higher risk of tumor involvement even in tumors mainly involving the left hepatic duct.
- The right hepatic duct and portal vein divide early into second-order branches. Consequently, complete resection with a wide margin and reconstruction of bile ducts and portal vein can be difficult. The left hepatic duct and portal vein have a longer extrahepatic course before branching.
- The left hepatic artery is rarely involved because it runs at the left periphery of the porta hepatis before entering the umbilical fissure.
- Segment I bile ducts enter the main bile ducts near the confluence of the left and right hepatic duct superior to the portal bifurcation and are therefore typically involved by direct tumor spread.[18]
- Biliary obstruction and portal vein involvement may cause lobar atrophy as shown by a shrunken lobe without regeneration capacity.[5]

Several prevalent anatomic variations may further affect the surgical strategy for liver resections:

- About 10% of patients have an infraportal right posterior duct compared with a supraportal course (**Fig. 2**). This variation allows a wider right posterior and anterior sectoral bile duct margin with a left hemihepatectomy.[19]
- About 10% of patients have a replaced or accessory right hepatic artery arising from the superior mesenteric artery.[20] Because this artery courses at the right and dorsal side of the hepatoduodenal ligament, it evades its normal close proximity to the biliary confluence.

Resectability

Centers in the Western and Eastern hemispheres disagree whether patients with stage IV PHC should undergo a resection. In Eastern series, patients with stage IVb PHC typically represent up to 10% of patients undergoing a resection.[19,21] Because survival of these patients is poor, most Western centers do not consider a resection for stage IV disease.

The goal of surgery is to completely remove all tumor tissue (R0 resection) maintaining an adequate FLR. An incomplete (R2) resection is probably futile and any potential benefit too small to justify the surgical risk. The biliary extent of PHC should allow an R0 resection and permit technically feasible biliary-enteric anastomoses. An adequate FLR includes at least 2 contiguous liver segments with arterial and portal inflow and venous outflow. An adequate FLR is typically defined as representing at least 25% of the total liver volume. However, the size of an adequate FLR also depends on the FLR function, which is determined by preexisting liver disease and biliary obstruction. Preoperative cholestasis and cholangitis are risk factors for postoperative liver failure and may require a larger FLR (ie, 30%–40%). PHC is unresectable if an R0 resection or an adequate FLR is not anticipated. In some patients a curative-intent resection is only possible with an arterial reconstruction. Clinicians at most Western centers think that

Table 1
Recent Eastern and Western patient series of resected PHC

Author	Accrual	N	Median Survival (mo)	Morbidity (%)	Mortality (%)	CL (%)	R0 (%)	L/R	Tri/Hemi/Min
Eastern Series									
Nagino et al[44]	2001–2010	386	36	47	2	100	78	219/148	121/245/20
Lee[78]	2000–2008	302	28–47	43	2	100	71	94/163	14/243/45
Song et al[36]	1995–2010	230	39	9	4	44	77	41/132	80/93/54
Shimizu et al[21]	1984–2008	224	±34	40	2–10	100	63–69	88/84	13/159/26
Esaki et al[26]	2000–2011	214, incl. IHC	38–45	56	3	100	53–72	119/46	30/182/2
Natsume et al[19]	2001–2010	201	24	33–59	1	100	70–85	—	86/115/—
Matsumoto et al[27]	2001–2012	174	±36	27–45	0–4	100	85 vs 82	—/174	33/141/—
Cheng et al[33]	2001–2010	171	29	26	3	80	78	122/41	28/131/12
Chen et al[31]	2000–2007	138	38	30	0	83	89	26/19	—/45/93
Kow et al[34]	1995–2010	127	35–64	6	3	55	88	34/83	45/72/—
Unno et al[79]	2001–2008	125	27	49	8	100	63	51/74	10/115/—
Hosokawa et al[28]	2001–2012	61	25–42	51	3	100	72	61/0	18/43/—
Xiong et al[47]	2005–2012	52	13–45	34–70	4	85	65–100	14/6	—/20/32
Lim et al[46]	2000–2012	52	19–23	31	0	100	73–100	6/13	1/18/26
Tamoto et al[43]	2005–2009	49	21	63	4	NR	82	0/49	49/—/—

Western Series

Nuzzo et al[10]	1992–2007	440, MC	NR	48	10	78	77	182/172	106/248/86
Farges et al[11]	1997–2008	366, MC	NR	67	11	Usually	NR	182/184	NR
De Jong[80]	1984–2010	305, MC	NR	NR	12	NR	65	95/114	68/141/96
Wahab et al[35]	1995–2010	159	36	52	6	50	55	104/55	—/159/—
Matsuo et al[13]	1991–2008	157	39	59	8	43	76	53/72	64/61/31
Neuhaus et al[42]	1990–2004	100	24–60	NR	8–9	100	NR	27/73	83/17/—
Hemming[81]	1999–2010	95	38	35	5	100	84	29/66	74/11/—
Ribero et al[32]	1989–2010	82	25	65	10	95	89	33/39	29/44/9
van Gulik et al[50]	2008–2010	41	NR	46	7	78	92	13/18	29/2/10
Total, n%/median, range	—	4251	34 (13–64)	42 (6–70)	5 (0–12)	100 (43–100)	78 (53–100)	1393/1825	981/2305/542
								43 vs 57%	26/60/14%

Search strategy: PubMed: (hilar OR perihilar) AND (cholangio*). Limits: English, humans. Case series published before 2008 or with fewer than 5 patients per year were excluded.

Abbreviations: CL, caudate lobectomy; Hemi, hemihepatectomy; IHC, intrahepatic cholangiocarcinoma; L/R, left-sided and right-sided liver resections; MC, multicenter study; Min, minor resection, including central liver resections and extrahepatic bile duct resections; NR, not reported; R0, R0 resection rate; Tri, trisectionectomy.

Data from Refs. 10,11,13,19,21,26–28,31–36,42–44,46,47,50,78–81

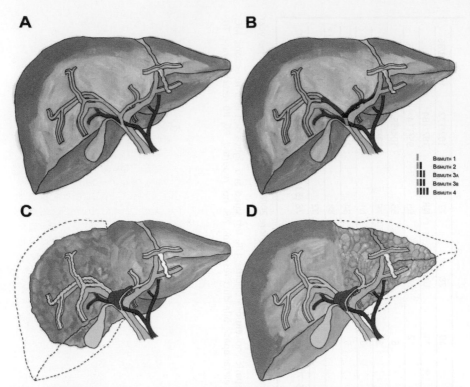

Fig. 1. Classification of PHC. (*A*) Key anatomic features. (*B*) Bismuth-Corlette staging system. Blumgart/Memorial Sloan Kettering Cancer Center (MSKCC) stage T1: tumor involving bile duct bifurcation and/or unilateral extension into second-order bile ducts. (*C*) Blumgart/ MSKCC stage T2, with unilateral vascular involvement and/or unilateral lobar atrophy. (*D*) Blumgart/MSKCC stage T3, with bilateral/contralateral involvement of second-order bile ducts, vascular involvement, and/or lobar atrophy. *Original artwork by Mrs. Elsbeth Leeffers.*

the increased postoperative mortality risk without proven survival benefit does not justify arterial reconstruction.[22]

Preoperative Biliary Drainage

Endoscopic or percutaneous biliary drainage of the FLR facilitates restoration of FLR function and regeneration. The contralateral lobe needs to be drained only in case of cholangitis. Whether biliary drainage should be pursued in each jaundiced patient with resectable PHC is still subject to debate, as is the optimal route of decompression. Risk of cholangitis caused by instrumentation of the bile ducts should be weighed against improvement of liver function and regeneration with biliary drainage. Most centers currently recommend preoperative biliary decompression with bilirubin levels greater than 2 mg/dL.[23] Eastern centers typically prefer nasobiliary decompression.[9] Western centers perform both endoscopic and percutaneous drainage. A phase III trial is currently recruiting patients to compare endoscopic and percutaneous drainage for patients with resectable PHC.[24]

Portal Vein Embolization

When the FLR is smaller than 40% of the total liver volume, portal vein embolization (PVE) of the contralateral portal vein is recommended to induce hypertrophy of the

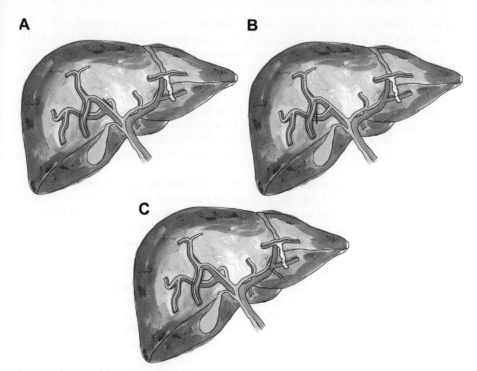

Fig. 2. Relation of the sectoral bile ducts to portal vein branches. (*A*) Supraportal course of right posterior bile duct. (*B*) Infraportal course of right posterior bile duct. (*C*) The umbilical portion of the left portal vein can be mobilized to the left, allowing transection of the bile ducts to segments II and III on the left side of the umbilical fissure. *Original artwork by Mrs. Elsbeth Leeffers.*

FLR.[25] Regenerative capacity of the liver is affected by bilious congestion, and biliary drainage of the FLR should therefore be performed before PVE. A downside of PVE is that the surgeon has to commit to a right-sided or left-sided resection. The preferred side for liver resection may change during exploratory laparotomy when the extent of the tumor differs from preoperative imaging (eg, contralateral hepatic artery involvement).

EXTENT OF LIVER RESECTION
Left or Right Hemihepatectomy

In patients eligible for resection, a choice should be made between a right-sided and a left-sided hepatectomy. Typically, the side of the liver with more extensive biliary disease (ie, involvement of second-order bile ducts or lobar atrophy) is resected. Both a left-sided and right-sided resection are possible in patients without lobar atrophy, second-order bile duct involvement, or right hepatic artery involvement. However, biliary drainage of the FLR and PVE of the resected liver regularly require that the decision between left-sided and right-sided resection is made before exploratory laparotomy.

In recent patient series, right-sided hepatectomies were performed slightly more often (58%) than left-sided resections (see **Table 1**). Three groups from Japan compared patients with left-sided and right-sided resections.[19,21,26,27] No difference was found in R0 resection rates, 5-year survival, and rate of portal vein reconstruction.

However, significantly more hepatic artery reconstructions were needed with a left hemihepatectomy (odds ratio [OR], 0.14; 95% confidence interval [CI], 0.06–0.31, $P<.001$) (Appendix 2: Fig. S1). The close anatomic relation of the right hepatic artery to the bile duct bifurcation may require more dissection near the tumor in left-sided approaches. One study accordingly found more positive periductal margins in left hemihepatectomies.[21]

A right-sided resection seems to allow for a wider margin because of the longer extrahepatic course of the left hepatic duct. However, detailed pathology study found small differences in the length of the resected right hepatic duct in left hemihepatectomy specimens (13.7 mm) and the left duct in right hemihepatectomy specimens (14.5 mm).[19,28]

In left-sided resections, wider margins can be obtained by extending the resection into the segmental ducts of the right anterior and posterior sector. However, in most patients (85%), the supraportal course of the right posterior sectoral duct limits the extent of bile duct resection: the right posterior sectoral duct quickly disappears behind the right anterior portal vein (see **Fig. 2**A).[29,30] In patients with a variant infraportal course of the right posterior sectoral duct (15%), a wide margin on the bile duct is facilitated with left hemihepatectomy (see **Fig. 2**B).[19] Theoretic advantages of left-sided and right-sided resections are summarized in **Table 2**.

In centers that do not commit to arterial reconstructions for PHC, establishing involvement of the right hepatic artery is a first crucial step before committing to a left hemihepatectomy. Left hepatic artery involvement is rare. **Fig. 3** presents a flowchart to guide selection of the type of liver resection in patients with PHC.

Trisectionectomy

A trisectionectomy is required if a hemihepatectomy may result in an incomplete resection. In patients with unilateral involvement of the second-order bile ducts (ie, Bismuth III) a trisectionectomy is required in the presence of contralateral atrophy or arterial involvement. For example, a right trisectionectomy can be considered for a patient with a Bismuth IIIb PHC and involvement of the right hepatic artery.

In patients with bilateral involvement of the second-order bile ducts (ie, Bismuth IV) a trisectionectomy is almost always required for a complete resection. One potential exception is patients with a variant infraportal course of the right posterior sectoral duct (15%), facilitating a wide margin when transecting the right sectoral ducts with a left hemihepatectomy (see **Fig. 2**B).[19]

Extended resections encompass 28% of resections for PHC in recent series (see **Table 1**). Four recent patient series studied the additional benefit of trisectionectomy versus hemihepatectomy in patients with PHC. Three studies included only left-sided resections and 1 study only right-sided resections. Pooled analysis showed that extended resections could be performed with no apparent additional risk of mortality

Table 2		
Advantages and disadvantages of left-sided and right-sided liver resections		
	Left-sided Resection	**Right-sided Resection**
FLR	Larger[78]	Smaller
Achieving negative bile duct margins	May be more difficult	May be more feasible
Portal vein reconstructions	More complex	Less complex
Arterial reconstruction required	More frequent	Rare
Trisectionectomy	More complex	Less complex

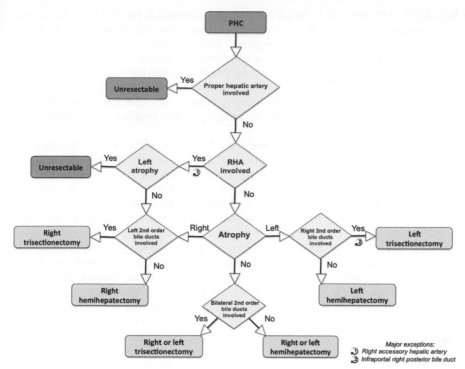

Fig. 3. Flowchart for surgical resection in PHC. RHA, right hepatic artery.

(2%–3%; OR, 0.65; 95% CI, 0.15–2.85; P = .6). However, a 2-fold increase in morbidity rate was found (up to 80%; OR, 2.37; 95% CI, 1.40–4.0; P = .001). These studies are all from Asian centers and may not be applicable to Western centers, which generally report higher mortalities.[10,11] Pooled analysis showed an increase in R0 resection rate with trisectionectomy (OR, 1.86; 95% CI, 1.18–2.94; P = .008) (Appendix 2: Fig. S2). No survival benefit was shown, although the trisectionectomy group contained more patients with advanced tumors.

Trisectionectomy seems justified to improve R0 resection rates in selected patients with PHC who are fit for major surgery with an anticipated adequate FLR (recommendation B2).

Caudate Lobectomy

The anatomic rationale for caudate lobectomy (CL) is that the segment I bile ducts enter the main bile ducts near the confluence of the left and right hepatic duct and are therefore prone to becoming involved by direct tumor spread. CL may increase the chance of an R0 resection by clearance of the caudate bile duct branches and surrounding hilar plate tissue. In 1990, Nimura and collagues[18] first described a case series of caudate lobe resection combined with partial hepatectomy. This report showed microscopic tumor involvement in the caudate branches in 44 out of 45 patients with PHC (98%). Two other reports show a much lower rate of involvement of 22% and 34%.[31,32]

In an analysis of 4 studies, representing 580 patients with Bismuth III to IV PHC, 61% underwent a concomitant CL. A 5-fold increased R1 rate was found when CL was omitted (OR, 0.20; 95% CI, 0.09–0.45; $P = .003$) (Appendix 2: Fig. S3).[33–36] CL was not an independent prognostic factor for overall survival in any individual study, and no increase in perioperative morbidity or mortality was reported.

CL can be technically challenging. The caudate lobe lies between the portal vein and the vena cava, beneath the gastrohepatic ligament. Caudate branches arising from the left and right hepatic arteries and portal vein are ligated and divided to control inflow to the caudate lobe. Transection of the lesser omentum exposes the caudate lobe. In right-sided resections an aberrant or accessory left hepatic artery should be preserved.

In right-sided resections, the right hepatic lobe is then mobilized and the retrohepatic veins are ligated and divided. The caudate lobe is now completely detached from the inferior vena cava (IVC), allowing division of the right hepatic vein. Next, at parenchymal transection the dorsal aspect of the middle hepatic vein is exposed, and the caudate lobe is pulled ventrally and detached from the left liver.

In left-sided resections, the retrohepatic veins are ligated and divided with a left-sided and inferior approach. Division of the ligamentum venosum exposes the common trunk of the left and middle hepatic veins, which is encircled and divided. The caudate lobe is then completely detached from the IVC en bloc with the left liver. Mobilization of the caudate lobe from the right side may be avoided to preserve the outflow vessels of the remnant liver. In these cases, an anterior approach (with hanging maneuver) can be considered to facilitate parenchymal transection with preservation of the outflow vessels of the remnant liver.[37,38]

En-bloc CL is recommended for resection of PHC (recommendation B1).

Extensive Resections

Several strategies have been proposed to decrease the risk of incomplete (R1 or R2) resections by extended hepatectomies or routine portal vein resections. A trade-off should be made between the oncological benefit of more extensive resection and the associated increased postoperative mortality.

Neuhaus and colleagues[39,40] (Berlin, Germany) proposed a hilar en-bloc resection involving a right trisectionectomy with en-bloc portal vein bifurcation, right hepatic artery, and extrahepatic bile ducts. The portal vein resection is performed in all patients without dissection near the tumor to determine involvement of the portal vein or right hepatic artery. The right hepatic artery is transected at its origin from the common hepatic artery. The left portal branch is isolated at the base of the umbilical portion, without dissecting out the portal bifurcation. After cross-clamping of the main and left portal veins, the portal vein is transected followed by an end-to-end reconstruction. In addition, the parenchyma is transected along the right side of the umbilical fissure. A similar technique was described by Hirano and colleagues[41] (Sapporo, Japan), combining routine portal vein resection with a right hemihepatectomy. This strategy is particularly appealing for patients with a high risk of portal vein involvement. In a retrospective study, this approach in 50 patients was compared with 50 conventional liver resections without routine portal vein resection.[42] The hilar en-bloc resection with routine portal vein resection conferred a survival benefit in R0 resected patients with similar postoperative mortality. However, a recent study failed to confirm the survival benefit associated with hilar en-bloc resection.[43] Therefore, routine portal vein resection is not recommended by consensus guidelines (recommendation C2).[23]

Nagino and colleagues[44] (Nagoya, Japan) introduced the anatomic right trisectionectomy. This approach extends the transection of the segmental bile ducts to the left side of the umbilical fissure to decrease the risk of a positive bile duct margin. In a right trisectionectomy, most surgeons divide the liver just to the right of the umbilical fissure to avoid injury to the blood supply and biliary drainage of segment II and III. Instead, with this strategy the branches to segment IV are divided within the umbilical fissure. Subsequently, the umbilical portion of the left portal vein can be pulled to the left, allowing transection of the bile ducts to segments II and III on the left side of the umbilical fissure (see **Fig. 2C**). With this approach, on average a 1-cm additional length of bile duct is resected.[27] This strategy is appealing in particular for patients with left-sided second-order bile duct involvement who require a right-sided resection. Rela and colleagues[45] (London, United Kingdom) introduced the Rex recess approach by combining the previous 2 strategies and adding a venous interposition graft for portal venous reconstruction.

Central Hepatectomy

Extended liver resections have a high incidence of postoperative liver failure and death. Consequently, a parenchymal-sparing central hepatectomy has been proposed. This partial hepatectomy involves anatomic or nonanatomic resection of only segments I and IV with en-bloc extrahepatic bile duct resection. The left bile duct is transected at the origin of the umbilical portion and at the right bile duct at the bifurcation of the anterior and posterior right bile ducts.[31,46] Multiple biliary-enteric reconstructions are typically required.

In 3 studies, a total of 150 patients undergoing central liver resection were compared with 91 patients with comparable tumor characteristics undergoing conventional major liver resection.[31,46,47] Most patients had Bismuth 1 or 2 tumors, and meta-analysis of the 3 studies showed more R0 resections with conventional major liver resection, although the OR was not statistically significant (OR, 0.20; 95% CI, 0.03–1.20; $P = .08$) (Appendix 2: Fig. S4). Infrequent concomitant CL may have biased these results toward lower R0 resection rates in central hepatectomies. Complication rates were 3-fold lower with central hepatectomies (OR, 0.35; 95% CI, 0.20–0.62; $P<.001$).

As in other resections for PHC, a central hepatectomy involves transection of the distal common bile duct and skeletonizing the portal vein and hepatic artery.[31,46,48,49] The caudate lobe is dissected free and its segmental arterial, portal, and retrohepatic branches are ligated and divided. Intraoperative ultrasonography guides the nonanatomic parenchymal resection of segment 4b a few centimeters away from the tumor. Alternatively, a wider dome-shaped central hepatectomy is performed, referred to as Taj Mahal resection (**Fig. 4**). This central hepatectomy consists of a base formed between the left side of the right hepatic vein and the medial side of the middle hepatic vein. At the liver dome the resection line narrows down toward the Cantlie line, which can be visualized by temporary vascular clamping.[48,49] The left hepatic duct is transected at the umbilical fissure and the right hepatic duct at or beyond the confluence of the right anterior and posterior bile ducts.

Central liver resections with CL can be considered for PHC with caution (recommendation B2). The main advantage is the reduced risk of postoperative liver failure and death. The main disadvantages are the concern for incomplete resection and the increased risk of biliary complications with multiple bilioenteric anastomoses. Alternative parenchymal-sparing techniques concern preservation of segment IVa and/or segment VIII with (extended) hemihepatectomies.[50] The decision to preserve segment IVa in a right trisectionectomy depends on the level where the segment IV sectoral duct enters the left hepatic duct.

Liver Transplantation

If a positive margin or inadequate FLR is anticipated, a total hepatectomy with liver transplant should be considered for PHC. A published multicenter study from the

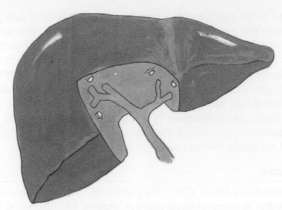

Fig. 4. Central liver resection including CL for PHC. *Original artwork by Mrs. Elsbeth Leeffers.*

United States presented a large cohort of 216 patients who underwent liver transplant for PHC after neoadjuvant (external beam) radiotherapy and chemotherapy.[51] Patients had unresectable early stage (I or II) PHC or underlying primary sclerosing cholangitis (63%). Posttransplant 5-year recurrence-free survival was 65%. Other groups have shown long-term survival in 30% to 45% of patients.[52,53] At present, PHC is an accepted indication for liver transplant in several countries worldwide, performed in study protocols with or without neoadjuvant therapy.[54]

INTRAOPERATIVE DECISION MAKING
Staging Laparoscopy

Up to 65% of patients who proceed to surgery for a curative-intent resection are found to have metastasis or unresectable tumors at surgical exploration.[55–58] Staging laparoscopy can avoid a laparotomy when peritoneal or liver metastases are found. In a pooled analysis (Appendix 2: Fig. S5) of 6 studies representing 546 patients with PHC, the authors found that the yield of staging laparoscopy was 27% (95% CI, 17%–37%).[55–60] However, the actual yield may be lower because of selection bias and improvement in preoperative imaging. After a negative staging laparoscopy an additional 1 out of 4 patients are found to harbor metastasis or are unresectable at exploratory laparotomy. Moreover, staging laparoscopy typically fails to detect nodal metastases beyond the hepatoduodenal ligament (N2) or unresectable disease because of biliary extent or vascular involvement.[61]

Laparoscopic examination for metastatic disease includes inspection of the peritoneum (including the diaphragm, falciform ligament, hepatoduodenal ligament, lesser sac, and pelvis), the liver (including the undersurface of segments 2/3 and 4b/5/6), and the greater omentum. The lesser omentum is opened to inspect the celiac lymph nodes. Enlarged lymph nodes may be sampled using a biopsy forceps.

Staging laparoscopy avoids unnecessary laparotomy in 1 out of 4 patients with PHC who are adequately staged by preoperative imaging techniques. It should be performed in all patients with PHC before exploratory laparotomy.

Frozen Sections

The risk of an R1 resection was about 25% in recent series of patients undergoing a curative-intent resection for PHC (see **Table 1**). Longitudinal tumor extension in bile ducts is difficult to assess with preoperative imaging as well as intraoperative ultrasonography. Frozen sections of the proximal and distal bile duct resection margins can ascertain tumor clearance. A pancreatoduodenectomy should be considered if a positive margin at the distal common bile duct is found and obtaining an additional margin is infeasible. Obtaining an additional proximal bile duct margin is often technically possible. Whether obtaining additional margins results in a survival benefit for patients with PHC has not been proved.[32,62,63] However, patients with a negative proximal bile duct margin after an initial positive frozen section have a better survival than those with an additional positive margin.[64] Frozen sections are tempting and performed by most liver surgeons, but probably do not improve survival. A positive margin is more likely a reflection of an advanced tumor than poor surgical judgment or technique.[65]

Intraoperative Assessment of Resectability

About 1 out of 6 patients with PHC with resectable disease on preoperative imaging is found to have (locally advanced) unresectable disease at exploratory laparotomy.[5] The most common findings precluding a curative-intent resection are the extent of bile duct involvement and unexpected involvement of the right hepatic artery. Preoperative imaging is imperfect in determining the biliary extent of the tumor. PHC is unresectable if a negative bile duct margin is not anticipated intraoperatively.

Unexpected involvement of the right hepatic artery may also preclude a resection; for example, in patients with left lobar atrophy. The right hepatic artery runs posterior to the common hepatic duct in 85% of patients. In this position posterior to the bile duct, extensive dissection in the liver hilum is required to evaluate involvement of the right hepatic artery. Early transection of the distal bile duct has been proposed to avoid dissection near the tumor and facilitate clearance of all tissue in the hepatoduodenal ligament.[66] The disadvantage of this strategy is that unresectable disease may be ascertained only after transecting the distal common bile duct.

Portal Vein Resection and Reconstruction

About 40% of patients with PHC have unilateral portal vein involvement.[64] In many patients, the involved left or right portal vein can be transected without vascular reconstruction. Portal vein reconstruction is required in patients with tumor involvement of the bifurcation or contralateral portal vein involvement. Reconstruction depends on the extent of resection: primary closure of a wedge resection, end-to-end anastomosis of a short segmental resection, and rarely reconstruction requiring patches or interposition grafts. In general, a left-sided hepatectomy requires a more complex portal vein reconstruction than right-sided hepatectomy, because of a shorter branch.[67] Portal vein reconstruction can be done before or after parenchymal transection. Several Eastern studies found no increase in morbidity and mortality with portal vein resections in patients with PHC.[22,68,69]

Lymphadenectomy

Regional lymph node metastases (N1) include nodes along the cystic duct, common bile duct, hepatic artery, and portal vein.[1,70,71] Involvement of periaortic, pericaval, and celiac nodes constitutes N2 and stage IV disease.[1] Lymphadenectomy of the hepatoduodenal ligament is recommended for all resections for PHC.[72] Lymphadenectomy is performed by skeletonizing the main portal vein and hepatic artery within the hepatoduodenal ligament. All lymphatic tissue can be resected en bloc with the extrahepatic bile duct.

A survival benefit of lymphadenectomy has not been shown. Lymphadenectomy is mainly useful for accurate staging. Lymph node status is the strongest independent prognostic factor in patients with PHC. In a series of 79 patients undergoing a resection for node-positive PHC, all patients eventually died of PHC.[73] No randomized controlled trial has been performed to investigate the benefit of extended lymphadenectomy for PHC. However, for pancreatic cancer, 5 randomized controlled trials found no benefit of extended lymphadenectomy.[74] A recent systematic review of the literature found that a lymph node count of more than 6 is adequate for prognostic staging of PHC.[75]

OUTCOMES OF CURATIVE-INTENT RESECTION FOR PERIHILAR CHOLANGIOCARCINOMA

A review of recent case series, representing more than 4000 patients with PHC who underwent surgery with curative intent, showed a median overall survival of 34 months. The aggregated morbidity and hospital mortality were 42% and 5%, respectively (see **Table 1**). These analyses include Eastern series with patients who underwent incomplete (R2) resections and resections for stage IV disease. Two large multicenter nationwide Western studies found a postoperative mortality of about 10%.[10,11]

Several prognostic factors may identify subgroups of patients with better survival. In patients with R0 resection median overall survival rates of 60 to 65 months are reported.[34,42,73] In addition, a negative lymph node status, lymph node count of more than 3, well-differentiated tumor grade, and papillary phenotype are independent predictors of favorable survival.[73,76] Lymph node metastases, present in 30% to 50% of patients, invariably lead to recurrence, with recurrence rates approaching 80% at 3-year follow-up and 100% at 7-year follow-up.[73,77] Despite these poor outcomes, a resection may still improve life expectancy and quality of life in patients with positive lymph nodes.

SUMMARY

Patients with stage IV disease (distant metastases or N2 nodal disease) and those unfit to tolerate major surgery are not eligible for surgical resection of PHC. Moreover, PHC is unresectable if an R0 resection with an adequate functional liver remnant is not feasible. Bilateral involvement of second-order bile ducts (ie, Bismuth IV) does not preclude an R0 resection. Patients requiring a hepatic artery reconstruction are considered unresectable in most Western centers. Selected patients with unresectable early stage tumors should be considered for liver transplant.

Preoperative decision making regarding biliary drainage and PVE is difficult. Preoperative biliary drainage of the FLR is intended to decrease the risk of postoperative liver failure. However, drainage may also cause cholangitis, which is strongly associated with postoperative death. PVE can increase the FLR volume beyond a minimum of 25% to 40%, but commits the surgeon to a left-sided or right-sided resection before exploratory laparotomy.

Lobar atrophy, involvement of the right hepatic artery, and involvement of second-order bile ducts guide the choice between left-sided and right-sided hepatectomies. The main advantages of a right-sided resection are less need for dissection near the tumor and the long left hepatic duct to avoid an incomplete resection. The main advantage of a left-sided resection is the larger size of the right posterior sector. A trisectionectomy may be required for a complete resection, but is associated with a substantial risk of liver failure and postoperative mortality. Resection for PHC should always include a CL.

A staging laparoscopy before exploratory laparotomy has a yield of about 1 in 4 patients with occult metastatic disease. The use of frozen section probably bears little significance on outcome, as does lymphadenectomy. However, adequate lymphadenectomy including at least 6 lymph nodes is recommended for proper staging.

Future studies should focus on reducing the high postoperative mortality in Western centers and finding better adjuvant treatments to reduce the high recurrence rate.

ACKNOWLEDGMENTS

The authors acknowledge the contribution from Mrs Elsbeth Leeffers for her excellent artwork.

REFERENCES

1. Edge S, Byrd DR, Compton CC, et al. AJCC Cancer Staging Manual. 7th edition. New York: Springer; 2010.
2. Bengmark S, Ekberg H, Evander A, et al. Major liver resection for hilar cholangiocarcinoma. Ann Surg 1988;207:120.
3. Gazzaniga GM, Filauro M, Bagarolo C, et al. Surgery for hilar cholangiocarcinoma: an Italian experience. J Hepatobiliary Pancreat Surg 2000;7:122.
4. Konstadoulakis MM, Roayaie S, Gomatos IP, et al. Aggressive surgical resection for hilar cholangiocarcinoma: is it justified? Audit of a single center's experience. Am J Surg 2008;196:160.
5. Jarnagin WR, Fong Y, DeMatteo RP, et al. Staging, resectability, and outcome in 225 patients with hilar cholangiocarcinoma. Ann Surg 2001;234:507.
6. Kambakamba P, DeOliveira ML. Perihilar cholangiocarcinoma: paradigms of surgical management. Am J Surg 2014;208:563.
7. Valle J, Wasan H, Palmer DH, et al. Cisplatin plus gemcitabine versus gemcitabine for biliary tract cancer. N Engl J Med 2010;362:1273.
8. Parodi A, Fisher D, Giovannini M, et al. Endoscopic management of hilar cholangiocarcinoma. Nat Rev Gastroenterol Hepatol 2012;9:105.
9. Nagino M, Ebata T, Yokoyama Y, et al. Evolution of surgical treatment for perihilar cholangiocarcinoma: a single-center 34-year review of 574 consecutive resections. Ann Surg 2013;258:129.
10. Nuzzo G, Giuliante F, Ardito F, et al. Improvement in perioperative and long-term outcome after surgical treatment of hilar cholangiocarcinoma: results of an Italian multicenter analysis of 440 patients. Arch Surg 2012;147:26.
11. Farges O, Regimbeau JM, Fuks D, et al. Multicentre European study of preoperative biliary drainage for hilar cholangiocarcinoma. Br J Surg 2013;100:274.
12. Bismuth H, Corlette MB. Intrahepatic cholangioenteric anastomosis in carcinoma of the hilus of the liver. Surg Gynecol Obstet 1975;140:170.
13. Matsuo K, Rocha FG, Ito K, et al. The Blumgart preoperative staging system for hilar cholangiocarcinoma: analysis of resectability and outcomes in 380 patients. J Am Coll Surg 2012;215:343.
14. Chaiteerakij R, Harmsen WS, Marrero CR, et al. A new clinically based staging system for perihilar cholangiocarcinoma. Am J Gastroenterol 2014;109:1881.
15. Corvera CU, Blumgart LH, Darvishian F, et al. Clinical and pathologic features of proximal biliary strictures masquerading as hilar cholangiocarcinoma. J Am Coll Surg 2005;201:862.
16. Juntermanns B, Kaiser GM, Reis H, et al. Klatskin-mimicking lesions: still a diagnostical and therapeutical dilemma? Hepatogastroenterology 2011;58:265.
17. Kloek JJ, van Delden OM, Erdogan D, et al. Differentiation of malignant and benign proximal bile duct strictures: the diagnostic dilemma. World J Gastroenterol 2008;14:5032.

18. Nimura Y, Hayakawa N, Kamiya J, et al. Hepatic segmentectomy with caudate lobe resection for bile duct carcinoma of the hepatic hilus. World J Surg 1990; 14:535.

19. Natsume S, Ebata T, Yokoyama Y, et al. Clinical significance of left trisectionectomy for perihilar cholangiocarcinoma: an appraisal and comparison with left hepatectomy. Ann Surg 2012;255:754.

20. Hiatt JR, Gabbay J, Busuttil RW. Surgical anatomy of the hepatic arteries in 1000 cases. Ann Surg 1994;220:50.

21. Shimizu H, Kimura F, Yoshidome H, et al. Aggressive surgical resection for hilar cholangiocarcinoma of the left-side predominance: radicality and safety of left-sided hepatectomy. Ann Surg 2010;251:281.

22. Abbas S, Sandroussi C. Systematic review and meta-analysis of the role of vascular resection in the treatment of hilar cholangiocarcinoma. HPB (Oxford) 2013;15:492.

23. Mansour JC, Aloia TA, Crane CH, et al. Hilar Cholangiocarcinoma: expert consensus statement. HPB (Oxford) 2015;17:691.

24. Wiggers JK, Coelen RJ, Rauws EA, et al. Preoperative endoscopic versus percutaneous transhepatic biliary drainage in potentially resectable perihilar cholangiocarcinoma (DRAINAGE trial): design and rationale of a randomized controlled trial. BMC Gastroenterol 2015;15:20.

25. Ebata T, Yokoyama Y, Igami T, et al. Portal vein embolization before extended hepatectomy for biliary cancer: current technique and review of 494 consecutive embolizations. Dig Surg 2012;29:23.

26. Esaki M, Shimada K, Nara S, et al. Left hepatic trisectionectomy for advanced perihilar cholangiocarcinoma. Br J Surg 2013;100:801.

27. Matsumoto N, Ebata T, Yokoyama Y, et al. Role of anatomical right hepatic trisectionectomy for perihilar cholangiocarcinoma. Br J Surg 2014;101:261.

28. Hosokawa I, Shimizu H, Yoshidome H, et al. Surgical strategy for hilar cholangiocarcinoma of the left–side predominance: current role of left trisectionectomy. Ann Surg 2014;259:1178.

29. Shimizu H, Sawada S, Kimura F, et al. Clinical significance of biliary vascular anatomy of the right liver for hilar cholangiocarcinoma applied to left hemihepatectomy. Ann Surg 2009;249:435.

30. Govil S, Reddy MS, Rela M. Surgical resection techniques for locally advanced hilar cholangiocarcinoma. Langenbecks Arch Surg 2014;399:707.

31. Chen XP, Lau WY, Huang ZY, et al. Extent of liver resection for hilar cholangiocarcinoma. Br J Surg 2009;96:1167.

32. Ribero D, Amisano M, Lo Tesoriere R, et al. Additional resection of an intraoperative margin-positive proximal bile duct improves survival in patients with hilar cholangiocarcinoma. Ann Surg 2011;254:776.

33. Cheng QB, Yi B, Wang JH, et al. Resection with total caudate lobectomy confers survival benefit in hilar cholangiocarcinoma of Bismuth type III and IV. Eur J Surg Oncol 2012;38:1197.

34. Kow AW, Wook CD, Song SC, et al. Role of caudate lobectomy in type III A and III B hilar cholangiocarcinoma: a 15-year experience in a tertiary institution. World J Surg 2012;36:1112.

35. Wahab MA, Sultan AM, Salah T, et al. Caudate lobe resection with major hepatectomy for central cholangiocarcinoma: is it of value? Hepatogastroenterology 2012;59:321.

36. Song SC, Choi DW, Kow AW, et al. Surgical outcomes of 230 resected hilar cholangiocarcinoma in a single centre. ANZ J Surg 2013;83:268.

37. Nanashima A, Tobinaga S, Abo T, et al. Left hepatectomy accompanied by a resection of the whole caudate lobe using the dorsally fixed liver-hanging maneuver. Surg Today 2011;41:453.
38. Hwang S, Lee SG, Lee YJ, et al. Modified liver hanging maneuver to facilitate left hepatectomy and caudate lobe resection for hilar bile duct cancer. J Gastrointest Surg 2008;12:1288.
39. Neuhaus P, Jonas S. Surgery for hilar cholangiocarcinoma–the German experience. J Hepatobiliary Pancreat Surg 2000;7:142.
40. Neuhaus P, Jonas S, Settmacher U, et al. Surgical management of proximal bile duct cancer: extended right lobe resection increases resectability and radicality. Langenbecks Arch Surg 2003;388:194.
41. Hirano S, Kondo S, Tanaka E, et al. No-touch resection of hilar malignancies with right hepatectomy and routine portal reconstruction. J Hepatobiliary Pancreat Surg 2009;16:502.
42. Neuhaus P, Thelen A, Jonas S, et al. Oncological superiority of hilar en bloc resection for the treatment of hilar cholangiocarcinoma. Ann Surg Oncol 2012; 19:1602.
43. Tamoto E, Hirano S, Tsuchikawa T, et al. Portal vein resection using the no-touch technique with a hepatectomy for hilar cholangiocarcinoma. HPB (Oxford) 2014; 16:56.
44. Nagino M, Kamiya J, Arai T, et al. "Anatomic" right hepatic trisectionectomy (extended right hepatectomy) with caudate lobectomy for hilar cholangiocarcinoma. Ann Surg 2006;243:28.
45. Rela M, Rajalingam R, Shanmugam V, et al. Novel en-bloc resection of locally advanced hilar cholangiocarcinoma: the Rex recess approach. Hepatobiliary Pancreat Dis Int 2014;13:93.
46. Lim JH, Choi GH, Choi SH, et al. Liver resection for Bismuth type I and Type II hilar cholangiocarcinoma. World J Surg 2013;37:829.
47. Xiong J, Nunes QM, Huang W, et al. Major hepatectomy in Bismuth types I and II hilar cholangiocarcinoma. J Surg Res 2015;194:194.
48. Kawarada Y, Isaji S, Taoka H, et al. S4a + S5 with caudate lobe (S1) resection using the Taj Mahal liver parenchymal resection for carcinoma of the biliary tract. J Gastrointest Surg 1999;3:369.
49. Miyazaki M, Kimura F, Shimizu H, et al. Extensive hilar bile duct resection using a transhepatic approach for patients with hepatic hilar bile duct diseases. Am J Surg 2008;196:125.
50. van Gulik TM, Ruys AT, Busch OR, et al. Extent of liver resection for hilar cholangiocarcinoma (Klatskin tumor): how much is enough? Dig Surg 2011;28:141.
51. Darwish Murad S, Kim WR, Harnois DM, et al. Efficacy of neoadjuvant chemoradiation, followed by liver transplantation, for perihilar cholangiocarcinoma at 12 US centers. Gastroenterology 2012;143:88.
52. Sudan D, DeRoover A, Chinnakotla S, et al. Radiochemotherapy and transplantation allow long-term survival for nonresectable hilar cholangiocarcinoma. Am J Transplant 2002;2:774.
53. Robles R, Figueras J, Turrion VS, et al. Spanish experience in liver transplantation for hilar and peripheral cholangiocarcinoma. Ann Surg 2004;239:265.
54. DeOliveira ML. Liver transplantation for cholangiocarcinoma: current best practice. Curr Opin Organ Transplant 2014;19:245.
55. Weber SM, DeMatteo RP, Fong Y, et al. Staging laparoscopy in patients with extrahepatic biliary carcinoma. Analysis of 100 patients. Ann Surg 2002;235:392.

56. Connor S, Barron E, Wigmore SJ, et al. The utility of laparoscopic assessment in the preoperative staging of suspected hilar cholangiocarcinoma. J Gastrointest Surg 2005;9:476.
57. Ruys AT, Busch OR, Gouma DJ, et al. Staging laparoscopy for hilar cholangiocarcinoma: is it still worthwhile? Ann Surg Oncol 2011;18:2647.
58. Barlow AD, Garcea G, Berry DP, et al. Staging laparoscopy for hilar cholangiocarcinoma in 100 patients. Langenbecks Arch Surg 2013;398:983.
59. Tilleman EH, de Castro SM, Busch OR, et al. Diagnostic laparoscopy and laparoscopic ultrasound for staging of patients with malignant proximal bile duct obstruction. J Gastrointest Surg 2002;6:426.
60. Goere D, Wagholikar GD, Pessaux P, et al. Utility of staging laparoscopy in subsets of biliary cancers : laparoscopy is a powerful diagnostic tool in patients with intrahepatic and gallbladder carcinoma. Surg Endosc 2006;20:721.
61. Jarnagin WR, Bodniewicz J, Dougherty E, et al. A prospective analysis of staging laparoscopy in patients with primary and secondary hepatobiliary malignancies. J Gastrointest Surg 2000;4:34.
62. Shingu Y, Ebata T, Nishio H, et al. Clinical value of additional resection of a margin-positive proximal bile duct in hilar cholangiocarcinoma. Surgery 2010; 147:49.
63. Endo I, House MG, Klimstra DS, et al. Clinical significance of intraoperative bile duct margin assessment for hilar cholangiocarcinoma. Ann Surg Oncol 2008;15: 2104.
64. Groot Koerkamp B, Wiggers JK, Gonen M, et al. Survival after resection of perihilar cholangiocarcinoma-development and external validation of a prognostic nomogram. Ann Oncol 2015;26:1930.
65. Cady B. Basic principles in surgical oncology. Arch Surg 1997;132:338.
66. Blumgart LH, Benjamin IS. Liver resection for bile duct cancer. Surg Clin North Am 1989;69:323.
67. Nagino M, Nimura Y, Nishio H, et al. Hepatectomy with simultaneous resection of the portal vein and hepatic artery for advanced perihilar cholangiocarcinoma: an audit of 50 consecutive cases. Ann Surg 2010;252:115.
68. Chen W, Ke K, Chen YL. Combined portal vein resection in the treatment of hilar cholangiocarcinoma: a systematic review and meta-analysis. Eur J Surg Oncol 2014;40:489.
69. Song GW, Lee SG, Hwang S, et al. Does portal vein resection with hepatectomy improve survival in locally advanced hilar cholangiocarcinoma? Hepatogastroenterology 2009;56:935.
70. Tsuji T, Hiraoka T, Kanemitsu K, et al. Lymphatic spreading pattern of intrahepatic cholangiocarcinoma. Surgery 2001;129:401.
71. Kitagawa Y, Nagino M, Kamiya J, et al. Lymph node metastasis from hilar cholangiocarcinoma: audit of 110 patients who underwent regional and paraaortic node dissection. Ann Surg 2001;233:385.
72. Razumilava N, Gores GJ. Cholangiocarcinoma. Lancet 2014;383:2168.
73. Groot Koerkamp B, Wiggers JK, Allen P, et al. Recurrence rate and pattern of perihilar cholangiocarcinoma after curative intent resection. J Am Coll Surg 2015;221(6):1041–9.
74. Dasari BV, Pasquali S, Vohra RS, et al. Extended Versus Standard Lymphadenectomy for Pancreatic Head Cancer: Meta-Analysis of Randomized Controlled Trials. J Gastrointest Surg 2015;19:1725.
75. Kambakamba P, Linecker M, Slankamenac K, et al. Lymph node dissection in resectable perihilar cholangiocarcinoma: a systematic review. Am J Surg 2015.

76. Popescu I, Dumitrascu T. Curative-intent surgery for hilar cholangiocarcinoma: prognostic factors for clinical decision making. Langenbecks Arch Surg 2014; 399:693.
77. Kobayashi A, Miwa S, Nakata T, et al. Disease recurrence patterns after R0 resection of hilar cholangiocarcinoma. Br J Surg 2010;97:56.
78. Lee SG, Song GW, Hwang S, et al. Surgical treatment of hilar cholangiocarcinoma in the new era: the Asan experience. J Hepatobiliary Pancreat Sci 2010;17:476.
79. Unno M, Katayose Y, Rikiyama T, et al. Major hepatectomy for perihilar cholangiocarcinoma. J Hepatobiliary Pancreat Sci 2010;17:463.
80. de Jong MC, Marques H, Clary BM, et al. The impact of portal vein resection on outcomes for hilar cholangiocarcinoma: a multi-institutional analysis of 305 cases. Cancer 2012;118:4737.
81. Hemming AW, Mekeel K, Khanna A, et al. Portal vein resection in management of hilar cholangiocarcinoma. J Am Coll Surg 2011;212:604.
82. Bismuth H. Revisiting liver anatomy and terminology of hepatectomies. Ann Surg 2013;257:383.
83. Guyatt GH, Oxman AD, Kunz R, et al. Going from evidence to recommendations. BMJ 2008;336:1049.
84. Open source software. Available at: http://www.cebm.brown.edu/open_meta/index.html. Accessed March 23, 2015.

APPENDIX 1: METHODS FOR LITERATURE REVIEW SECTIONS

A literature search was conducted in PubMed, using search terms "(hilar OR perihilar) AND (cholangio*)," including only human studies, written in English. A total of 1226 references were screened based on title and abstract and relevant selections filed into subtopics (eg, case series, staging laparoscopy, lymphadenectomy, frozen section, and liver transplantation). Case series published before 2008 or with fewer than 5 patients per year were excluded. In case series diluted with cases of intrahepatic or distal cholangiocarcinoma, data pertaining to patients with PHC were extracted. Meta-analysis was performed for case series reporting results of right versus left hemihepatectomy, trisectionectomy versus hemihepatectomy, and concomitant versus no CL. Quality assessment of studies was performed using the GRADE (Grading of Recommendations Assessment, Development and Evaluation [short GRADE] Working Group) tool.[82,83] Data are presented as ORs or proportions. Meta-analysis was performed using OpenMeta [Analyst] 10.10[84] and random-effects model (DerSimonian Laird) was used.

APPENDIX 2: SUPPLEMENTARY FIGURES

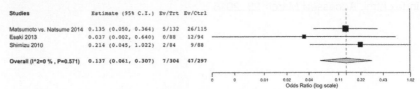

Fig. S1. Forest plot for proportion of hepatic artery reconstructions in right versus left hemihepatectomy. OR less than 1 favors right hemihepatectomy.

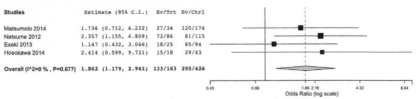

Fig. S2. R0 resection rate in trisectionectomies versus hemihepatectomies. OR greater than 1.0 favors trisectionectomies.

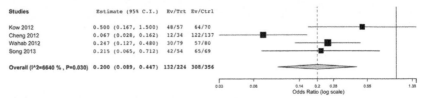

Fig. S3. Forest plot caudate lobectomies. OR for obtaining negative resection margins (R0). OR less than 1.0 favors CL.

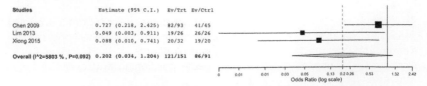

Fig. S4. R0 resection rates in major liver resection (MLR) versus central liver resections. OR less than 1.0 favors MLR.

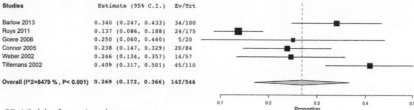

Fig. S5. Yield of staging laparoscopy.

Technical Aspects of Orthotopic Liver Transplantation for Hepatocellular Carcinoma

 CrossMark

Lung-Yi Lee, MD[a], David P. Foley, MD[a,b,*]

KEYWORDS

- Liver transplantation • Surgery • Hepatocellular carcinoma • Piggyback technique
- Portal vein thrombosis

KEY POINTS

- In the majority of cases, patients with cirrhosis and hepatocellular carcinoma (HCC) who undergo liver transplantation are transplanted based on their higher Model for End-Stage Liver Disease (MELD) exception score and not their physiologic MELD score; this usually results in fewer physiologic derangements during liver transplantation.
- Patients who have previously undergone locoregional therapy or liver resection for HCC can develop significant perihepatic adhesions that increase the complexity of the hepatectomy during transplant.
- Implantation strategy of the inferior vena cava (IVC) during liver transplant may need to be modified based on location of previously treated HCC.
- Patients who undergo transarterial chemoembolization for pretransplant HCC therapy may have higher rates of hepatic artery thrombosis after liver transplant; therefore, aorto-hepatic bypass grafting with donor iliac artery may be required for arterial in flow to the liver allograft.
- Patients with portal vein (PV) thrombosis with a bland thrombus and a patent superior mesenteric vein (SMV) can undergo successful liver transplant through either PV thrombectomy and standard end-to-end PV-PV anastomosis, or the use of SMV-PV bypass graft with donor iliac vein.

[a] Department of Surgery, University of Wisconsin School of Medicine and Public Health, Clinical Sciences Center, H4/766, 600 Highland Avenue, Madison, WI 53792-3284, USA; [b] Veterans Administration Surgical Services, William S. Middleton Memorial Veterans Hospital, 2500 Overlook Terrace, Madison, WI 53705, USA
* Corresponding author. Clinical Science Center, H4/766, 600 Highland Avenue, Madison, WI 53792-7375.
E-mail address: foley@surgery.wisc.edu

Surg Clin N Am 96 (2016) 269–281
http://dx.doi.org/10.1016/j.suc.2015.11.004
0039-6109/16/$ – see front matter Published by Elsevier Inc.

surgical.theclinics.com

INTRODUCTION

Hepatocellular carcinoma (HCC) remains a significant worldwide malignancy. Liver cancer, primarily HCC, is the fifth most common cancer in men, the ninth most common cancer in women, and the second leading cause of cancer death in the world.[1] In the United States, HCC ranks tenth in new estimated cancers but represents the fifth leading cause of cancer death.[2] Most cases of HCC develop in the setting of cirrhosis secondary to viral hepatitis (hepatitis B virus [HBV] and hepatitis C virus [HCV]) and alcohol overuse.[3] However, there has been a rising association between obesity, metabolic syndrome, nonalcoholic fatty liver disease (NAFLD), and HCC.[4,5] In fact, more reports have described an increased incidence of HCC in noncirrhotic patients with NAFLD or nonalcoholic steatohepatitis (NASH).[6] Due to the ongoing obesity epidemic, it is likely that the incidence of NAFLD and NASH will increase, as will the presence of HCC in these patients.

There are multiple therapies aimed at treating patients with HCC. Locoregional therapies for HCC include radiofrequency ablation,[7] microwave ablation,[8] cryotherapy,[9] transarterial embolization,[10] and radioembolization.[11] The decision to use a specific therapy is based on multiple factors, including but not limited to tumor size, biology, location, and number, as well as institutional expertise. Surgical resection of HCC can be a viable option for patients with compensated hepatic function.[12] The decision to perform resection is based upon the location of the tumor, absence of macrovascular invasion and extrahepatic disease, size of the remnant liver, severity of portal hypertension, and the lack of significant comorbidities.

Patients who are not candidates for surgical resection can be considered candidates for liver transplantation. However, careful selection of the appropriate candidate is critical for obtaining optimal outcomes after transplantation. This article discusses the selection of candidates with HCC for liver transplantation and the technical aspects of orthotopic liver transplantation for HCC.

PATIENT SELECTION

All patients with cirrhosis who are evaluated for liver transplantation undergo an extensive workup to be sure that they can tolerate the complexities of the surgical procedure. Some of these tests include, but are not limited to, noninvasive cardiac stress test, cardiac catheterization, 2-dimensional echocardiogram, and abdominal imaging to assess the hepatic vascular anatomy and the presence of tumors. When a diagnosis of HCC is made, the Milan criteria are used to determine which patients with HCC are suitable candidates for liver transplantation. The Milan criteria were established from a prospective study performed by Mazzaferro and colleagues[13] in 1996. In this report, the eligibility criteria for transplantation were the presence of a tumor 5 cm or less in diameter in patients with a single HCC, and no more than 3 tumor nodules each 3 cm or less in diameter in patients with multiple tumors. Recipients who met these criteria had overall and tumor-free 4-year survival rates of 85% and 92%, while patients with greater tumor burden had survival rates of 50% and 59%, respectively.

Because these survival rates were similar to those in liver transplant recipients without HCC, the Milan criteria became and have remained the standard tumor acceptance criteria for patients with HCC undergoing liver transplantation. However, in the past, some had felt that the Milan criteria were too restrictive, meaning that that patients with tumor burden outside Milan criteria may be suitable for liver transplantation. In 2001, Yao and colleagues[14] established the University of San Francisco (UCSF) criteria by studying patients with expanded criteria. These criteria included single tumors of no more than 6.5 cm or no more than 3 tumors, with each tumor being no more than 4.5 cm, with a sum tumor diameter of no more than 8 cm. When these patients were transplanted, their 5-year survival after liver transplantation was 75%. These data suggested that the selection of patients with tumor burden that is outside Milan criteria but within UCSF criteria may have acceptable outcomes after liver transplantation.

Despite these favorable results in patients within UCSF criteria, the allocation of deceased donor livers for patients with HCC depends upon the Model for End-Stage Liver Disease (MELD) score and the Milan criteria. The MELD scoring system was implemented in 2003 as a predictor of mortality for patients on the liver transplant waiting list. The physiologic MELD score is based on the patient's creatinine, total bilirubin, and international normalized ratio (INR), and it is predictive of 90-day waitlist mortality.[15] In many cases, patients with HCC have compensated liver function with low physiologic MELD scores, and they are less likely to be transplanted in a timely manner. If liver allocation were solely based on their physiologic scores, there would be a high likelihood of tumor growth outside of Milan criteria, thus making the patient ineligible for liver transplant. In order to create equipoise for these patients on the list, MELD exception scores are given to HCC patients to increase their likelihood of being transplanted.

With the implementation of MELD exception points for patients with HCC, there has been an increase in the number of patients transplanted with HCC exception scores over time. According to the most recent Scientific Registry for Transplant Recipients Annual Report, the number of liver transplants per 100 wait-list years performed in 2012 was three times higher among active adult candidates with HCC exceptions compared with those candidates without HCC exceptions.[16] In most instances, wait-listed patients with cirrhosis and HCC have MELD exception scores that are higher than their physiologic MELD scores. Therefore, these exception scores become their allocation scores.

From a technical standpoint, liver transplantation is generally less complicated for patients with HCC due to the fact that they are usually receiving livers based on their MELD exception scores that are higher than their physiologic MELD scores. Because of compensated liver function in most of these patients, the authors have generally observed less coagulopathy, reduced portal hypertension, and preserved renal function during liver transplant. For these reasons, the hepatectomy and liver transplant are usually more straightforward. However, there are exceptions in these patients that can make the liver transplant in the setting of HCC more technically challenging. This article will discuss the technical aspects of orthotopic liver transplantation for patients with cirrhosis and HCC.

SURGICAL TECHNIQUE
Preoperative Planning

If patients with HCC do not have a potential living donor, they can be placed on the deceased donor waiting list. If their tumor burden is initially within Milan criteria and remains there for 6 months, they receive a MELD exception score of 28. As long as they remain within Milan criteria, they receive a 10% increase for each subsequent 3-month interval until their score is capped at 34. Patients who are within UCSF criteria are not eligible for an automatic exception score but can be downstaged into Milan criteria with locoregional therapy. A recent analysis revealed that successful downstaging with locoregional therapy into Milan criteria resulted in low rates of HCC recurrence and excellent liver transplant outcomes.[17] After a subsequent period of observation to rule out aggressive tumor biology, transplant centers usually request a MELD exception score through the United Network for Organ Sharing (UNOS) Regional Review Board.

While on the transplant list, patients with HCC routinely undergo locoregional therapy to treat HCC and bridge them to transplant. The goal of this therapy is to arrest tumor growth and keep patients within Milan criteria. The choice of therapy usually depends on location of tumor, size of tumor, tumor biology, and institutional expertise. Locoregional treatment serving as bridging therapy has been shown to increase the likelihood of patients with HCC undergoing transplant.[18]

SURGICAL APPROACH
Recipient Hepatectomy

The first stage of any liver transplant procedure involves the recipient hepatectomy. The essential aspects of the recipient hepatectomy include the division of the hepatic ligaments resulting in mobilization of the liver, dissection and isolation of the structures within the porta hepatis, and IVC dissection. Because most patients with cirrhosis have portal hypertension, the dissection of the perihepatic tissue can lead to significant bleeding. During the dissection of the liver, it is critical to control small vessel bleeding as one progresses in the operation in order to minimize blood loss. Large amounts of blood loss during the hepatectomy can lead to significant coagulopathy and prolonged bleeding after reperfusion of the liver allograft.

After the abdomen is opened and the retractors placed, a frequently present recannulized umbilical vein is ligated with silk ties and divided. The falciform ligament is divided down to the hepatic veins with cautery. If the patient has significant portal hypertension, it may be best to proceed with porta hepatis dissection at this point and avoid further perihepatic dissection. If bleeding is not significant, then one can safely proceed to dividing the left and right triangular ligaments toward the IVC. In patients with large left lateral segments that are contiguous to the spleen, one can defer this dissection until after the portal vein is ligated to minimize bleeding from the left lateral segment. The cirrhotic segment can then be dissected off the spleen by cutting into the liver parenchyma and thus minimizing the risk of splenic injury. The hepatogastric and hepatoduodenal ligaments are then divided up to the level of the IVC. If a replaced left hepatic artery is seen within the hepatogastric ligament, it is ligated with silk ties and divided.

In patients who have undergone locoregional therapy for HCC prior to transplant, the location of the tumor can impact the potential complications during hepatectomy. Centrally located tumors that have been treated usually do not adversely impact the hepatectomy. However, more peripherally located tumors that have been treated may increase the degree of inflammation and scar around adjacent structures. Previously treated tumors located in segments V and VIII can result in extensive scar tissue and potential diaphragmatic injury during hepatectomy. This would require primary diaphragmatic repair and usually does not lead to significantly adverse sequelae. Previously treated tumors in segments II and III can be in proximity to a large spleen. Dissection of the inflamed liver edge can lead to potential splenic injury. Tumors in segment VI and VII can cause more adhesions near the adrenal gland and kidney, making this dissection more challenging. Caudate lobe tumors that have been treated with either radiofrequency ablation (RFA) or microwave ablation can increase scar tissue adjacent to the IVC, increasing the risk of IVC injury during dissection.

Patients who have had previous liver resections for the management of HCC have greater amounts of scar tissue surrounding the areas of resection, thus obliterating the natural tissue planes and making the dissection more difficult. This becomes more problematic in the setting of portal hypertension, severe coagulopathy, and thrombocytopenia. Any dissection that results in disruption of Glisson capsule before portal vein ligation can lead to significant parenchymal bleeding that may not be amenable to argon beam coagulation. Nonanatomic resections that did not require porta hepatis dissection are usually less problematic during the hepatectomy provided that the adjacent tissue does not involve the gastric or duodenal walls or major vascular structures. However, in patients who have previously undergone formal left or right hemihepatecomies for HCC and required dissection of the porta hepatis, one needs to be extremely cautious to avoid vascular injury. For these reasons, HCC therapy used to bridge patients to liver transplantation usually include less invasive approaches such as ablational or transarterial therapies. Liver resection surgery for the treatment of HCC is generally used as a method of destination therapy in selected patients.

Porta Hepatis Dissection

The goal during dissection of the porta hepatis is to isolate each of the major structures (hepatic artery, portal vein, and common bile duct) and dissect them from the liver edge down to the duodenum. The authors prefer arterial dissection first with isolation of the proper, right, and left hepatic arteries. These vessels are identified and dissected proximally to the level of the gastroduodenal artery (GDA). In a large retrospective single center study analyzing vascular complications after liver transplantation, vascular control of the common hepatic artery (CHA) at the beginning of portal dissection resulted in a significantly decreased incidence of arterial thrombosis and reduced by 3-fold the requirement for an aortohepatic arterial conduit.[19] Based on their experience and these data, the authors prefer to place an atraumatic bulldog clamp on the proximal CHA to mitigate the risk of arterial damage during dissection.

Once the artery is dissected freely from surrounding structures, the anterior wall of the portal vein is identified. The interface between the posterior surface of the common bile duct (CBD) and the anterior wall of the portal vein is identified and dissected. The proximal CBD is encircled, ligated with silk ties, and divided. The cystic duct is also dissected and ligated with silk ties and divided. The CBD is then dissected from surrounding structures to the level of the duodenum. Careful attention is made to avoid disruption of the longitudinal arteries of the CBD and possible devascularization. In 10% to 15% of the cases, a replaced right hepatic artery is identified running posterior to the CBD and lateral to the portal vein. When this is identified, the artery is encircled with a vessel loop and controlled proximally with an atraumatic bulldog clamp. The vessel is then ligated and divided distally. In many instances, this artery is sufficient to use for arterial inflow to the allograft. Careful attention to avoid injury to this artery when encircling the CBD is thus critical.

The portal vein is then skeletonized from the bifurcation proximally to the superior portion of the duodenum. The posterior attachments to the portal vein are dissected and divided with cautery. Meticulous technique during this dissection is critical in order to avoid proximal, retroduodenal injury to the portal vein. Injury to the portal vein in this region can lead to significant, hemorrhage that is difficult control and can be fatal.

The timing of portal vein ligation depends partly on the degree of portal hypertension and presence of collateral veins. In patients with significant portal hypertension, the portal vein can be divided at this point to help facilitate the mobilization of the liver and IVC dissection. In patients with venous collaterals, prolonged portal venous clamping should not result in marked bowel edema. However, in patients with HCC who do not have sufficient venous collaterals, early ligation of the portal vein can lead to marked swelling and congestion of the bowel and impair adequate exposure during implantation. If the portal vein needs to be divided early in the dissection, a temporary end-to-side portal–caval shunt can be created to allow for venous decompression, avoid bowel congestion, and diminish portal hypertensive bleeding during IVC dissection.

The challenge of porta hepatis dissection arises in the setting of a previous surgical procedure involving the hilum of the liver. These can include previous hemi-hepatectomy for HCC, open cholecystectomy, or liver transplant. In these settings, there are extensive adhesions surrounding the porta hepatis structures. In addition, the adhesions make the extrahepatic portal vein length foreshortened, resulting in a shorter recipient vein to complete the portal venous anastomosis. It is critical to start this dissection close to the liver and move in a distal to proximal direction. If a portal venous injury occurs, then one can quickly gain proximal control with a Pringle maneuver and proceed with the dissection. If the bleeding from the hepatic parenchyma is extensive before the major structures are dissected freely, then clamping of the entire porta hepatis may be necessary. The porta hepatis is then transected close to the liver. After the IVC dissection and hepatectomy, the structures can then be dissected individually in preparation for implantation. This approach is not ideal, but it is helpful in extreme situations.

Inferior Vena Cava Dissection

Once the porta hepatis dissection is complete and the portal vein is divided, the authors then proceed to dissection of the IVC. The management of the recipient IVC during hepatectomy depends on the anticipated strategy for donor IVC implantation. If the piggyback technique (**Fig. 1**A or B) is planned, then the recipient liver is dissected off the IVC from an inferior-to-superior direction. Venous branches draining the posterior segments of the liver are ligated and divided. Dissection continues up to the level of the hepatic veins. A large vascular clamp is then placed below the hepatic veins, thus partially occluding the IVC. The hepatic parenchyma is dissected off the proximal hepatic veins creating maximal venous length. The hepatic veins are then transected, and the liver is passed off the table. A common orifice is made between the right, middle, and left hepatic veins in preparation for implantation of the new liver. This approach allows for a large hepatic venous opening and thus minimizes the risk of a venous outflow stenosis after implantation.

An alternative approach is to transect the right hepatic vein with a vascular stapler during the IVC dissection prior to placement of the hepatic venous vascular clamp. The advantage of this approach is to facilitate mobilization of the right hemi-liver and to complete the posterior dissection of the middle and left hepatic veins. This approach is favorable when matching the size of a smaller donor IVC to the common orifice of the hepatic vein ostia. With the right vein stapled, a common opening is created between the left and middle hepatic veins and a portion of the IVC inferior to the staple line.

If the decision to perform IVC replacement (**Fig. 1**C) is made, the dissection of the IVC from the native liver is not required. Proximal and distal control of the IVC is obtained with umbilical tapes. At this point it is necessary to assess the hemodynamic stability of the recipient and the patient's response to complete clamping of the IVC. If the patient has had significant blood loss and is unstable on multiple vasopressors, IVC clamping may not be tolerated due to the high dependency on preload from the IVC. If this occurs, then putting the patient on veno-venous bypass would be preferred.

Veno-venous bypass requires the placement of perfusion cannulas in the femoral and internal jugular veins. The circuit allows for blood drawn from the femoral vein

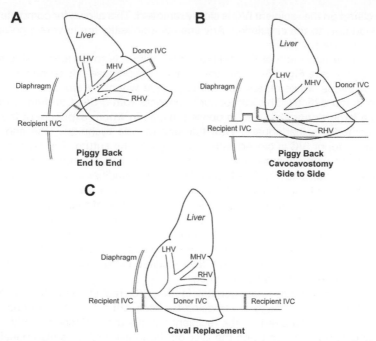

Fig. 1. Implantation of donor IVC. (*A*) Piggyback technique. The donor IVC is connected to the confluence of the recipient hepatic veins in an end-to-end manner. (*B*) Piggyback technique with side-to-side cavocavostomy. The suprahepatic donor IVC and the recipient hepatic vein ostia are sutured close. Longitudinal venotomies are then made in the donor and recipient IVC for side-to-side anastomosis. (*C*) Caval replacement. After gaining vascular control, the recipient retrohepatic IVC is removed with recipient hepatectomy. Donor suprahepatic IVC and infrahepatic IVC are then anastomosed to the recipient IVC in an end-to-end manner.

to pass through an external centrifugal pump and return to the internal jugular vein during IVC clamping. This allows for sufficient venous return and improved hemodynamic stability during implantation. If the patient is hemodynamically stable and does not have a significant drop in blood pressure with IVC test clamping, one can usually proceed without bypass as long as the implantation occurs quickly.

In patients who have undergone locoregional therapy for tumors that are close to the IVC, one needs to assess the degree of scar tissue around the IVC when planning for hepatectomy and implantation of the hepatic allograft. Previous ablation therapy can lead to scarring and narrowing of the native IVC, making the dissection more difficult. Therefore, IVC replacement may be the preferred technique in these instances.

IMPLANTATION OF THE DONOR LIVER
Inferior Vena Cava Anastomosis

The first step in implantation of the liver is to perform the IVC anastomosis. If the piggyback technique (see **Fig. 1**A) is performed, the end of the donor suprahepatic IVC is sutured to the confluence of the hepatic veins with a running prolene suture. A vascular clamp is then placed on the donor side of the anastomosis, and the vascular clamp on the recipient IVC is slowly removed. This allows for complete return of IVC blood flow to the circulation. Any anastomotic leaks are now recognized and repaired as needed.

An alternative approach of the piggyback technique is to perform a side-to-side cavocavostomy (see **Fig. 1**B). Some transplant surgeons use this technique as their primary technique, while others use the technique when the standard end-to-side technique is too difficult. This can occur in patients with a deep abdomen who are receiving a large donor liver, and in obese patients in whom exposure of the upper IVC anastomosis is inadequate. With the side-to-side technique, the end of the suprahepatic donor IVC is closed with a running prolene suture. The recipient right, left, and middle vein ostia are also closed with a running prolene suture. After the recipient IVC is clamped proximally and distally, longitudinal venotomies are made in the midportion of the donor and recipient IVC. The venous anastomosis is performed with running prolene sutures (see **Fig. 1**B). Either of these piggyback techniques can be used in patients with HCC. The decision is primarily based on the location of previously treated tumors. In patients who have undergone liver resection in the past, one needs to determine if the previous dissection and the resultant hepatectomy at the time of transplant have resulted in any damage to the IVC that would favor one technique over the other.

Another option for IVC management is the IVC replacement technique (see **Fig. 1**C). The main advantage of replacing the recipient IVC with the donor IVC is to minimize the time required for the recipient hepatectomy. Resection of the recipient IVC is quicker than removing the liver off the native IVC. It is also beneficial in patients with previously treated HCC near the IVC, as the dissection of scar tissue in this area is avoided, or if there is evidence of a narrowed IVC. A disadvantage of this technique is that it may result in increased hemodynamic instability during clamping and implantation of the allograft. It may also require the use of venovenous bypass to re-establish hemodynamic stability. When chosen IVC replacement technique proceeds with end-to-end anastomosis of the suprahepatic donor IVC to the recipient IVC using a running prolene suture. This is followed by the end-to-end anastomosis of the infrahepatic donor and recipient IVC with a running prolene suture.

Portal Venous Anastomosis

After the IVC anastomosis is completed, the liver is flushed through the portal vein with chilled lactated ringers and albumin solution. This flushes the University of Wisconsin solution with high potassium levels out of the liver through the infrahepatic IVC prior to reperfusion. With the piggyback technique, the infrahepatic IVC is then ligated with silk ties. With the caval replacement technique, the anastomosis of the infrahepatic IVC is then completed with the running prolene suture. The donor and recipient portal veins are then cut to the appropriate length to avoid the redundancy or venous kinking after the retractors are removed. The standard approach is to proceed with end-to-end anastomosis between the recipient and donor portal veins (**Fig. 2**A). A 1-cm air knot is created when tying the running prolene suture to allow for expansion of the portal vein after reperfusion and to avoid an anastomotic stricture.

In patients with HCC who present with portal vein thrombosis, preoperative imaging is required to determine the location of the tumor in relation to the thrombus. If the thrombosis is suspected to be tumor thrombus, then the patient is not a transplant candidate. If the tumor is at a noncontiguous site from the thrombus, the thrombus may be benign and the patient may be considered a transplant candidate. One can

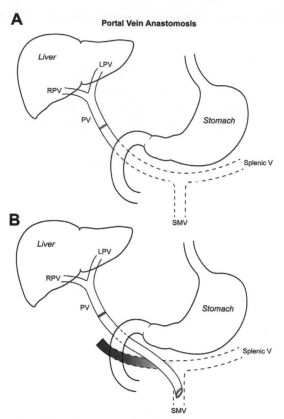

Fig. 2. Techniques of portal vein anastomosis. (*A*) Standard approach. The recipient and donor portal veins are cut to appropriate length, and an end-to-end anastomosis is performed. (*B*) SMV to portal vein bypass graft. In patients with nonmalignant portal vein thrombi precluding the standard portal venous anastomosis, donor iliac vein can be used as a jump graft between donor portal vein and the patent recipient SMV.

confirm the presence of a malignant thrombus by identifying vascular flow within the thrombus by duplex ultrasound. Percutaneous ultrasound-guided biopsy of the thrombus can also be performed to identify tumor cells. If a nonmalignant thrombus is present in the main portal vein, then abdominal imaging is required to confirm the patency of the superior mesenteric vein (SMV). A patent SMV is required for transplant candidacy so that the use of an SMV to portal venous jump graft for venous in-flow is feasible. Most portal vein thrombi that are located distal to the bifurcation of the SMV and splenic vein can be removed via thrombectomy at the time of transplant. However, when chronic thrombosis with cavernous transformation and portal vein calcifications are present, venous thrombectomy is usually unsuccessful and not attempted. In those instances, the use of a donor iliac vein for the SMV to portal venous bypass graft is the technique of choice (**Fig. 2B**).

After the portal venous anastomosis is completed, the hepatic venous vascular clamp is removed, followed by the portal venous clamp. During reperfusion of the allograft, the patient is at risk of electrolyte abnormalities and hemodynamic instability that contribute to postreperfusion syndrome. This syndrome can be short-lived or prolonged depending on the degree of ischemia reperfusion injury of the donor liver. After surgical bleeding is controlled, attention is brought to the creation of the hepatic arterial anastomosis.

Hepatic Arterial Anastomosis

There are multiple strategies that can be used for the construction of the hepatic arterial anastomosis. Most commonly, the recipient CHA is used for arterial in-flow (**Fig. 3**A). A common arterial cuff can be made at the bifurcation of the right and left hepatic arteries or at the bifurcation of the proper hepatic artery and the

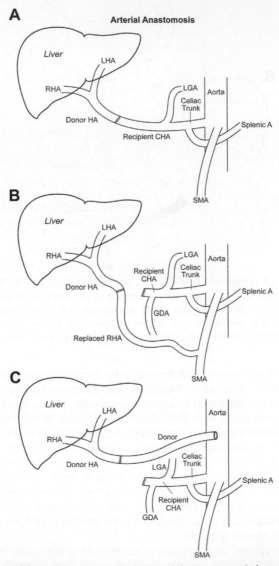

Fig. 3. Techniques of hepatic artery anastomosis. (*A*) Anastomosis between the recipient CHA and donor HA. (*B*) Anastomosis between the recipient replaced RHA and donor HA. (*C*) Aortohepatic bypass graft between the recipient aorta and donor HA using donor iliac arterial conduit.

gastroduodenal (GDA) artery. On the donor side, a branch patch can be configured at the junction of the GDA and the proper hepatic artery. Shortening the arteries to this degree minimizes the chance of arterial kinking when the retractors are removed. In recipients who have a replaced right hepatic artery that has sufficient diameter and flow, this artery can serve as the arterial in-flow to the allograft (**Fig. 3**B). The donor artery is trimmed back to sufficient length so that there is minimal redundancy and tension on the anastomosis.

If there is insufficient flow in the recipient CHA or replaced RHA, an aortohepatic arterial conduit is necessary for arterial in-flow. The arterial conduit that is used is the iliac artery from the deceased donor. The proximal portion of the conduit can be connected to either the supraceliac or infrarenal aorta. The position that is chosen depends on the presence of aortic calcifications, size of the patient, and personal preference. If the supraceliac aorta is used for the in-flow, the proximal anastomosis should be performed during the anhepatic phase as opposed to after the liver is reperfused through the portal vein. During the anhepatic phase, the exposure is better, and clamping of the aorta will not impact portal venous flow, a condition one would see if the liver were already reperfused. The distal anastomosis is then performed to a portion of the donor hepatic artery with the best size match and length (**Fig. 3**C). Although the aortohepatic bypass graft provides excellent arterial in-flow to the liver, this technique is a significant risk factor for the development of hepatic artery thrombosis (HAT).[19]

There have been questions in the literature as to whether patients with HCC who undergo transarterial chemoembolization (TACE) prior to liver transplant have a higher rate of hepatic arterial thrombosis. One retrospective study reported a 2.3-fold increase risk of HAT in patients who underwent TACE.[19] Others have shown that preoperative chemoembolization for treatment of HCC does not increase overall hepatic arterial complications after liver transplantation[20] but has been associated with increased hepatic artery stenosis.[21] In patients who have had preoperative TACE, one needs to review the arterial anatomy and the previous interventional procedures to aid in the determination of arterial inflow to the new liver.

Biliary Anastomosis

After the vascular anastomoses are completed, and hemostasis is attained, the attention is focused on the biliary anastomosis. The standard options for the biliary anastomosis are either an end-to-end choledochocholedochostomy (EE-CC) or a Roux-en-Y hepaticojejunostomy (R-HJ). The EE-CC is usually the preferred approach. However, an R-HJ is recommended in recipients with primary sclerosing cholangitis or a devascularized recipient CBD and in patients in whom there is a significant size mismatch between the donor and recipient CBDs. This is especially true when the diameter of the donor CBD is significantly greater than that of the recipient CBD.

For EE-CC, the ends of the recipient and donor bile ducts are cut back to assure adequate arterial flow from the longitudinal arteries. The anastomosis can be performed with either a running or interrupted monofilament absorbable suture. There does not appear to be significant differences in anastomotic leaks or strictures when interrupted versus running sutures are compared.[22] The use of internal biliary stenting has been described in attempt to mitigate biliary complications.[23] However, retrospective studies do not demonstrate that internal stenting results in a reduction the risk of post-transplant biliary complications.[24] In previous years, T-tubes were used routinely with EE-CC to decrease the risk of biliary complications. These are no longer the standard of care due to studies that demonstrate no added benefit[25] and documented increases in complications with their use.[26] However, they can be used with small CBDs when EE-CC is the preferred approach. The authors routinely perform EE-CC without internal stenting but use T-tubes selectively.

For construction of the R-HJ, a jejunojejunostomy (JJ) is created approximately 20 cm from the ligament of Treitz to create a Roux limb of approximately 40 cm. A side-to-side JJ is created with a GIA stapler, and the remaining opening is closed in 2 layers with interrupted silk sutures. The Roux limb is then brought up to the liver in a retrocolic fashion. The distal jejunal staple line is oversewn with interrupted silk sutures. The end-to-side HJ is then performed without an internal stent with interrupted absorbable monofilament sutures. As is the case with EE-CC, the use of a transanastomotic internal stent for R-HJ has not been shown to decrease the incidence of biliary complications after liver transplantation.[27]

The biliary reconstruction in HCC patients is no different than that seen in patients with other indications for liver transplantation. Routine treatment of HCC with locoregional therapy does not appear to affect biliary complication rates after liver transplantation. The presence of HCC in the explanted liver does not impact the intraoperative decision to perform either EE-CC or R-HJ for the biliary reconstruction.

SUMMARY

HCC in the setting of cirrhosis remains a common indication for liver transplantation. The decision to proceed with transplant depends on multiple factors including the inability to perform a safe or beneficial surgical resection, Milan criteria, and the absence of both macrovascular invasion and extrahepatic disease. Pretransplant locoregional therapies aimed at downstaging the patient into Milan criteria or bridging the patient to transplant on the waitlist can impact the intraoperative decisions during liver transplant. Modification of the technical strategies may be necessary to obtain optimal outcomes after liver transplantation for patients with HCC.

REFERENCES

1. Torre LA, Bray F, Siegel RL, et al. Global cancer statistics, 2012. CA Cancer J Clin 2015;65(2):87–108.
2. Siegel RL, Miller KD, Jemal A. Cancer statistics, 2015. CA Cancer J Clin 2015; 65(1):5–29.
3. El-Serag HB. Hepatocellular carcinoma. N Engl J Med 2011;365(12):1118–27.
4. Vanni E, Bugianesi E. Obesity and liver cancer. Clin Liver Dis 2014;18(1): 191–203.
5. Sanyal A, Poklepovic A, Moyneur E, et al. Population-based risk factors and resource utilization for HCC: US perspective. Curr Med Res Opin 2010;26(9): 2183–91.
6. Yasui K, Hashimoto E, Komorizono Y, et al. Characteristics of patients with nonalcoholic steatohepatitis who develop hepatocellular carcinoma. Clin Gastroenterol Hepatol 2011;9(5):428–33 [quiz: e50].
7. Cabibbo G, Maida M, Genco C, et al. Survival of patients with hepatocellular carcinoma (HCC) treated by percutaneous radio-frequency ablation (RFA) is affected by complete radiological response. PLoS One 2013;8(7):e70016.
8. Zhang NN, Lu W, Cheng XJ, et al. High-powered microwave ablation of larger hepatocellular carcinoma: evaluation of recurrence rate and factors related to recurrence. Clin Radiol 2015;70(11):1237–43.
9. Rong G, Bai W, Dong Z, et al. Cryotherapy for cirrhosis-based hepatocellular carcinoma: a single center experience from 1595 treated cases. Front Med 2015; 9(1):63–71.

10. Hodavance MS, Vikingstad EM, Griffin AS, et al. Effectiveness of transarterial embolization of hepatocellular carcinoma as a bridge to transplantation. J Vasc Interv Radiol 2015. http://dx.doi.org/10.1016/j.jvir.2015.08.032.

11. Biederman DM, Titano JJ, Lee KM, et al. Yttrium-90 glass-based microsphere radioembolization in the treatment of hepatocellular carcinoma secondary to the hepatitis B virus: safety, efficacy, and survival. J Vasc Interv Radiol 2015;26(11):1630–8.

12. Hsu CY, Liu PH, Lee YH, et al. Aggressive therapeutic strategies improve the survival of hepatocellular carcinoma patients with performance status 1 or 2: a propensity score analysis. Ann Surg Oncol 2015;22(4):1324–31.

13. Mazzaferro V, Regalia E, Doci R, et al. Liver transplantation for the treatment of small hepatocellular carcinomas in patients with cirrhosis. N Engl J Med 1996;334(11): 693–9.

14. Yao FY, Ferrell L, Bass NM, et al. Liver transplantation for hepatocellular carcinoma: expansion of the tumor size limits does not adversely impact survival. Hepatology 2001;33(6):1394–403.

15. Wiesner R, Edwards E, Freeman R, et al, United Network for Organ Sharing Liver Disease Severity Score Committee. Model for end-stage liver disease (MELD) and allocation of donor livers. Gastroenterology 2003;124(1):91–6.

16. Kim WR, Smith JM, Skeans MA, et al. OPTN/SRTR 2012 annual data report: liver. Am J Transplant 2014;14(Suppl 1):69–96.

17. Yao FY, Mehta N, Flemming J, et al. Downstaging of hepatocellular cancer before liver transplant: long-term outcome compared to tumors within milan criteria. Hepatology 2015;61(6):1968–77.

18. Sheth RA, Patel MS, Koottappillil B, et al. Role of locoregional therapy and predictors for dropout in patients with hepatocellular carcinoma listed for liver transplantation. J Vasc Interv Radiol 2015;26(12):1761–8.

19. Duffy JP, Hong JC, Farmer DG, et al. Vascular complications of orthotopic liver transplantation: experience in more than 4,200 patients. J Am Coll Surg 2009; 208(5):896–903 [discussion: 903–5].

20. Li H, Li B, Wei Y, et al. Preoperative transarterial chemoembolization does not increase hepatic artery complications after liver transplantation: a single center 12-year experience. Clin Res Hepatol Gastroenterol 2015;39(4):451–7.

21. Goel A, Mehta N, Guy J, et al. Hepatic artery and biliary complications in liver transplant recipients undergoing pretransplant transarterial chemoembolization. Liver Transpl 2014;20(10):1221–8.

22. Castaldo ET, Pinson CW, Feurer ID, et al. Continuous versus interrupted suture for end-to-end biliary anastomosis during liver transplantation gives equal results. Liver Transpl 2007;13(2):234–8.

23. Johnson MW, Thompson P, Meehan A, et al. Internal biliary stenting in orthotopic liver transplantation. Liver Transpl 2000;6(3):356–61.

24. Mathur AK, Nadig SN, Kingman S, et al. Internal biliary stenting during orthotopic liver transplantation: anastomotic complications, post-transplant biliary interventions, and survival. Clin Transpl 2015;29(4):327–35.

25. Verran DJ, Asfar SK, Ghent CN, et al. Biliary reconstruction without T tubes or stents in liver transplantation: report of 502 consecutive cases. Liver Transpl Surg 1997;3(4):365–73.

26. Koivusalo A, Isoniemi H, Salmela K, et al. Biliary complications in one hundred adult liver transplantations. Scand J Gastroenterol 1996;31(5):506–11.

27. Wang GS, Yang Y, Jiang N, et al. Routine use of a transanastomotic stent is unnecessary for hepatojejunostomy in liver transplantation. Chin Med J (Engl) 2012;125(14):2411–6.

Vascular Reconstruction in Hepatic Malignancy

Jennifer Berumen, MD*, Alan Hemming, MD

KEYWORDS

- Vascular reconstruction • Ex vivo liver surgery • Portal vein reconstruction
- IVC reconstruction

KEY POINTS

- Increased experience with vascular resection to achieve negative margins with hepatic malignancies has improved short-term outcomes.
- High-quality preoperative imaging with triphasic computed tomography or contrast MRI is required for appropriate planning and decision making.
- Vascular reconstruction requires careful assessment, planning of clamp placement, and a strategy to reconstruct the artery or vein with appropriate grafts if needed.
- Ideally future liver remnant (FLR) volume of 40% of total liver volume is recommended when vascular resection is planned. Portal vein embolization can be used to increase FLR before resection.
- Cold perfusion, whether in situ, ante situm, or ex vivo, are options for resection in otherwise unresectable tumors involving the inferior vena cava and/or hepatic veins.

INTRODUCTION

The best, if not only, option for cure and long-term survival with malignancy in hepatic surgery has always been surgical resection with negative margins. Patients who are unresectable and undergo chemotherapy and/or interventional procedures have substantially worse survival than those who can be resected. Although interpretation of available data has inherent bias that is included in the selection of patients for surgery, it is clear that there remains some truth in the adage that a chance to cut is a chance to cure.

In the past many surgeons have considered liver tumors with vascular invasion or involvement to be unresectable or at least that the risk involved with the surgery outweighs the benefit. Over the last several years there has been an evolution in surgical

Disclosure statement: The authors have nothing to disclose.
Division of Transplantation and Hepatobiliary Surgery, University of California San Diego, 9300 Campus Point Drive, #7745, La Jolla, CA 92037, USA
* Corresponding author.
E-mail address: jberumen@ucsd.edu

thought. Many surgeons now consider vascular resection in order to achieve negative margins for resection of hepatic malignancies, including hilar cholangiocarcinoma, as well as other primary or secondary liver malignancies. Resections may include resection of the portal vein (PV), hepatic artery, inferior vena cava (IVC), or hepatic veins and may require conduits for vessel reconstruction.[1] Techniques to control hepatic vascular inflow and outflow must be used; adequate preoperative imaging needs to be obtained to ensure appropriate uninvolved vasculature can be found for clamp placement, anastomosis, and subsequent reestablishment of flow. Improving outcomes has made vascular resection in hepatic malignancy more frequent and successful at centers with experience in these techniques.[2]

General guidelines for liver resections suggest a future liver remnant (FLR) of greater than 20% be obtained to avoid complications of postoperative liver dysfunction.[3] Volumetric assessment of the FLR by preoperative imaging is a key component in planning resections that include vascular reconstruction. With vascular resection and the potential increased ischemic injury to the remnant liver, an FLR of 40% is preferred, though not always obtainable.[4] Preoperative PV embolization (PVE) is an important adjunct to improve outcomes. In cases with borderline FLR or when extremely complex vascular reconstructions may be required, PVE of the side of the liver ipsilateral to the tumor should be performed 4 to 6 weeks before resection to allow hypertrophy of the remaining liver.[5] In many cases that require vascular reconstruction, PVE is not necessary, however, because the involvement of vessels by tumor may create an atrophy/hypertrophy complex that favors resection. The role of preoperative biliary drainage of the FLR in cases with biliary obstruction is controversial.[6–9] The authors' own practice in cases of biliary obstruction is to drain the FLR until bilirubin is less than 2 mg/dL before proceeding with resection; however, this practice may increase the risk of perioperative infectious complications and is not uniform across centers.

PORTAL VEIN RESECTION

- It was first described in the West in 1990 by Blumgart for hilar cholangiocarcinoma.[10]
- Variations in anatomy of the PV can make reconstruction challenging, so thorough assessment with preoperative imaging is necessary.
- Vein grafts can come from the left renal vein, gonadal vein, saphenous vein panel grafts, or resected hepatic veins from the side of the liver removed.

PV resection with hepatectomy was first described in the West in 1990 as a method to achieve negative margins and complete tumor resection for hilar cholangiocarcinoma by Blumgart.[11] This method was met with skepticism at that time as surgeons thought that the risk of such a procedure did not justify the outcome. Over time, more centers published successful results with combined hepatectomy with PV resection; the technique was used to obtain complete resection and increase the number of resectable patients with cholangiocarcinoma or gallbladder adenocarcinoma. In 1997 Klempnauer and colleagues[12] reported the first combined right trisectionectomy and PV resection in the West, and later in 1999 Neuhaus and colleagues[13,14] described a no-touch en bloc resection technique for hilar cholangiocarcinoma including PV resection with excellent outcomes. PV resection is now the most common vascular resection performed for hilar cholangiocarcinoma and has become an accepted if not uniformly applied technique.

Outcomes with PV resection in current studies are similar to hepatic resection without PV resection with comparable morbidity and mortality.[15,16] The most recent reports have shown improvements in perioperative mortality from 8% to 33% in early studies in the 1990s and early 2000s to reports of mortality of 0% to 2% more recently.[15,17–27] The reasons for improvement in outcome are multifactorial and include not only improved surgical planning and technique but also improved perioperative management, including the use of PVE. The primary goal in obtaining a successful oncologic outcome is the achievement of an R0 resection with or without PV resection. It is clear that survival in patients resected, even should they require PV reconstruction, is longer than those who are deemed unresectable. The use of vascular resection has increased the number of resectable and, therefore, curable patients, both by virtue of patients undergoing resection of the PV as well as those patients who are initially thought to require PV resection but are found at surgery to be resectable without vascular reconstruction. Without the surgeon being at least prepared to perform the vascular resection, those patients would not have been offered surgery. Long-term survival when using PV resection depends entirely on the ability to achieve negative margins. Earlier studies comparing PV resection to resection alone showed a decrease in long-term survival, but these results seemed more related to the ability to achieve negative margins than the issue of PV resection alone.[19] Several studies demonstrate patients undergoing combined hepatectomy and PV resection with negative margins have similar outcomes to patients with negative margins undergoing hepatic resection alone.[11,13,16,28] However, the presence of intraluminal tumor or positive margins does have a negative effect on survival.[26]

The potential for resection must be assessed preoperatively with imaging, including either a triphasic computed tomography (CT) or MRI to assess the extent of vessel involvement and confirm that there is an accessible PV segment above and below the tumor for anastomosis. Intraoperatively the distal PV on the liver remnant side must be free of tumor before anastomosis. In general, a minimum of 0.8 to 1.0 cm of PV before segmental branching of the left PV is required after right hepatectomy or trisectionectomy in order to have room for clamp placement and anastomosis. For left-sided resections, the right PV may be the target for anastomosis; but often the resection requires extension, and the right posterior sectoral branch becomes the target for anastomosis. Portal venous anatomy as well as the position of the hepatic artery segmental branches in relation to the PV branches is more variable on the right, and the surgeon must be very aware of the relative positions or risk catastrophe.[29–31] Preoperative imaging along with intraoperative identification of vessel position is a key part of the procedure.

Primary end-to-end PV anastomosis is preferred rather than the use of grafts if possible. Complete mobilization of the proximal main PV down to the level of the pancreas during the lymphadenectomy facilitates later resection and anastomosis. Anastomosis of the main to left PV can almost always be performed without the use of a graft (**Figs. 1** and **2**), frequently before liver transection because the course of the left PV is accessible before liver division. However, if there is likely to be undue tension or there is difficulty with access, the vein resection and anastomosis can be performed after the liver is transected. After transection and specimen removal, the access is excellent and the liver can be rotated down to take tension off of the anastomosis. On a left-sided resection with reconstruction of the right PV or right posterior sectoral branch of the PV, it has been the authors' experience that the liver requires transection before the portal venous resection and reconstruction. If primary anastomosis is not possible, many potential autologous conduits are available, including left renal vein, superficial femoral vein, hepatic vein (from resected liver), jugular veins, or saphenous vein modified to a spiral graft.[17–21,32,33] If the native vein is unable to be used, synthetic or cryopreserved grafts can be used but, if possible, are avoided because of the risk of thrombosis and infection.

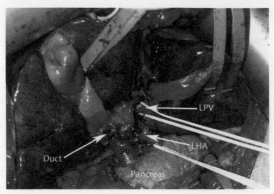

Fig. 1. In hilar cholangiocarcinoma, the left PV can be dissected out above the tumor with the main PV dissected out and mobilized to the pancreas. Duct, common bile duct; LHA, left hepatic artery; LPV, left PV; PV, main PV.

HEPATIC ARTERY RESECTION

- This method is growing in frequency with improved techniques in arterial reconstruction from live-donor liver experience as well as utilization of arterial reconstruction in pancreaticoduodenectomy (PD) for malignancy.
- Similar to early reports of portal venous resection, there is increased morbidity with the procedure with no proven survival benefit.
- Increasing experience and improved techniques with the addition of microsurgery have improved short-term outcomes and may make arterial resection a valuable part of achieving long-term survival.

Although not yet considered mainstream, improving options for chemotherapy have increased the interest in hepatic arterial resection and reconstruction for malignancy in PD, whereby technical issues of reconstruction of the proximal hepatic artery at the level of the gastroduodenal artery are less challenging but the biological behavior of the tumor has remained dismal. In the pancreas setting, technical success of arterial

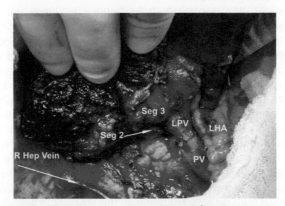

Fig. 2. The tumor in **Fig. 1** has been resected with a right trisectionectomy with bile duct resection and PV resection. The main PV has been anastomosed to the left PV. The segment (Seg) 2 and segment 3 ducts will later be implanted into a Roux-en-Y limb. LHA, left hepatic artery; LPV, left PV; PV, main PV; R Hep Vein, right hepatic vein.

reconstruction is less of an issue because of the size of the vessels reconstructed and also because there is a lesser physiologic insult that occurs more with PD than occurs with extensive liver resection. Improvement in chemotherapeutic options for hilar cholangiocarcinoma has not been as robust, but now hepatic artery resection is slowly being integrated into aggressive resection options for hepatic malignancies to try an increase negative margins during resection.[28,34] Most commonly, cases of combined liver and hepatic arterial resection are performed for involvement of the hepatic artery at its bifurcation and are often performed in combination with PV resection with or with PD.

Preoperative imaging assessment is essential for planning both the need and options for reconstruction. Planned arterial resection with reconstruction of either the right or left hepatic artery or posterior branch of the right hepatic artery requires assessment of potential proximal and distal control sites and assessment of options for obtaining suitable grafts or swinging alternative inflow to the liver. If end-to-end primary anastomosis is attempted, the artery must be fully mobilized to avoid tension on the anastomosis. Alternative inflow, such as the gastroduodenal or left hepatic artery,[35] are options; however, careful attention to anatomic variation and preservation of length of those vessels is required during the initial portal dissection. Interposition grafts, including radial artery, splenic artery, or the saphenous vein, can be used (**Fig. 3**).[36] Microsurgical techniques may be used when dealing with small sectoral (1–2 mm) arteries. Arterial reconstruction should follow PV reconstruction and typically is easier when done after liver transection and specimen removal has been completed.

When hepatic artery resection is required for tumor clearance, but technically reconstruction is simply not feasible, PV arterialization has been described as a final option.[37] Direct end-to-side anastomosis of the hepatic artery to the PV or inferior mesenteric artery to the inferior mesenteric vein anastomosis can be performed. This method is not uncomplicated, however, and is associated with an increased risk of biliary complications, including biliary abscesses and portal hypertension. It has been advocated that if PV arterialization is used, later selective transcatheter embolization of the hepatic artery several weeks after the surgery should be done to prevent long-term issues of portal hypertension and future biliary complications.[5]

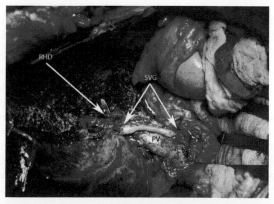

Fig. 3. An extended left hepatectomy for hilar cholangiocarcinoma has been done. The hepatic artery has been resected with a saphenous vein graft placed from the proper hepatic artery to the right hepatic artery several millimeters before its division into anterior and posterior divisions. PV, main PV; RHD, right hepatic duct; SVG, saphenous vein graft.

Because of the increased risk of complications, PV arterialization is only performed when no other options are available.[38]

Initial studies involving arterial resection did not demonstrate improved long-term survival: in contradistinction, long-term survival was worse, with a high mortality secondary to the operation itself and no survivors after 3 years. Reports of operative mortality ranged from 33.3% to 55.6%, with 1-year survival of only 17%.[15,39,40] These outcomes were confirmed in a recent meta-analysis of 24 articles involving vascular resection for hilar cholangiocarcinoma that concluded with an increased morbidity and no proven survival benefit for arterial resection.[41] However, centers with experience continue to push the boundaries of the possible and have now shown acceptable outcomes when combining arterial resection even with the addition of PV resection. In the largest current reported series Nagino and colleagues[18] reported a cohort of 50 patients who underwent combined PV and arterial resections. Negative margins were obtained in 66% of these patients, with only one perioperative mortality. The 1-, 3-, and 5-year survival rates were 78.9%, 36.3%, and 30.3%, respectively. Microsurgical techniques for anastomosis were used, including 32 end-to-end anastomoses, 11 greater saphenous vein or radial artery interpositions, and 2 using the left or right gastric artery. Three patients were unable to be reconstructed.

Improved surgical techniques and experience, particularly with microsurgery, seem to have potential to improve these short-term outcomes, however improvement in long-term survival awaits improvements in adjuvant therapies. In the authors' own practice, they will consider arterial resection and reconstruction in very select patients with hilar cholangiocarcinoma or gallbladder carcinoma. The authors' unpublished results to date, in a mixed cohort of patients with hilar cholangiocarcinoma and gallbladder adenocarcinoma, demonstrate that the procedure can be done with technical success with an acceptable 4% operative mortality but that long-term survival remains elusive with a 5-year survival of only 21% (Alan Hemming, MD, unpublished data). Arterial resection in the setting of hepatic malignancy should likely be considered in only select patients at experienced centers. Widespread utilization of this approach awaits improvements in adjuvant therapy.

HEPATIC VEIN/INFERIOR VENA CAVA RESECTION

- IVC and high hepatic vein involvement have traditionally been contraindications to resection.
- Resection with vascular reconstruction has improved outcomes over chemotherapy.
- Techniques for complex resection include in situ cold perfusion, ante situm, and ex vivo resection.

Patients with tumors involving the IVC or hepatic veins have limited options for treatment with chemotherapy or interventional radiology. Survival without surgical treatment is typically less than 1 year. However, with techniques ported from liver transplant along with improved techniques for liver resection and perioperative management, tumors involving the IVC and hepatic veins are now considered resectable in select patients with acceptable morbidity and mortality.[1] Including venous resection/reconstruction with liver resection is now accepted for most liver tumors, including hepatocellular carcinoma, cholangiocarcinoma, and colorectal metastasis, although the extent of vascular reconstruction and need for cold perfusion techniques remain open for discussion.

The technique for resection depends on the extent of involvement of the IVC or hepatic veins and location of the tumor.[42,43] Options for vena caval involvement alone include primary resection, patch reconstruction, or complete replacement of the vena cava with a synthetic or biological graft. If there is minimal IVC involvement, a side-biting clamp can be used to preserve caval flow and reconstruction can be done primarily or with a patch.[44–47] For larger degrees of involvement, that is, not involving the hepatic veins or IVC at the hepatic vein confluence, the vena cava can be clamped below the level of the hepatic veins to occlude flow through the retro hepatic IVC, while preserving portal inflow and hepatic venous outflow. In this technique, most of the liver parenchymal transection can be completed and the hepatic veins of the planned resection side of the liver segment divided, exposing the IVC below. Once the IVC above and below the tumor involvement is exposed, clamps are placed and the liver resection completed along with caval resection, leaving the IVC ready for reconstruction. Resection of portions of the IVC up to approximately 3 to 4 cm can be resected with primary end-to-end repair still possible. Larger defects can be reconstructed using 20-mm Gore-Tex (W.L. Gore & Associates, Inc, Newark, DE) graft, autologous peritoneum,[14] or bovine pericardium if needed (**Fig. 4**).[48]

Tumors that involve the IVC at the hepatic confluence require total vascular exclusion (TVE) with occlusion of both portal venous and hepatic arterial inflow as well as occluding the IVC above and below the hepatic veins. TVE is considered to be more damaging to the liver than simply portal inflow clamping, given the lack of hepatic venous backflow from the IVC and hepatic veins.[49] In order to avoid ischemic damage to the liver, as much of the liver resection and exposure of the IVC that can be done should be done before placing the clamps for TVE. The clamp placement sequence for TVE is in the sequence of infrahepatic cava, then PV and hepatic artery,

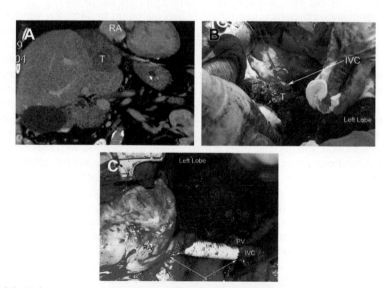

Fig. 4. (*A*) CT demonstrating tumor extending to the IVC at the hepatic vein confluence. RA, right atrium; T, tumor. (*B*) Intraoperative picture of the patient shown in (*A*). The liver has been divided exposing the tumor around the IVC. Control of the suprahepatic IVC required sternotomy with intrapericardial control. Left lobe, left hepatic lobe; T, tumor. (*C*) The case in (*B*) with 20-mm ringed Gore-Tex graft used to reconstruct the IVC. Left lobe, left lobe of liver; RA, right atrium. (*From* [*B*] Hemming AW, Mekeel KL, Zendejas I, et al. Resection of the liver and inferior vena cava for hepatic malignancy. J Am Coll Surg 2013;217(1):117, with permission; and [*C*] Hemming AW, Mekeel KL, Zendejas I, et al. Resection of the liver and inferior vena cava for hepatic malignancy. J Am Coll Surg 2013;217(1):118, with permission.)

and lastly suprahepatic IVC. Clamps can be repositioned as needed on the IVC to isolate only hepatic veins if only hepatic veins require reconstruction.

For tumors involving the hepatic vein confluence and vena cava where simple resection is not possible, options include in situ cold perfusion, ante situm, and ex vivo techniques. These procedures involve TVE and potentially require the use of venovenous bypass or alternate strategies to maintain cardiac return if patients cannot tolerate clamping of the vena cava after volume resuscitation. In situ cold perfusion may be used if the length of ischemia is expected to extend past 45 minutes to an hour. Cold perfusion may be done in situ or ex vivo and improves the ability of the liver to tolerate ischemia and allows resection to be completed in a bloodless field.[43,50–52] For better exposure of the area around the hepatic veins, in situ cold perfusion can be modified to an ante situm technique in which the suprahepatic vena cava is divided and movement and rotation of the liver forward allows better access to the hepatic venous/caval confluence.[53] This method can be combined with division of the infrahepatic IVC below for even more rotation of the liver up into the operative field and improved access. Compared with TVE alone, cold perfusion of the liver decreases the ischemic injury.

Ex vivo resection gives the ideal access and can also be performed for tumor involvement of vascular structures requiring complex reconstruction. The ex vivo technique interrupts and transects major inflow and outflow, as well as the bile duct, to remove the liver from the abdomen for cold perfusion on the back table. The resection is completed on the back table before reimplantation of the liver, similar to a partial liver graft transplant.[38] In ex vivo cases, the IVC may be reconstructed with a Gore-Tex graft with hepatic vein branches reimplanted into the Gore-Tex.

When venovenous bypass is used during caval clamping to decrease venous pressure and maintain cardiac return, outflow cannulas are placed in the femoral vein and PV and inflow into the right jugular or axillary vein. Cannulas can be placed via the open or percutaneous technique, depending on surgeon preference. An alternative to venovenous bypass to maintain cardiac return and portal venous decompression is to place both an IVC graft and temporary portacaval shunt during the time that the liver is ex vivo. The resected/reconstructed liver can then be implanted into the Gore-Tex graft and the temporary shunt taken down to perform the portal venous anastomosis. In cases when the tumor has no IVC involvement and needs only hepatic vein reconstruction, the hepatic veins are controlled and divided with maintenance of IVC flow. A temporary portacaval shunt is created to decompress the splanchnic circulation and avoid bypass. The use of bypass does increase potential complications, including venous thromboembolic events and increased length of stay, and has the potential for vascular complications or air embolus with increased need for blood transfusions. Bypass does not, however, seem to increase the risk of renal injury or need for dialysis over clamping and may help in more complex cases.[54–57]

The in situ cold perfusion techniques offer the advantage of keeping the PV and hilum intact as compared with ex vivo perfusion.[43] Perfusion is instituted through a small incision in the PV above the portal clamp or via the PV branch on the resection side. During the infusion of the cold perfusate, the effluent is removed via a venotomy in the IVC or hepatic veins that can be repaired after completion of the resection/reconstruction before restoration of flow.

Cold perfusion is given with standard preservations solutions, including University of Wisconsin (UW) solution or histidine-tryptophan-ketoglutarate. UW solution has high potassium content, and should be flushed out of the liver before reperfusion of the liver. At the authors' institution, they use UW as their perfusion solution and then flush with chilled 5% albumin or Ringers lactate solution.

For tumors that involve more extensive sections of the hepatic veins, or have hepatic confluence and hilar involvement, ex vivo resection is used. Before removal of the liver, the tumor must be assessed for resectability. A sternotomy with opening of the pericardium may be needed for better visualization of the IVC and tumor. Once a tumor is deemed resectable, the hilum is dissected and cholecystectomy performed. The infrahepatic IVC is dissected down to the renal veins, and the liver is mobilized. The suprahepatic IVC is then dissected free, and phrenic veins are divided. Depending on tumor involvement, clamps are placed in sequence: the artery is transected typically at the level of the gastroduodenal artery, PV 1.5 to 2.0 cm below the bifurcation, and the bile duct taken sharply at 1.0 to 1.5 cm below the bifurcation. The suprahepatic IVC may be transected below the diaphragm or clamped in the intrapericardial portion if more distance from the tumor is needed. The IVC is then transected leaving as much length behind as possible, and the liver is taken to the back table.

After the liver is removed, it is placed in an ice bath and cold perfusion initiated via the PV. The hepatic artery and bile duct are also hand flushed with preservation solution. The resection is then performed using standard liver resection techniques or can be done sharply with a knife. Flushing the liver after resection helps identify potential leaks that are repaired before reimplantation. Complex reconstructions can be performed in multiple methods depending on what remains after resection (**Fig. 5**).

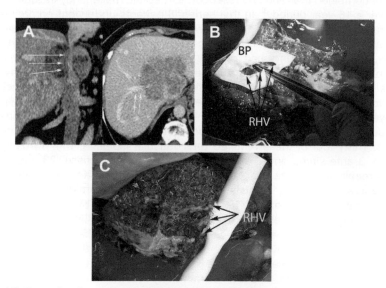

Fig. 5. (*A*) Centrally placed cholangiocarcinoma involving IVC and all hepatic veins. Note that tumor extends to branches of right hepatic vein (RHV) that will need reconstruction. The 2 arrows show the tumor extending to branch point of RHV; 3 arrows show the tumor involvement of IVC. (*B*) Bovine pericardial fence placed to plastied branches of RHV during ex vivo procedure. BP, bovine pericardium. (*C*) Bovine pericardial fence implanted into Gore-Tex IVC graft that will subsequently be reimplanted in the patient. Three arrows show branches of RHV. (*From* [*A*] Hemming AW, Mekeel KL, Zendejas I, et al. Resection of the liver and inferior vena cava for hepatic malignancy. J Am Coll Surg 2013;217(1):117, with permission; and [*B*] Hemming AW, Mekeel KL, Zendejas I, et al. Resection of the liver and inferior vena cava for hepatic malignancy. J Am Coll Surg 2013;217(1):119, with permission.)

Hepatic veins are reimplanted into the IVC, reconstructed with multiple vein grafts, or plastied together in groups for reconstruction.[58] If needed, the IVC is typically replaced using a 20-mm Gore-Tex tube graft.

After completion of resection and reconstruction, the resultant liver segment is reimplanted. The anastomoses are performed in a similar fashion to a standard partial liver transplant. The suprahepatic caval anastomosis is completed first, followed by the infrahepatic anastomosis. Before completion of the infrahepatic anastomosis, the liver is flushed free of UW solution if used. The portal venous anastomosis is completed next; the liver is reperfused sequentially starting first with the suprahepatic clamp removal and then the infrahepatic clamp removal; then the portal flow is reestablished. The arterial anastomosis is performed typically after the liver has been reperfused with portal flow and hemostasis has been obtained. The last anastomosis completed is the biliary anastomosis, done either duct to duct or with a Roux-en-Y choledochojejunostomy if the duct ends do not come together without tension.

It is clear in multiple studies that caval and hepatic vein resection, particularly with ex vivo resection and subsequent auto transplantation of the liver, has definite increased morbidity and mortality.[38,52,58–64] However, for these patients resection is the only possibility for cure. Additionally, those patients who are resected have longer median survival than those who are not resected. Successful long-term survival in a small number of patients is possible,[52,60] although patient selection is important to minimize postoperative mortality.[65–68] The largest series to date of combined liver and IVC resection for hepatic malignancy includes 60 patients over a 16-year period.[38] In that series, 8 patients underwent primary reconstruction, including 3 with hepatic vein reimplantation, one of which required an ex vivo approach to reimplant the hepatic veins, though the IVC was reconstructed primarily. Fourteen patients had defects greater than 5 cm that were repaired with a patch of autologous vein, bovine pericardium, or Gore-Tex. Thirty-eight patients required full reconstruction of the IVC with a Gore-Tex graft, including 5 ex vivo resections and 8 with cold perfusion. Perioperative mortality was 8% and 3-year survival 35%.[38] In another similar series published by Malde and colleagues,[58] 35 patients underwent combined liver and IVC resection over 15 years. Thirty-four of these required total vascular isolation, with 13 using cold perfusion, 3 ante situm, and 6 ex vivo techniques. Among these, 23 had primary or patch repair of the cava and 12 had reconstruction with an interposition graft. The perioperative mortality in this series was 11.4% and morbidity 40.0% with an actuarial 5-year survival of 37.7%. Another recent study by Azoulay and colleagues[51] published a series of 391 patients who underwent TVE with venovenous bypass for complex liver resections. Seventy-seven of these had in situ cold perfusion, and 35 had hepatic vein or IVC reconstructions. The 90-day mortality was 19.5% (15 patients) and seemed to be significantly related to a maximum tumor size of greater than 10 cm, Charlson Comorbidity Index of 3 or more, and postoperative liver insufficiency on multivariate analysis. The 5-year survival rate in this group was 30.4%.

Table 1 shows several series and reports of hepatic and IVC resections involving ex situ liver surgery. The reported 5-year survival for these groups was 20% to 30%, if long-term survival was achieved and reported. Several of the patients in early studies did require salvage liver transplantation for liver failure, which carried a high mortality rate; all but one patient reported had tumor recurrence within 1 year after transplant. Salvage liver transplantation is, therefore, not recommended (see **Table 1**).[42,60,69–74]

Table 1
Studies involving hepatic vein and IVC reconstruction and including ex vivo liver resections

Author	Dates	Indications	TVE	HV/IVC Resection	In Situ Perfusion	Ante Situ	Ex Vivo	90-d Mortality Overall	1-y Survival	3-y Survival	5-y Survival
Oldhafer[69]	1988–1998	1° or 2° malignancy, FNH	24	5	0	0	23	8	NR, only FNH pts alive at 5 and 9 y		
Lodge[70]	1995–1998	CLM	6	8	0	0	4	2	NR		
Hemming[38]	1996–2012	CLM, HCC, CHL, GIST, HPBST, SCC	60	60	8	NR	6	5	89%	NR	35%
Zhang[73]	1999–2008	Hemangioma, CHL	3	3	0	0	3	1	2 pts still alive at publication		
Forni[71]	NR	CLM, RCC	4	—	0	0	4	3	Fourth pt died of recurrence at 16 mo		
Malde[58]	1995–2010	CLM, HCC, CHL	34	35	13	3	6	4	75.9%	58.7%	19.6%
Gruttandauria[72]	2003–2004	CLM	2	2	0	0	2	0	First pt alive at 23 mo, second NR		
Wang[74]	2008–2010	Echinococcal cyst	6	6	0	0	6	1	83.3%	NR	

Abbreviations: CHL, cholangiocarcinoma; CLM, colorectal liver metastasis; FNH, focal nodular hyperplasia; GIST, gastrointestinal stromal tumor; HCC, hepatocellular carcinoma; HPBST, hepatoblastoma; NR, none reported; pt, patient; RCC, renal cell carcinoma; SCC, squamous cell carcinoma.
Data from Refs.[43,48,59,61,69–72]

SUMMARY

- Vascular resection is a growing trend in hepatic surgery for malignancy with improved outcomes over time.
- One must be able to achieve adequate margins for success, which may involve PV, hepatic artery, IVC, or hepatic vein resection and reconstruction with multiple techniques.
- In situ cold perfusion, ante situm, and ex vivo resections offer a technically challenging option to tumor resection in select patients.

   With current relatively ineffective options for chemotherapy and nonsurgical intervention for patients with vascular involvement of hepatic tumors, vascular resection has become an increasingly used option in combination with hepatic resection to obtain tumor clearance. Preoperative imaging is essential to determine the potential for complete resection and for operative planning for vessel reconstruction. With increasing experience, a small number of centers have significantly improved outcomes and decreased mortality in the last 2 decades. Although vascular reconstruction is associated with an increased morbidity and mortality, it allows a potential curative approach in otherwise incurable patients and should be considered in select patients.

REFERENCES

1. Hemming AW, Reed AI, Fujita S, et al. Role for extending hepatic resection using an aggressive approach to liver surgery. J Am Coll Surg 2008;206(5):870–5.
2. Mekeel K, Hemming A. Evolving role of vascular resection and reconstruction in hepatic surgery for malignancy. Hepatic Oncol 2014;1(1):53–65.
3. Shindoh J, Tzeng CW, Aloia TA, et al. Safety and efficacy of portal vein embolization before planned major or extended hepatectomy: an institutional experience of 358 patients. Gastrointest Surg 2014;18(1):45–51.
4. Hemming AW, Reed AI, Howard RJ, et al. Preoperative portal vein embolization for extended hepatectomy. Ann Surg 2003;237(5):686–91 [discussion: 691–3].
5. Sano T, Shimizu Y, Senda Y, et al. Assessing resectability in cholangiocarcinoma. Hepatic Oncol 2014;1(1):39–51.
6. Nimura Y. Preoperative biliary drainage before resection for cholangiocarcinoma (Pro). HPB (Oxford) 2008;10(2):130–3.
7. Neuhaus P, Thelen A. Radical surgery for right-sided Klatskin tumor. HPB (Oxford) 2008;10(3):171–3.
8. Nimura Y. Radical surgery: vascular and pancreatic resection for cholangiocarcinoma. HPB (Oxford) 2008;10(3):183–5.
9. Hemming A, Mekeel K, Khanna A, et al. Portal vein resection in the management of hilar cholangiocarcinoma. J Am Coll Surgeons 2011;212(4):604–13.
10. Hadjis NS, Blenkharn JI, Alexander N, et al. Outcome of radical surgery in hilar cholangiocarcinoma. Surgery 1990;107(6):597–604.
11. Hidalgo E, Asthana S, Nishio H, et al. Surgery for hilar cholangiocarcinoma: the Leeds experience. Eur J Surg Oncol 2008;34(7):787–94.
12. Klempnauer J, Ridder GJ, Werner M, et al. What constitutes long-term survival after surgery for hilar cholangiocarcinoma? Cancer 1997;79(1):26–34.
13. Neuhaus P, Thelen A, Jonas S, et al. Oncological superiority of hilar en bloc resection for the treatment of hilar cholangiocarcinoma [Comparative Study Evaluation Studies]. Ann Surg Oncol 2012;19(5):1602–8.
14. Neuhaus P, Jonas S, Bechstein WO, et al. Extended resections for hilar cholangiocarcinoma. Ann Surg 1999;230(6):808–18 [discussion: 19].

15. Miyazaki M, Kato A, Ito H, et al. Combined vascular resection in operative resection for hilar cholangiocarcinoma: does it work or not? Surgery 2007;141(5):581–8.
16. Kurosaki I, Hatakeyama K, Minagawa M, et al. Portal vein resection in surgery for cancer of biliary tract and pancreas: special reference to the relationship between the surgical outcome and site of primary tumor. J Gastrointest Surg 2008;12(5): 907–18.
17. Lee SG, Song GW, Hwang S, et al. Surgical treatment of hilar cholangiocarcinoma in the new era: the Asan experience. J Hepatobiliary Pancreat Sci 2010;17(4): 476–89.
18. Nagino M, Nimura Y, Nishio H, et al. Hepatectomy with simultaneous resection of the portal vein and hepatic artery for advanced perihilar cholangiocarcinoma: an audit of 50 consecutive cases. Ann Surg 2010;252(1):115–23.
19. Igami T, Nishio H, Ebata T, et al. Surgical treatment of hilar cholangiocarcinoma in the "new era": the Nagoya University experience. J Hepatobiliary Pancreat Sci 2010;17(4):449–54.
20. Hemming AW, Kim RD, Mekeel KL, et al. Portal vein resection for hilar cholangio-carcinoma. Am Surg 2006;72(7):599–604 [discussion: 604–5].
21. de Jong MC, Marques H, Clary BM, et al. The impact of portal vein resection on outcomes for hilar cholangiocarcinoma: a multi-institutional analysis of 305 cases. Cancer 2012;118(19):4737–47.
22. Gerhards MF, van Gulik TM, de Wit LT, et al. Evaluation of morbidity and mortality after resection for hilar cholangiocarcinoma–a single center experience. Surgery 2000;127(4):395–404.
23. Shimada H, Endo I, Sugita M, et al. Hepatic resection combined with portal vein or hepatic artery reconstruction for advanced carcinoma of the hilar bile duct and gallbladder. World J Surg 2003;27(10):1137–42.
24. Ebata T, Nagino M, Kamiya J, et al. Hepatectomy with portal vein resection for hilar cholangiocarcinoma: audit of 52 consecutive cases. Ann Surg 2003;238(5):720–7.
25. Dinant S, Gerhards MF, Rauws EA, et al. Improved outcome of resection of hilar cholangiocarcinoma (Klatskin tumor). Ann Surg Oncol 2006;13(6):872–80.
26. Young AL, Prasad KR, Toogood GJ, et al. Surgical treatment of hilar cholangiocar-cinoma in a new era: comparison among leading Eastern and Western centers, Leeds. J Hepatobiliary Pancreat Sci 2010;17(4):497–504.
27. Miyazaki M, Kimura F, Shimizu H, et al. One hundred seven consecutive surgical resections for hilar cholangiocarcinoma of bismuth types II, III, IV between 2001 and 2008. J Hepatobiliary Pancreat Sci 2010;17(4):470–5.
28. Bachellier P, Rosso E, Lucescu I, et al. Is the need for an arterial resection a contraindication to pancreatic resection for locally advanced pancreatic adenocarcinoma? A case-matched controlled study. J Surg Oncol 2011; 103(1):75–84.
29. Shimizu H, Sawada S, Kimura F, et al. Clinical significance of biliary vascular anatomy of the right liver for hilar cholangiocarcinoma applied to left hemihepa-tectomy. Ann Surg 2009;249(3):435–9.
30. Yamanaka N, Yasui C, Yamanaka J, et al. Left hemihepatectomy with microsur-gical reconstruction of the right-sided hepatic vasculature. A strategy for preser-ving hepatic function in patients with proximal bile duct cancer. Langenbecks Arch Surg 2001;386(5):364–8.
31. Madariaga JR, Iwatsuki S, Todo S, et al. Liver resection for hilar and peripheral cholangiocarcinomas: a study of 62 cases. Ann Surg 1998;227(1):70–9.
32. Lee SG, Lee YJ, Park KM, et al. One hundred and eleven liver resections for hilar bile duct cancer. J Hepatobiliary Pancreat Surg 2000;7(2):135–41.

33. Mollberg N, Rahbari NN, Koch M, et al. Arterial resection during pancreatectomy for pancreatic cancer: a systematic review and meta-analysis [Comparative Study Meta-Analysis Review]. Ann Surg 2011;254(6):882–93.

34. Ota T, Araida T, Yamamoto M, et al. Operative outcome and problems of right hepatic lobectomy with pancreatoduodenectomy for advanced carcinoma of the biliary tract. J Hepatobiliary Pancreat Surg 2007;14(2):155–8.

35. de Santibañes E, Ardiles V, Alvarez FA, et al. Hepatic artery reconstruction first for the treatment of hilar cholangiocarcinoma bismuth type IIIB with contralateral arterial invasion: a novel technical strategy. HPB (Oxford) 2012;14(1):67–70.

36. Kondo S, Hirano S, Ambo Y, et al. Arterioportal shunting as an alternative to microvascular reconstruction after hepatic artery resection. Br J Surg 2004; 91(2):248–51.

37. Bhangui P, Salloum C, Lim C, et al. Portal vein arterialization: a salvage procedure for a totally de-arterialized liver. The Paul Brousse Hospital experience. HPB (Oxford) 2014;16(8):723–38.

38. Hemming AW, Mekeel KL, Zendejas I, et al. Resection of the liver and inferior vena cava for hepatic malignancy. J Am Coll Surgeons 2013;217(1):115–24.

39. Shimada K, Sano T, Sakamoto Y, et al. Clinical implications of combined portal vein resection as a palliative procedure in patients undergoing pancreatico-duodenectomy for pancreatic head carcinoma. Ann Surg Oncol 2006;13(12): 1569–78.

40. Abbas S, Sandroussi C. Systematic review and meta-analysis of the role of vascular resection in the treatment of hilar cholangiocarcinoma. HPB (Oxford) 2013;15(7):492–503.

41. Sakamoto Y, Sano T, Shimada K, et al. Clinical significance of reconstruction of the right hepatic artery for biliary malignancy. Langenbecks Arch Surg 2006; 391(3):203–8.

42. Azoulay D, Andreani P, Maggi U, et al. Combined liver resection and reconstruction of the supra-renal vena cava: the Paul Brousse experience. Ann Surg 2006; 244(1):80–8.

43. Sarmiento JM, Bower TC, Cherry KJ, et al. Is combined partial hepatectomy with segmental resection of inferior vena cava justified for malignancy? Arch Surg 2003;138(6):624–30 [discussion: 630–1].

44. Johnson ST, Blitz M, Kneteman N, et al. Combined hepatic and inferior vena cava resection for colorectal metastases [Comparative Study]. J Gastrointest Surg 2006;10(2):220–6.

45. Delis SG, Madariaga J, Ciancio G. Combined liver and inferior vena cava resection for hepatic malignancy. J Surg Oncol 2007 1;96(3):258–64.

46. Bower TC, Nagorney DM, Cherry KJ Jr, et al. Replacement of the inferior vena cava for malignancy: an update. J Vasc Surg 2000;31(2):270–81.

47. Azoulay D, Eshkenazy R, Andreani P, et al. In situ hypothermic perfusion of the liver versus standard total vascular exclusion for complex liver resection. Ann Surg 2005;241(2):277–85.

48. Pulitanó C, Crawford M, Ho P, et al. Hepatocellular carcinoma with intracavitary cardiac involvement: a case report and review of the literature. HPB (Oxford) 2013;15(8):628–32.

49. Saiura A, Yamamoto J, Sakamoto Y, et al. Safety and efficacy of hepatic vein reconstruction for colorectal liver metastases. Am J Surg 2011;202(4):449–54.

50. Dubay D, Gallinger S, Hawryluck L, et al. In situ hypothermic liver preservation during radical liver resection with major vascular reconstruction. Br J Surg 2009;96(12):1429–36.

51. Azoulay D, Lim C, Salloum C, et al. Complex liver resection using standard total vascular exclusion, venovenous bypass, and in situ hypothermic portal perfusion: an audit of 77 consecutive cases. Ann Surg 2015;262(1):93–104.
52. Yamamoto Y. Ante-situm hepatic resection for tumors involving the confluence of hepatic veins and IVC. J Hepatobiliary Pancreat Sci 2013;20(3):313–23.
53. Gurusamy KS, Koti R, Pamecha V, et al. Veno-venous bypass versus none for liver transplantation. Cochrane Database Syst Rev 2011;(3):CD007712.
54. Glebova NO, Hicks CW, Piazza KM, et al. Outcomes of bypass support use during inferior vena cava resection and reconstruction. Ann Vasc Surg 2016;30:12–3.
55. Jackson P, Jankovic Z. Veno-venous bypass catheters for hepatic transplant risk unique complications. Anaesth Intensive Care 2007;35(5):805–6.
56. Khoury GF, Mann ME, Porot MJ, et al. Air embolism associated with veno-venous bypass during orthotopic liver transplantation. Anesthesiology 1987;67:848–51.
57. Smyrniotis V, Kostopanagiotou G, Lolis E, et al. Effects of hepatovenous back flow on ischemic reperfusion injuries in liver resections with the Pringle maneuver. J Am Coll Surg 2003;197(6):949–54.
58. Malde DJ, Khan A, Prasad KR, et al. Inferior vena cava resection with hepatectomy: challenging but justified. HPB (Oxford) 2011;13(11):802–10.
59. Hemming AW, Reed AI, Langham MR Jr, et al. Combined resection of the liver and inferior vena cava for hepatic malignancy. Ann Surg 2004;239(5):712–9.
60. Lin DX, Zhang QY, Li X, et al. An aggressive approach leads to improved survival in hepatocellular carcinoma patients with portal vein tumor thrombus. J Cancer Res Clin Oncol 2011;137(1):139–49.
61. Kondo K, Chijiiwa K, Kai M, et al. Surgical strategy for hepatocellular carcinoma patients with portal vein tumor thrombus based on prognostic factors. J Gastrointest Surg 2009;13(6):1078–83.
62. Xu JF, Liu XY, Wang S, et al. Surgical treatment for hepatocellular carcinoma with portal vein tumor thrombus: a novel classification. World J Surg Oncol 2015;13:86.
63. Shi J, Lai EC, Li N, et al. Surgical treatment for hepatocellular carcinoma with portal vein tumor thrombus. Hepatogastroenterology 2006;53(69):415–9.
64. Peng ZW, Guo RP, Zhang YJ, et al. Hepatic resection versus transcatheter arterial chemoembolization for the treatment of hepatocellular carcinoma with portal vein tumor thrombus. Cancer 2012;118(19):4725–36.
65. Wu CC, Hsieh SR, Chen JT, et al. An appraisal of liver and portal vein resection for hepatocellular carcinoma with tumor thrombi extending to portal bifurcation [Research Support, Non-U.S. Gov't]. Arch Surg 2000;135(11):1273–9.
66. Dokmak S, Aussilhou B, Sauvanet A, et al. Peritoneum as an autologous substitute for venous reconstruction in hepatopancreatobiliary surgery. Ann Surg 2015; 262(2):366–71.
67. Nuzzo G, Giuliante F, Ardito F, et al. Improvement in perioperative and long-term outcome after surgical treatment of hilar cholangiocarcinoma: results of an Italian multicenter analysis of 440 patients [Multicenter Study Research Support, Non-U.S. Gov't]. Arch Surg 2012;147(1):26–34.
68. Hirano S, Kondo S, Tanaka E, et al. Safety of combined resection of the middle hepatic artery in right hemihepatectomy for hilar biliary malignancy. J Hepatobiliary Pancreat Surg 2009;16(6):796–801.
69. Oldhafer KJ, Lang H, Schlitt HJ, et al. Long-term experience after ex situ liver surgery. Surgery 2000;127(5):520–7.
70. Lodge JP, Ammori BJ, Prasad KR, et al. Ex vivo and in situ resection of inferior vena cava with hepatectomy for colorectal metastases. Ann Surg 2000;231(4): 471–9.

71. Forni E, Meriggi F. Bench surgery and liver autotransplantation. Personal experience and technical considerations. G Chir 1995;16(10):407–13.
72. Gruttadauria S, Marsh JW, Bartlett DL, et al. Ex situ resection techniques and liver autotransplantation: last resource for otherwise unresectable malignancy. Dig Dis Sci 2005;50(10):1829–35.
73. Zhang KM, Hu XW, Dong JH, et al. Ex-situ liver surgery without veno-venous bypass. World J Gastroenterol 2012;18(48):7290–5.
74. Wang H, Liu Q, Wang Z, et al. Clinical outcomes of Ex Vivo liver resection and liver autotransplantation for hepatic alveolar echinococcosis. J Huazhong Univ Sci Technolog Med Sci 2012;32(4):598–600.

Minimally Invasive Hepatic Surgery

Lee M. Ocuin, MD[a], Allan Tsung, MD[b],*

KEYWORDS

- Minimally invasive • Laparoscopic • Robotic-assisted • Resection • Hepatectomy

KEY POINTS

- Minimally invasive hepatectomy is safe and feasible in properly selected patients.
- Preoperative workup, anesthetic management, and postoperative management are similar to open hepatectomy.
- Minimally invasive hepatectomy is associated with fewer perioperative complications and shorter hospital length of stay.
- Short- and long-term oncologic outcomes are similar between minimally invasive and open hepatectomy done for malignancy.
- Minimally invasive hepatectomy is best performed by surgeons who are trained in open liver surgery and at high-volume hepatopancreaticobiliary centers.

INTRODUCTION

The application of minimally invasive techniques has transformed the surgical landscape over the past 20 years. This approach has demonstrated benefit in surgical subspecialties, including colorectal surgery,[1,2] gynecology,[3] urology,[4] and thoracic surgery.[5] Multiple studies have demonstrated reduced postoperative pain, reduced morbidity, decreased length of stay, improved cosmesis, and improved overall cost-effectiveness without compromising oncologic outcomes.[1,2,6–8] These complex procedures require advanced laparoscopic skills, including suturing, knot-tying, and bimanual tissue manipulation. Limitations of conventional laparoscopic techniques include reduced visualization, amplification of physiologic tremor, and suboptimal ergonomics. Range of motion is restricted to 4 degrees of freedom, compared with the 7 degrees of freedom of the human wrist.[9,10] These limitations become increasingly

[a] Division of Surgical Oncology, Department of Surgery, University of Pittsburgh Medical Center, 5150 Centre Avenue, Suite 414, Pittsburgh, PA 15232, USA; [b] Division of Hepatobiliary and Pancreatic Surgery, Department of Surgery, Liver Cancer Center, University of Pittsburgh Medical Center, UPMC Kauffman Building, 3471 Fifth Avenue, Suite 300, Pittsburgh, PA 15213, USA
* Corresponding author.
E-mail address: tsunga@upmc.edu

Surg Clin N Am 96 (2016) 299–313
http://dx.doi.org/10.1016/j.suc.2015.12.004
0039-6109/16/$ – see front matter © 2016 Elsevier Inc. All rights reserved.

surgical.theclinics.com

apparent as the complexity of the procedure increases, translating to a steep learning curve, and have likely slowed the application of minimally invasive approaches to hepatopancreaticobiliary procedures, which are generally performed at high-volume tertiary care centers.

As the comfort and understanding of hepatopancreaticobiliary surgery have grown, minimally invasive approaches have been applied with increasing frequency to the field.[11–21] Laparoscopic liver surgery affords the same universal benefits of minimally invasive surgery elsewhere, including reduced postoperative pain and decreased length of hospital stay, and it has demonstrated safety in experienced hands.[7] However, the laparoscopic approach to the liver is challenging due to complex vascular and biliary anatomy, risk of bleeding, fragile parenchyma, and difficult exposure secondary to size and deep, posterior retroperitoneal attachments. The minimally invasive approach is being used more frequently, but mainly for nonanatomic resections. The learning curve is approximately 60 cases.[22] In a large review by Nguyen and colleagues[7] of more than 2800 laparoscopic liver resections, nonanatomic wedge resections and left lateral sectionectomy comprised nearly two-thirds of cases, whereas fewer than 10% of cases were formal right or left hepatic lobectomies.

In an effort to standardize and summarize the current position on laparoscopic liver surgery, an international conference was held in Louisville, Kentucky in 2008.[23] Consensus recommendations included the following: (1) the best indications for laparoscopic liver resection are in patients with solitary lesions, 5 cm or less, located in peripheral liver segments II to VI; (2) the laparoscopic approach to left lateral sectionectomy should be considered standard practice; and (3) although all types of liver resection can be performed laparoscopically, major liver resections (right or left hepatectomy) should be reserved for experienced surgeons already skilled at more complex laparoscopic hepatic resections. Lesions adjacent to major vessels or near the liver hilum were not considered appropriate for laparoscopic resection because of the potential risk of massive bleeding and need for biliary reconstruction. However, surgeons at high-volume centers may choose to operate beyond these criteria, provided that the surgeon is comfortable with minimally invasive methods to achieve hemostasis should significant bleeding be encountered. Despite the technical limitations of laparoscopy, malignant tumors are not a contraindication to minimally invasive resection as demonstrated in many comparative studies, and laparoscopic resection does not appear to compromise the oncologic integrity of the procedure with regards to margin status and local recurrence rate when compared with the open approach.[7,17,24,25]

The inherent visual and ergonomic limitations of laparoscopy have played a major role in the development of robotic surgery, which allows surgeons to perform advanced laparoscopic procedures with greater ease. Currently, the da Vinci Surgical System (Intuitive Surgical, Inc, Sunnyvale, CA, USA) is the only commercially available robotic surgical system approved by the US Food and Drug Administration for use in surgery. Advantages include articulating instruments that re-create the 7 degrees of freedom of the human wrist, 3-dimensional view of the operative field in high-definition, and complex algorithms that minimize physiologic tremor. These features allow for precise dissection and intracorporeal suturing, thus expanding the scope and complexity of procedures that can be performed in a minimally invasive fashion. Disadvantages include high cost, loss of haptic feedback, inability to operate in multiple fields, and need for a skilled bedside assistant. The lack of haptic feedback is generally overcome by enhanced 3-dimensional visualization, which allows the operating surgeon to "see" how much tension or force is being applied to tissues and suture within the operative field.[26] The first major series reporting the use of robotics in general surgery was by Giulianotti and colleagues[27] in 2003. The report included 207 procedures such as fundoplication, cholecystectomy, esophagectomy, colectomy, pancreatectomy, and hepatectomy. Morbidity and mortality rates were acceptable (8.3% and 1.5%, respectively), and the conversion rate was 2.1%. This report established that robotic surgery was both safe and feasible. Over the past decade, robotic-assisted surgery has been applied broadly in urologic, gynecologic, hepato-pancreaticobiliary, and cardiac surgery.[20,28–30] The platform has controls and ergonomics that closely mimic the movements of open surgery, has improved 3-dimensional visualization, and appears to shorten the learning curve for complex cases compared with conventional laparoscopy.[27,31,32] The multitude of technically challenging hepatopancreaticoobiliary procedures provides an ever-expanding and ideal application of this technology.[18,20,33,34]

PREOPERATIVE PLANNING

All patients should undergo a comprehensive history and physical examination. Although not absolute contraindications, multiple prior abdominal surgeries or the presence of underlying comorbidities, such as chronic obstructive pulmonary disease or congestive heart failure, should be kept in mind when choosing patients for minimally invasive hepatectomy.

Standard workup of patients with primary or metastatic hepatic malignancies includes a triphasic computed tomographic (CT) scan (noncontrast, arterial, and portal venous phase) or contrast-enhanced MRI examination of the abdomen and pelvis. These imaging studies should be recent (within 4–6 weeks of surgery) and allow for evaluation of tumor size and location, extent of hepatic disease, assessment of the background liver for cirrhosis and hepatic steatosis, and the size of the future liver remnant. In addition, preoperative imaging should be used to identify the pertinent vascular and biliary anatomy of the liver and the presence of any anatomic variants. If diagnostic uncertainty exists, tissue sampling by ultrasound or CT-guided core-needle biopsy may be performed. Tissue sampling of uninvolved liver can be used to assess the degree of background steatosis or cirrhosis. Evaluation for extrahepatic disease can be accomplished with a CT scan of the chest or CT/PET imaging. Routine laboratory tests include complete blood count, coagulation panel, and hepatic function panel. Serum tumor markers, including α-fetoprotein, chromogranin A, carcinoembryonic antigen, and cancer antigen 19-9, should be sent based on the suspected underlying malignancy. These tumor markers are useful as part of the diagnostic workup and postoperative surveillance.

Similar to open hepatectomy, the authors favor a low central venous pressure (CVP) anesthesia approach when performing minimally invasive hepatic resections.[35] A CVP anesthesia approach avoids distention of the inferior vena cava (IVC), facilitating mobilization of the liver and dissection of the retrohepatic cava and major hepatic veins. Low CVP anesthesia decreases bleeding during parenchymal transection and simplifies control of inadvertent venous injury. The incidence of gas embolism is rare during laparoscopic liver resection.[36]

SURGICAL TECHNIQUE

Techniques for minimally invasive hepatopancreaticobiliary surgery include pure laparoscopic, hand-assisted laparoscopic, hybrid (laparoscopic mobilization with open parenchymal transection), and robotic-assisted approach.[37–39] The choice of technique is surgeon-specific. Preferences are influenced by a combination of surgeon experience and comfort with each technique and patient factors (tumor size, tumor location, body habitus, prior abdominal surgery), which contribute to the technical challenges of a planned extirpation. Regardless of approach, the key steps of each procedure are essentially the same. The minimally invasive techniques used for both major and minor hepatic resections are described in later discussion.

For all laparoscopic cases, the patient is placed in the supine position with both arms tucked (**Fig. 1**A). For robotic-assisted cases, the patient is supine with arms tucked and legs split (**Fig. 1**B). Pressure points should be padded appropriately, and the patient should be secured to the operative table with safety straps or pads and tape. An orogastric tube and Foley catheter should be placed. The patient's chest and abdomen are prepared anteriorly from the nipples to the symphysis pubis, and laterally to the midaxillary lines.

Minimally Invasive Right Hepatic Lobectomy

The key steps are summarized in **Box 1** and are described in later discussion. For right-sided hepatic resections, the surgeon stands on the patient's left, and the assistant stands on the patient's right.

Creation of pneumoperitoneum and port placement

The authors access the peritoneum using a 5-mm optical separator at the right mid-clavicular (MCL) line on laparoscopic cases or the left MCL line on robotic-assisted cases. They insufflate to 12 mm Hg and place the remaining ports using a 5-mm 30° laparoscope. A 10-mm 30° camera in the right paramedian position is used for visualization throughout the procedure, regardless of approach. For hand-assisted cases, they access the peritoneum through an 8-cm vertical incision in the supraumbilical position. **Fig. 2** depicts the usual port placement for laparoscopic, hand-assisted laparoscopic, and robotic-assisted right hepatectomy. Once the ports are placed, the patient is placed in reverse Trendelenburg and rotated so the right side is up. The abdomen is inspected for evidence of extrahepatic disease.

Dissection of the ligamentous attachments and mobilization of the right hemiliver

Using either cautery or a bipolar sealing device, the round and falciform ligaments are divided and dissection is carried posteriorly to the anterior surface of the hepatic

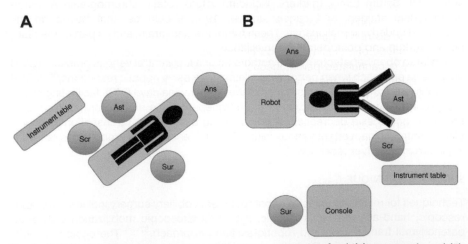

Fig. 1. Standard operating room setup and patient positioning for (*A*) laparoscopic and (*B*) robotic-assisted hepatectomy. Ans, anesthesia; Ast, assistant; Scr, scrub; Sur, surgeon.

Box 1
Key steps of minimally invasive right hepatectomy

1. Creation of pneumoperitoneum
2. Port placement
3. Mobilization of the right hemiliver off of the ligamentous attachments
4. Intraoperative ultrasound
5. Dissection of the retrohepatic cava and ligation of the short hepatic veins
6. Cholecystectomy and portal dissection
7. Outflow dissection and ligation of the right hepatic vein
8. Parenchymal transection
9. Specimen retrieval and inspection of the cut surface

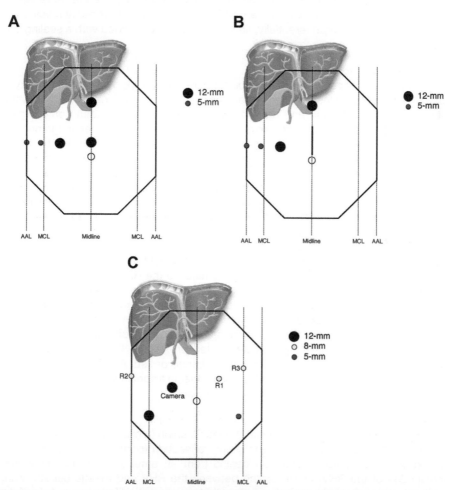

Fig. 2. Typical port placement for minimally invasive right hepatic lobectomy: (A) pure laparoscopic, (B) hand-assisted, and (C) robotic-assisted. AAL, anterior axillary line; MCL, midclavicular line.

veins. Using the gallbladder (if present) as a handle, the liver is reflected anteromedially to facilitate dissection of the right triangular ligament, and inferiorly to expose and dissect the right coronary ligament, thus mobilizing the liver off of its retroperitoneal attachments.

Intraoperative ultrasound
A 10-mm laparoscopic ultrasound probe is placed through the subxiphoid port, and the relevant target anatomy is confirmed. The relationship of the tumor to hepatic inflow and outflow structures is characterized to confirm the planned resection is appropriate. In addition, the future liver remnant is examined to ensure no unexpected lesions are present that would preclude resection or require a change in the operative plan. If robotic assistance is planned, the authors dock the robot following intraoperative ultrasound.

Dissection of the retrohepatic vena cava and ligation of the short hepatic veins
Using long graspers through the 2 right-sided assistant ports, the liver is reflected anteriorly and cephalad to expose the retrohepatic IVC. The short hepatic veins are identified, dissected circumferentially, ligated with clips, or divided with a sealing device up to the right hepatic vein (RHV).

Cholecystectomy and portal dissection
If the gallbladder is present, the authors perform the initial steps of cholecystectomy in standard laparoscopic fashion. Once the critical view of safety is obtained, the cystic duct and artery are ligated and divided. Maintaining cephalad traction on the gallbladder, cautery dissection then proceeds across the hepatoduodenal ligament to expose the right-sided portal structures. The right hepatic artery (RHA) is the most anterolateral structure and is encountered first. The authors proceed to dissect it circumferentially. They perform a test clamp on the RHA and confirm flow to the left hemiliver on intraoperative Doppler and then divide the RHA using an endoscopic stapler with a vascular (2.5 mm) load. The right portal vein lies immediately posterior to the RHA, and it should be dissected from the surrounding tissue and isolated. The authors prefer to pass a silk tie behind the vein in order to retract it superiorly and anterolaterally, which allows them to pass an endoscopic stapler across it with greater ease. The stapler is placed through the subxiphoid port and the right portal vein is divided. The right hepatic duct usually lies superior and anterior to the RHA. With vascular inflow now divided, a line of demarcation should begin to develop between the specimen side and future liver remnant. They then locate the right external portion of the right hepatic duct. The common bile duct identified medial and anterior to the RHA, and it is traced distally to the bifurcation. The right hepatic duct is dissected free from surrounding tissue, ligated distally, and transected proximally. Once bile is seen, the proximal end of the right hepatic duct can be clipped or tied. At this point, they complete the cholecystectomy and place the gallbladder in a specimen retrieval bag. It can be removed now or together with the final specimen.

Outflow dissection and ligation of the right hepatic vein
The RHV can be ligated in either an extrahepatic fashion (formal right hepatectomy) or an intrahepatic manner during parenchymal transection (partial right hepatectomy). For extrahepatic ligation, dissection begins from an anterior approach along the medial edge of the RHV, in the crotch between the RHV and middle hepatic vein. The liver is then reflected anteriorly and the RHV is approached from the undersurface of the liver, completing the window. A flexible grasper is placed through the window; the liver is placed back in normal anatomic position, and a vessel loop is placed into

the flexible graspers, which are pulled through the window from anterior to posterior, encircling the RHV. Using the vessel loop for traction as well as a guide, a vascular stapler is introduced through the window, and the RHV is ligated and divided.

Parenchymal transection

The authors place large stay sutures on the specimen side and future liver remnant side across the line of ischemic demarcation. They define the line of transection using the hook cautery and repeat intraoperative ultrasound to confirm that the target lesion is included within the specimen. They use a sealing device to come through the parenchyma. Larger structures (including the RHV if not taken extrahepatically) are divided between titanium clips (<5 mm) or locking clips (<15 mm), or with a vascular stapler.

Specimen retrieval and evaluation of the cut surface

With parenchymal transection complete, the authors re-establish euvolemia with crystalloid and colloid (5% albumin) resuscitation. The specimen is placed in a plastic retrieval bag and is removed by enlarging the supraumbilical port site incision (pure laparoscopic), by the hand port (hand-assisted cases), or through the right lower quadrant assistant port (robotic-assisted cases). The abdomen is reinsufflated and the cut surface of the liver is inspected for hemostasis and bile leak. The argon beam coagulator should not be used for hemostasis during minimally invasive hepatic resections because of the risk of gas embolism. Saline and contrast cholangiograms can be performed through the cystic duct stump to confirm the absence of biliary leak. They leave a 19-French round, fluted closed suction drain in the resection bed and bring it out through the 5-mm port site at the right MCL. The operative field is irrigated with saline, and the fascia of the 12-mm ports is closed under visualization. The remaining ports are removed, and hemostasis is confirmed. The skin is then closed.

Minimally Invasive Left Hepatic Lobectomy

Room setup and patient positioning are similar to right hepatectomy (see **Fig. 1**). Port placement is depicted in **Fig. 3**. The surgeon stands on the patient's left and the assistant on the right for the initial mobilization and portal dissection. The surgeon moves to the patient's right for parenchymal transection. For robotic-assisted cases, the assistant stands between the patient's legs following laparoscopic mobilization. Key steps are summarized in **Box 2** and are described in later discussion.

Creation of pneumoperitoneum and port placement

The authors access the peritoneum using a 5-mm optical separator in the left upper quadrant, and the abdomen is insufflated to 12 mm Hg. The camera is placed through a 12-mm port in the right paramedian position in line with the porta hepatis. Remaining port placement is depicted in **Fig. 2**. Just as for right hepatic lobectomy, the abdomen is thoroughly inspected for extrahepatic disease. The patient is then placed in the reverse Trendelenburg position with the left side up.

Mobilization of the left hemiliver and intraoperative ultrasound

Using cautery or a bipolar sealing device, the round and falciform ligaments are divided, and dissection proceeds posterior to the anterior surface of the hepatic veins. The round ligament should be left long enough to be used as a handle for traction. Next, the left coronary and triangular ligaments are divided back to the left hepatic vein (LHV). Intraoperative ultrasound is then performed in a similar fashion to right hepatectomy. If robotic assistance is planned, the authors dock the robot at this point.

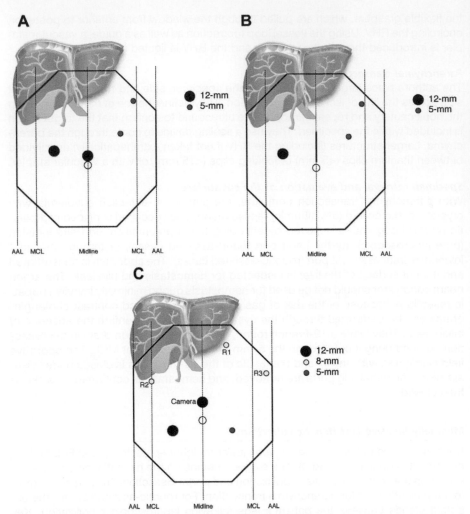

Fig. 3. Typical port placement for minimally invasive left hepatic lobectomy or left lateral sectionectomy: (*A*) pure laparoscopic, (*B*) hand-assisted, and (*C*) robotic-assisted.

Dissection of the gastrohepatic ligament and portal dissection

The liver is reflected anteriorly to expose the undersurface of the left lateral section. The pars flaccida is divided with hook cautery or a sealing device, staying close to the undersurface of the liver and away from the lesser curvature of the stomach. If an accessory left hepatic artery (LHA) is encountered, it should be ligated and divided. If a parenchymal bridge exists between the left lateral and medial sections, it should be divided. Next, a cholecystectomy is performed to aid with exposure of the porta hepatis.

The ligamentum teres should be grasped and retracted anteriorly and cephalad to expose the base of umbilical fissure. The peritoneum at the base of the umbilical fissure is scored with hook cautery, and the LHA should be encountered first, in the most anterior position. The authors dissect it circumferentially, and following a test clamp and confirmation of flow to the right hemiliver, transect the LHA with silk ties

---

Box 2
Key steps of minimally invasive left hepatectomy

1. Creation of pneumoperitoneum
2. Port placement
3. Mobilization of left hemiliver off of the ligamentous attachments
4. Intraoperative ultrasound
5. Dissection of the gastrohepatic ligament
6. Portal dissection and inflow control
7. Outflow dissection and control
8. Parenchymal transection
9. Specimen retrieval and inspection of the cut surface

---

and clips, or with an endoscopic vascular stapler. Next, the left portal vein (LPV) is identified posterior to the LHA and fully defined with blunt and cautery dissection. A vessel loop or silk tie is passed behind the vein to facilitate leftward traction and passage of vascular stapler, staying away from the bifurcation of the main portal vein. The LPV is divided, and a line of ischemic demarcation should begin to form between the right and left hemilivers.

Depending on the oncologic indications of the procedure, attention is then turned to the left hepatic duct, which has a long extrahepatic course and runs superior and anterior to the LPV. Once fully dissected, it is ligated between clips and ties and divided. Alternatively, it can be divided in an intrahepatic manner during parenchymal transection.

Outflow dissection

The LHV can be taken by either an extrahepatic or an intrahepatic approach. If an extrahepatic approach is chosen, the anterior surface of the common trunk of the middle and LHVs is exposed. The lobe is then reflected to the right to expose the Arantius ligament.[40] The ligament is scored with cautery, and dissection is carried anteriorly, exposing the inferior border of the LHV. The space between the LHV and middle hepatic vein is developed, and a vessel loop is passed around the LHV, which is then divided with a vascular stapler.

Parenchymal transection

Using cautery, a line of transection is defined along the line of ischemic demarcation. Intraoperative ultrasound is performed to ensure the target lesion is included within the specimen. As in a right hepatectomy, the authors place stay sutures on either side of the transection line. Parenchyma is divided inferior to superior, and anterior to posterior. They use a combination of cautery, bipolar sealing device, clips, and vascular staplers depending on structure size and surgeon preference. If the LHV was not divided in extrahepatic fashion, it is encountered posteriorly and superiorly and should be divided intrahepatically with a vascular stapler.

Inspection of the cut surface and specimen retrieval

Similar to right hepatectomy, the patient is resuscitated to euvolemia following parenchymal transection. The cut surface is inspected for hemostasis and bile leakage. Saline and contrast cholangiograms via the cystic duct remnant are optional but not routinely performed. The specimen is placed in an endoscopic retrieval bag and is removed through the supraumbilical (pure laparoscopic or hand-assisted approach) or the right lower quadrant (robotic-assisted) port sites. A 19-mm round, fluted closed suction drain is placed adjacent to the resection bed and is brought out through the left upper quadrant port site. The fascia and skin are then closed.

Minimally Invasive Left Lateral Sectionectomy

Port placement and patient positioning are identical to formal left hepatectomy (see **Fig. 3**). Key steps are summarized in **Box 3** and described in later discussion.

Establishment of pneumoperitoneum and port placement
As for left hepatectomy, the peritoneum is accessed through the left upper quadrant using a 5-mm optical separator. The remaining ports are placed under direct visualization following insufflation to 12 mm Hg.

Mobilization of the left lateral section and intraoperative ultrasound
Just as during left hepatectomy, the round, falciform, left coronary, and left triangular ligaments are divided using cautery or a bipolar sealing device. The pars flaccida of the hepatogastric ligament is divided close to the undersurface of the liver, and a replaced accessory LHA should be ligated and divided if encountered. Portal dissection is not routinely performed. Intraoperative ultrasound is performed to ensure the target lesion is within the left lateral section and no unexpected masses are within the future liver remnant.

Parenchymal transection
Staying to the left of the falciform ligament, the line of transection is defined using the hook cautery. A bipolar sealing device is then used to come through the parenchyma in an inferior-to-superior, anterior-to-posterior direction. The portal pedicles to segments II and III are identified and defined using blunt dissection. These crossing pedicles can be ligated with clips and ties, the bipolar sealing device, or an endoscopic vascular stapler. Posteriorly and superiorly, the pedicle of the LHV will be encountered and should be divided with a vascular stapler.

Inspection of the cut surface and specimen retrieval
The surgical field is irrigated and the cut surface is inspected for hemostasis and bile leakage, and bleeding or bile leaks should be controlled with cautery or suture ligation. The patient should be resuscitated to euvolemia. The specimen is placed in a retrieval bag and is removed by enlarging the periumbilical port site. A closed suction drain may be left adjacent to the resection bed as for left hepatectomy. The fascia and skin are closed.

Box 3
Key steps of minimally invasive left lateral sectionectomy

1. Creation of pneumoperitoneum
2. Port placement
3. Mobilization of the left lateral section
4. Intraoperative ultrasound
5. Parenchymal transection
6. Specimen retrieval and inspection of the cut surface

POSTOPERATIVE CARE

The orogastric tube should be removed. The patient may be observed in the intensive care unit or a monitored floor bed depending on the patient's overall health, operative duration, intraoperative complications, and surgeon preference. The authors start subcutaneous heparin prophylaxis on the evening of the day of surgery. A clear liquid diet is routinely started on the first postoperative day and advanced as tolerated. Central venous catheters, if present, are removed between the first and third postoperative day, depending on surgeon preference and patient status. Foley catheters are removed on the first postoperative day if the patient has made adequate urine and there are no significant deviations in the expected postoperative course. They trend complete blood counts, electrolytes, hepatic function panels, and coagulation studies daily for the first 3 postoperative days.

RESULTS

Minimally invasive hepatectomy is being performed with increasing frequency. In the largest review of laparoscopic liver resections to date, Nguyen and colleagues[7] analyzed case series totaling more than 2800 cases. The overall findings suggested that minimally invasive liver resection is both safe and feasible. Nearly 75% of the cases were performed purely laparoscopically; 17% were performed with hand assistance, and 2% were performed in hybrid fashion. The overall conversion rate was 4%. Nearly 50% of resections were for malignancy. As mentioned earlier, most cases (65%) were minor resections, including wedge hepatectomy or left lateral sectionectomy. Formal lobectomy was performed in 15% of cases, and fewer than 1% of the cases were extended lobectomies. The overall morbidity and mortality were acceptable. Perioperative death occurred in 0.3% of the patients. The overall complication rate was 11%, with the most common complications being bile leak (1.5%) and transient hepatic dysfunction (1%).

Several series have compared laparoscopic to open major liver resection.[41–44] Laparoscopic resections appear to be associated with less blood loss, fewer postoperative complications, and shorter hospital length of stay, with the tradeoff being slightly longer operative times. Short- and long-term oncologic outcomes of laparoscopic liver resections are comparable to disease-matched open outcomes.[45,46]

There are 8 series in the literature that statistically compare robotic liver resection to laparoscopic liver resection.[18,34,47–52] Data are summarized in **Table 1**. The largest experience belongs to the group of Tsung and colleagues[18] at the University of Pittsburgh. Each of the 57 patients who underwent robotic hepatectomy were retrospectively matched in a 1:2 ratio to patients that underwent laparoscopic liver resection, with an emphasis on background liver disease, extent of resection, diagnosis, American Society of Anesthesiologists score, age, body mass index, and gender. There was no difference in estimated blood loss (EBL), transfusion requirements, conversion rate, complication rate, or length of stay. Robotic-assisted procedures took significantly longer (253 vs 199 min). There appeared to be a learning curve effect when comparing the initial 13 robotic procedures to the subsequent 44, because there were significant reductions in EBL (300 vs 100 mL), operative times (381 vs 232 min), and length of stay (5 vs 4 days). However, the comparison of robotic-assisted to surgery to conventional laparoscopy may not be worthwhile, because the robotic platform should be looked at as an advanced tool to overcome the inherent limitations of conventional laparoscopy, thus expanding the repertoire of complex minimally invasive procedures that can be applied to the liver, pancreas, and biliary tract.

Table 1
Perioperative outcomes of robotic-assisted hepatectomy versus laparoscopic hepatectomy

	Tsung et al,[18] 2014			Tranchart et al,[49] 2014			Troisi et al,[50] 2013			Wu et al,[51] 2014			Yu et al,[52] 2014			Spampinato et al,[48] 2014			Packiam et al,[34] 2012			Berber et al,[47] 2010		
	LA	RA	P	LA	RA	P	LA	RA	P	LA	RA	P	LA	RA	P	LA	RA	P	LA	RA	P	LA	RA	P
Major resection (n)	42	21	NS	0	0	NS	37	0	<.05	10	20	NR	11	3	NR	25	25	NS	0	0	NR	0	0	NR
Minor resection (n)	72	36		28	28		186	40	NR	59	32	NR	6	10		0	0	NS	18	11	NR	23	9	NS
Operative time (min)	199	253	<.05	176	210	NS	262	271	NS	227	380	<.05	241	292	NS	360	430	NS	188	175	NS	234	259	NS
EBL (mL)	100	200	NS	150	200	NS	174	330	<.05	173	325	<.05	343	389	NS	400	250	NS	30	30	NS	155	136	NS
Transfusion (%)	7	4	NS	4	14	NS		NR			NR		0	0	NS	44	16	<.05	0	0	NS		NR	
Conversion (%)	9	7	NS	7	14	NS	8	20	<.05	12.2	5	NS	0	0	NS	4	4	NS	0	0	NS	0	11	NR
Morbidity (%)	26	20	NS	18	18	NS	13	13	NS	10	8	NS	12	0	NS	36	16	NS	0	27	<.05	17	11	NR
Length of stay (d)	4	4	NS	6	6	NS	6	6	NS	7	8	NS	10	8	NS	7	8	NS	3	4	<.05		NR	

Abbreviations: LA, laparoscopic-assisted; NR, not reported; NS, not significant; RA, robotic-assisted.
Data from Refs.[18,34,47–52]

A learning curve is required for all of the minimally invasive approaches. All 3 techniques have comparable outcomes to the open approach; pure laparoscopy affords the best cosmesis; hand-assisted hepatic resection is associated with the most favorable perioperative outcomes, and the hybrid approach provides better outcomes in difficult cases by offering the benefits of minimally invasive surgery without compromising patient safety.[36]

SUMMARY

The literature demonstrates that in properly selected patients, minimally invasive liver resection is a feasible and safe option, best performed by surgeons trained in open liver surgery who are skilled in minimally invasive techniques. Available data suggest that open, laparoscopic, and robotic approaches have similar perioperative outcomes, but the robotic approach comes at a higher cost. Short- and long-term oncologic outcomes appear to be equivalent. Currently, most minimally invasive hepatectomies are nonanatomic resections, and therefore, there is no clear-cut advantage to the robotic approach over laparoscopy in minor hepatectomy. There are no high-quality, prospective data analyzing minimally invasive hepatectomy. Therefore, it is difficult to draw any definitive conclusions at this time with regards to overall efficacy and benefits in both immediate (length of stay, postoperative pain, morbidity, mortality, and cost-effectiveness) and long-term (quality of life, oncologic recurrence) patient outcomes. Existing data are promising and warrant further investigation.

REFERENCES

1. Clinical Outcomes of Surgical Therapy Study Group. A comparison of laparoscopically assisted and open colectomy for colon cancer. N Engl J Med 2004; 350(20):2050–9.
2. Guillou PJ, Quirke P, Thorpe H, et al. Short-term endpoints of conventional versus laparoscopic-assisted surgery in patients with colorectal cancer (MRC CLASICC trial): multicentre, randomised controlled trial. Lancet 2005;365(9472):1718–26.
3. Ghezzi F, Cromi A, Ditto A, et al. Laparoscopic versus open radical hysterectomy for stage IB2-IIB cervical cancer in the setting of neoadjuvant chemotherapy: a multi-institutional cohort study. Ann Surg Oncol 2013;20(6):2007–15.
4. Trabulsi EJ, Hassen WA, Touijer AK, et al. Laparoscopic radical prostatectomy: a review of techniques and results worldwide. Minerva Urol Nefrol 2003;55(4): 239–50.
5. Luketich JD, Pennathur A, Awais O, et al. Outcomes after minimally invasive esophagectomy: review of over 1000 patients. Ann Surg 2012;256(1):95–103.
6. Martel G, Boushey RP. Laparoscopic colon surgery: past, present and future. Surg Clin North Am 2006;86(4):867–97.
7. Nguyen KT, Gamblin TC, Geller DA. World review of laparoscopic liver resection—2,804 patients. Ann Surg 2009;250(5):831–41.
8. Jayne DG, Guillou PJ, Thorpe H, et al. Randomized trial of laparoscopic-assisted resection of colorectal carcinoma: 3-year results of the UK MRC CLASICC Trial Group. J Clin Oncol 2007;25(21):3061–8.
9. Berguer R, Rab GT, Abu-Ghaida H, et al. A comparison of surgeons' posture during laparoscopic and open surgical procedures. Surg Endosc 1997;11(2): 139–42.
10. Cadiere GB, Himpens J, Germay O, et al. Feasibility of robotic laparoscopic surgery: 146 cases. World J Surg 2001;25(11):1467–77.

11. Wakabayashi G, Cherqui D, Geller DA, et al. Recommendations for laparoscopic liver resection: a report from the second international consensus conference held in Morioka. Ann Surg 2015;261(4):619–29.
12. Croome KP, Farnell MB, Que FG, et al. Pancreaticoduodenectomy with major vascular resection: a comparison of laparoscopic versus open approaches. J Gastrointest Surg 2015;19(1):189–94.
13. Croome KP, Farnell MB, Que FG, et al. Total laparoscopic pancreaticoduodenectomy for pancreatic ductal adenocarcinoma: oncologic advantages over open approaches? Ann Surg 2014;260(4):633–8 [discussion: 638–40].
14. Kendrick ML. Laparoscopic and robotic resection for pancreatic cancer. Cancer J 2012;18(6):571–6.
15. Kendrick ML, Cusati D. Total laparoscopic pancreaticoduodenectomy: feasibility and outcome in an early experience. Arch Surg 2010;145(1):19–23.
16. Kendrick ML, Sclabas GM. Major venous resection during total laparoscopic pancreaticoduodenectomy. HPB (Oxford) 2011;13(7):454–8.
17. Nguyen KT, Marsh JW, Tsung A, et al. Comparative benefits of laparoscopic vs open hepatic resection: a critical appraisal. Arch Surg 2011;146(3):348–56.
18. Tsung A, Geller DA, Sukato DC, et al. Robotic versus laparoscopic hepatectomy: a matched comparison. Ann Surg 2014;259(3):549–55.
19. Zeh HJ 3rd, Bartlett DL, Moser AJ. Robotic-assisted major pancreatic resection. Adv Surg 2011;45:323–40.
20. Zureikat AH, Moser AJ, Boone BA, et al. 250 robotic pancreatic resections: safety and feasibility. Ann Surg 2013;258(4):554–9 [discussion: 559–62].
21. Zureikat AH, Nguyen KT, Bartlett DL, et al. Robotic-assisted major pancreatic resection and reconstruction. Arch Surg 2011;146(3):256–61.
22. Vigano L, Laurent A, Tayar C, et al. The learning curve in laparoscopic liver resection: improved feasibility and reproducibility. Ann Surg 2009;250(5):772–82.
23. Buell JF, Cherqui D, Geller DA, et al. The international position on laparoscopic liver surgery: the Louisville Statement, 2008. Ann Surg 2009;250(5):825–30.
24. Cai XJ, Yang J, Yu H, et al. Clinical study of laparoscopic versus open hepatectomy for malignant liver tumors. Surg Endosc 2008;22(11):2350–6.
25. Mirnezami R, Mirnezami AH, Chandrakumaran K, et al. Short- and long-term outcomes after laparoscopic and open hepatic resection: systematic review and meta-analysis. HPB (Oxford) 2011;13(5):295–308.
26. Amodeo A, Linares Quevedo A, Joseph JV, et al. Robotic laparoscopic surgery: cost and training. Minerva Urol Nefrol 2009;61(2):121–8.
27. Giulianotti PC, Coratti A, Angelini M, et al. Robotics in general surgery: personal experience in a large community hospital. Arch Surg 2003;138(7):777–84.
28. Coelho RF, Rocco B, Patel MB, et al. Retropubic, laparoscopic, and robot-assisted radical prostatectomy: a critical review of outcomes reported by high-volume centers. J Endourol 2010;24(12):2003–15.
29. O'Neill M, Moran PS, Teljeur C, et al. Robot-assisted hysterectomy compared to open and laparoscopic approaches: systematic review and meta-analysis. Arch Gynecol Obstet 2013;287(5):907–18.
30. Tatooles AJ, Pappas PS, Gordon PJ, et al. Minimally invasive mitral valve repair using the da Vinci robotic system. Ann Thorac Surg 2004;77(6):1978–82 [discussion: 1982–4].
31. Bokhari MB, Patel CB, Ramos-Valadez DI, et al. Learning curve for robotic-assisted laparoscopic colorectal surgery. Surg Endosc 2011;25(3):855–60.
32. Buchs NC, Pugin F, Bucher P, et al. Learning curve for robot-assisted Roux-en-Y gastric bypass. Surg Endosc 2012;26(4):1116–21.

33. Daouadi M, Zureikat AH, Zenati MS, et al. Robot-assisted minimally invasive distal pancreatectomy is superior to the laparoscopic technique. Ann Surg 2013;257(1):128–32.
34. Packiam V, Bartlett DL, Tohme S, et al. Minimally invasive liver resection: robotic versus laparoscopic left lateral sectionectomy. J Gastrointest Surg 2012;16(12): 2233–8.
35. Cunningham JD, Fong Y, Shriver C, et al. One hundred consecutive hepatic resections. Blood loss, transfusion, and operative technique. Arch Surg 1994; 129(10):1050–6.
36. Lin NC, Nitta H, Wakabayashi G. Laparoscopic major hepatectomy: a systematic literature review and comparison of 3 techniques. Ann Surg 2013;257(2):205–13.
37. Kitisin K, Packiam V, Bartlott DL, et al. A current update on the evolution of robotic liver surgery. Minerva Chir 2011;66(4):281–93.
38. Koffron AJ, Kung RD, Auffenberg GB, et al. Laparoscopic liver surgery for everyone: the hybrid method. Surgery 2007;142(4):463–8 [discussion: 468.e1–2].
39. Nitta H, Sasaki A, Fujita T, et al. Laparoscopy-assisted major liver resections employing a hanging technique: the original procedure. Ann Surg 2010;251(3):450–3.
40. Di Giuro G, Lainas P, Franco D, et al. Laparoscopic left hepatectomy with prior vascular control. Surg Endosc 2010;24(3):697–9.
41. Martin RC, Scoggins CR, McMasters KM. Laparoscopic hepatic lobectomy: advantages of a minimally invasive approach. J Am Coll Surg 2010;210(5):627–34, 634–6.
42. Cai XJ, Wang YF, Liang YL, et al. Laparoscopic left hemihepatectomy: a safety and feasibility study of 19 cases. Surg Endosc 2009;23(11):2556–62.
43. Dagher I, Di Giuro G, Dubrez J, et al. Laparoscopic versus open right hepatectomy: a comparative study. Am J Surg 2009;198(2):173–7.
44. Abu Hilal M, Di Fabio F, Teng MJ, et al. Single-centre comparative study of laparoscopic versus open right hepatectomy. J Gastrointest Surg 2011;15(5):818–23.
45. Takahara T, Wakabayashi G, Beppu T, et al. Long-term and perioperative outcomes of laparoscopic versus open liver resection for hepatocellular carcinoma with propensity score matching: a multi-institutional Japanese study. J Hepatobiliary Pancreat Sci 2015;22(10):721–7.
46. Beppu T, Wakabayashi G, Hasegawa K, et al. Long-term and perioperative outcomes of laparoscopic versus open liver resection for colorectal liver metastases with propensity score matching: a multi-institutional Japanese study. J Hepatobiliary Pancreat Sci 2015;22(10):711–20.
47. Berber E, Akyildiz HY, Aucejo F, et al. Robotic versus laparoscopic resection of liver tumours. HPB (Oxford) 2010;12(8):583–6.
48. Spampinato MG, Coratti A, Bianco L, et al. Perioperative outcomes of laparoscopic and robot-assisted major hepatectomies: an Italian multi-institutional comparative study. Surg Endosc 2014;28(10):2973–9.
49. Tranchart H, Ceribelli C, Ferretti S, et al. Traditional versus robot-assisted full laparoscopic liver resection: a matched-pair comparative study. World J Surg 2014;38(11):2904–9.
50. Troisi RI, Patriti A, Montalti R, et al. Robot assistance in liver surgery: a real advantage over a fully laparoscopic approach? Results of a comparative bi-institutional analysis. Int J Med Robot 2013;9(2):160–6.
51. Wu YM, Hu RH, Lai HS, et al. Robotic-assisted minimally invasive liver resection. Asian J Surg 2014;37(2):53–7.
52. Yu YD, Kim KH, Jung DH, et al. Robotic versus laparoscopic liver resection: a comparative study from a single center. Langenbecks Arch Surg 2014;399(8): 1039–45.

Hepatic Tumor Ablation

Timothy J. Ziemlewicz, MD[a],*, Shane A. Wells, MD[a],
Meghan G. Lubner, MD[a], Christopher L. Brace, PhD[a,b], Fred T. Lee Jr, MD[a,b],
J. Louis Hinshaw, MD[a]

KEYWORDS

- Liver • Percutaneous • Microwave • Radiofrequency • Hepatocellular carcinoma
- Metastasis

KEY POINTS

- Hepatic tumor ablation allows for local control of tumors that are not amenable to surgical resection, increasing potentially curative treatment options.
- For hepatocellular carcinoma, tumor ablation is the preferred treatment of patients within the Milan criteria who are not surgical candidates and the first-line treatment of tumors less than 2 cm in patients ineligible for transplant.
- Adjunctive techniques should be used to ensure an adequate safety margin, while allowing maximum energy delivery.
- Multiapplicator synergy can be utilized to maximize treatment effectiveness.
- Optimal applicator placement to create margins of at least 5 mm in hepatocellular carcinoma (HCC) and 10 mm in metastatic disease is key to a successful ablation.

 Video content accompanies this article at http://www.surgical.theclinics.com

INTRODUCTION

Tumor ablation is a safe and effective technique for managing both primary and metastatic liver tumors that are not amenable to surgical resection. In the Barcelona Clinic Liver Cancer (BCLC) staging system for HCC, which has been adopted by the American Association for the Study of Liver Diseases (AASLD), tumor ablation is considered curative and the treatment of choice for patients with Stage 0 and Stage A HCC not amenable to resection or transplantation.[1] The newest BCLC staging system has

Disclosures: None (T.J. Ziemlewicz, S.A. Wells, M.G. Lubner); Stockholder, Consultant for Neu-Wave Medical (C.L. Brace); Patent holder, receives royalties from Covidien; Stockholder, Member of the Board of Directors, NeuWave Medical (F.T. Lee Jr); Stockholder, Member of the Board of Medical Advisors, NeuWave Medical (J.L. Hinshaw).
^a Department of Radiology, University of Wisconsin School of Medicine and Public Health, 600 Highland Avenue MC 3252, Madison, WI 53792, USA; ^b Department of Biomedical Engineering, University of Wisconsin, 1415 Engineering Drive, Madison, WI 53706, USA
* Corresponding author.
E-mail address: tziemlewicz@uwhealth.org

been updated to recommend tumor ablation over resection for patients with stage 0 HCC who are not eligible for transplantation.[2] Ablation is also successful in bridging patients to transplantation, decreasing patient drop-off from the wait list.[3,4] In the setting of metastatic disease, ablation is a treatment strategy available in the multidisciplinary management of oligometastatic disease that is not amenable to surgical resection or in conjunction with a resection when all sites of disease can be controlled.[5]

Ablation covers a wide range of treatment modalities that allow focal destruction of tumors utilizing a needle-like device to deliver energy or chemicals to the targeted tissue. Chemical ablation is most frequently performed via the injection of ethanol, although other substances have been used and are currently under research. Energy-based treatment is most frequently used in modern tumor ablation practice; the largest reported experiences have been using thermal modalities (radiofrequency [RF] ablation, microwave [MW] ablation, and cryoablation). Other modalities with early clinical data include noninvasive high-intensity focused ultrasound (HIFU) and irreversible electroporation (IRE) via electrode applicators.

This article reviews the approach to hepatic tumor ablation, including patient selection, procedure planning, procedure technique with associated adjunctive maneuvers, and outcomes.

PREPROCEDURE PLANNING
Patient Selection

Hepatocellular carcinoma
The AASLD and European Association for the Study of the Liver (EASL) have adopted the BCLC staging and treatment algorithm in their guidelines for the treatment of HCC.[1,6] Within this strategy, patients with very early (stage 0, Child-Pugh A liver function, Eastern Cooperative Oncology Group [ECOG] performance status of 0, and a single HCC less than 2 cm) and early (stage A, Child-Pugh A-B liver function, ECOG performance status of 0, and single HCC up to 5 cm or less than 3 tumors that are smaller than 3 cm) are recommended to undergo RFA for curative treatment when a patient is not eligible for surgical resection or transplantation. Studies comparing RFA and resection for stage 0 HCC have been mixed, although overall demonstrating equivalent survival with an improved safety profile for ablation, leading to a recent update to the BCLC treatment algorithm recommending ablation over resection for this stage.[2,7–9] RFA has also been shown successful at bridging patients to transplantation by preventing tumor progression that would place a patient beyond the Milan criteria.[3,4] Because the mechanisms of action for tissue destruction with RF and MW are identical, tissue heating with MW is more efficient, the literature for MW treatment of HCC is rapidly expanding (and compares favorably to RF), and the procedures are virtually identical, the use of MW for treating stage 0 and an HCC is a reasonable alternative to RF.[10,11]

Metastatic disease
Patients with oligometastatic disease who have unresectable tumors, who are not surgical candidates or who have recently undergone resection, or who will have inadequate liver reserve after resection are appropriate candidates for tumor ablation.[5] National Comprehensive Cancer Network guidelines for colorectal and neuroendocrine malignancies include ablation among the treatment options. For colorectal metastasis, all sites of disease should be amenable to either ablation or resection for ablation to be considered. Recent guidelines from an expert panel of interventional oncologists suggest treating 3 tumors or fewer with the largest treated tumor up to 3 cm as the preferred patient population, although up to 5 tumors and tumors up to

5 cm can be considered in the appropriate settings.[5] In cases of neuroendocrine metastasis, ablation can be performed to control all sites of disease or can be performed to decrease the tumor burden in symptomatic patients.[12,13] It is reasonable to treat up to 10 tumors in patients with symptomatic neuroendocrine tumors, provided all but the largest 3 tumors are smaller than 2 cm. Treatment of hepatic metastatic disease from other primaries, such as breast, melanoma, and sarcoma, has been described.[14–16] Any patient with isolated metastatic disease to the liver that is not responding to therapy or is progressing without extrahepatic progression may be appropriate for ablation depending on treatment goals.

Benign disease

Most patients with benign hepatic tumors do not require any intervention; however, there is a subset in which intervention may be indicated due to pain, risk for hemorrhage, or risk of malignant degeneration. Percutaneous tumor ablation is an excellent treatment modality for these entities due to its low complication profile. Hemangiomas causing pain or nausea have been successfully treated with ablation.[17–19] Hepatic adenomas may be indicated for treatment if they do not regress after removal of hormone therapy, are larger than 5 cm, or have atypical pathologic findings.[20,21]

Ablation Modality Selection

Selecting the appropriate modality for the planned ablation can improve the efficacy and safety of the procedure. The authors have previously described their approach to modality selection.[22]

Chemical

Ethanol ablation was one of the earliest techniques of tumor ablation, performed via injection of 95% ethanol directly into a tumor, frequently over multiple sessions.[23] Ethanol induces coagulative necrosis via cellular dehydration and protein denaturation of the target cells as well as thrombosis of blood vessels within the tumor. The use of acetic acid has also been reported. Heterogeneity in chemical distribution limits treatment efficacy, however, so chemical ablation has largely been replaced by thermal ablation as a monotherapy. Ethanol injection currently has a role in treating tumors near critical structures, either alone for HCC less than 2 cm or in combination with a thermal modality (**Fig. 1**).[24]

Radiofrequency

RFA is the application of alternating electrical current to agitate ions and generate heat in tissues adjacent to an electrode. RFA has the largest amount of data of any of the thermal ablation modalities and is specifically referred to in the AASLD and EASL guidelines for the treatment of HCC. It has a role in treating tumors less than 3 cm; however, effectiveness is substantially reduced for tumors larger than 3 cm, where multiple overlapping ablations are often required to obtain an adequate treatment, even with the advent of multitined applicators. RFA may also be susceptible to the heat sink of adjacent blood vessels.[25]

Microwave

MW ablation is the production of heat by electromagnetic waves that propagate from an antenna, rapidly oscillating water molecules in the adjacent tissue. This mechanism of energy delivery is more robust than electrical current, allowing faster and greater heat generation than RFA.

MW ablation has a long history, although adoption of early systems was limited by inconsistent and frequently small ablation zone sizes as well as unacceptable rates of

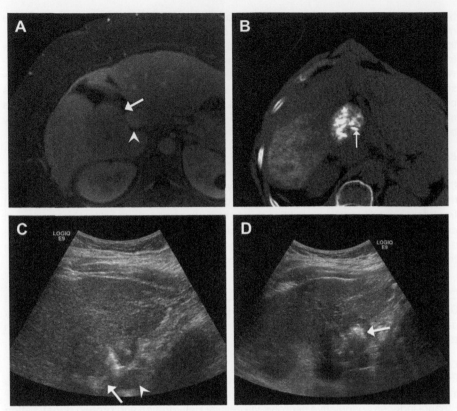

Fig. 1. Ethanol injection performed immediately prior to MW ablation of an HCC. (*A*) HCC adjacent to the common duct (*arrow*) and portal vein (*arrowhead*). (*B*) Ethiodol from previous TACE within tumor; 20-gauge needle (*arrow*) is pointed at the duct/portal vein. (*C*) US image of needle adjacent to duct (*arrow*) and portal vein (*arrowhead*); note echogenic material near needle tip representing gas formation postethanol injection. (*D*) Further gas formation within tumor (*arrow*) after additional ethanol injection.

complications. Modern MW systems allow for the production of larger ablations, both with single-applicator and multiapplicator capable systems.[26] As a result, MW is replacing RF as the leading ablation modality in the liver. In the authors' experience, tumors amenable to RFA are also amenable to MW ablation and it is possible to treat some tumors with MW ablation that would not be treatable with RFA.

Cryoablation

Cryoablation is the cooling of tissues adjacent to a cryoprobe to extremely low temperatures. The mechanism of cell death varies by cooling rate and temperature; rapid formation of intracellular ice causes mechanical disruption of the cell membrane whereas extracellular ice produced during slower freeze/thaw cycles creates osmotic shifts and local hypertonicity. Repeated freezing also interrupts metabolism, causes apoptosis, and produces vascular thrombosis, resulting in coagulative necrosis.

Cryoablation has been used to treat a variety of tumors in the liver and via multiapplicator capability can be utilized to treat large tumors. It has a role in treating metastatic disease, especially for tumors adjacent to the diaphragm or body wall because the ice has an anesthetic effect. This may allow treatment of tumors in patients who are not sedation candidates. The use of cryoablation in large tumors and in patients with cirrhosis should be approached with caution. Large zones of cryoablation have been associated with ice fracture, leading to bleeding complications during the thaw cycle. In addition, large-volume cryoablations in the liver, especially cirrhotic liver, can cause a systemic inflammatory response (cryoshock) that has been associated with postprocedure morbidity and mortality.[27]

Irreversible electroporation

IRE is the use of high-voltage direct current electrical pulses between parallel electrodes to create pores in cell membranes of sufficient size that the cell cannot recover. This mechanism is nonthermal, although thermal damage and resultant coagulative necrosis can occur with IRE.[28] IRE has been used to treat primary and metastatic tumors of the liver, with the primary indication being tumors adjacent to critical structures, such as bile ducts, that might be adversely affected by a thermal modality. There is a paucity of data on the use of IRE to date and little adoption due to the limited indications relative to heat-based ablation modalities.

Technical Considerations

Imaging

Available imaging should be reviewed to evaluate the appropriateness of a tumor for ablation. Adjacent structures within the liver, such as bile ducts and blood vessels, should be evaluated to determine if the proximity to bile ducts require ethanol ablation, combination ethanol ablation/thermal ablation (see **Fig. 1**), or deferring to a nonablative modality, such as transarterial chemoembolization (TACE) or radioembolization, if more than a single margin abuts a critical structure.

Tumors that abut adjacent structures, such as bowel, gallbladder, pancreas, and the body wall, need to be considered for adjunctive techniques for percutaneous procedures. Determination of need for hydrodissection, positioning, or needle leverage maneuvers prior to the procedure allows immediate availability of necessary equipment.

In the authors' practice, all patients who are referred for percutaneous hepatic tumor ablation undergo an US prior to the procedure, often in a separate visit. This US visit allows review of patient history and relevant laboratory data, a directed physical examination, discussion of the procedure details with the patient, a time separate from the immediacy of the procedure to obtain informed consent, and a US examination assessing the following:

- Patient positioning for the procedure
- Visualization of the tumor by US
- Tumor depth to determine length of applicator
- Proximity of the tumor to adjacent structures in the planned position

Anesthesia considerations

Laparoscopic and open ablations require general anesthesia. Percutaneous ablation can be performed under general anesthesia, deep sedation monitored by anesthesia, or conscious sedation monitored by the performing physician. Advantages to general anesthesia with a percutaneous approach include the ability to immobilize the diaphragm in reproducible positions during needle placement and to eliminate the pain response to needle placement and ablation. The accurate placement of needles, which is improved with a motionless liver, is a key component of a successful ablation. The lack of pain response with general anesthesia ensures that the full, planned ablation can be carried out without interruption in energy delivery, another step to ensuring a successful ablation. For these reasons, general anesthesia is the standard of care for percutaneous hepatic ablations performed in the authors' practice.

Conscious sedation or deep sedation monitored by anesthesia has the advantages of decreased procedure time and anesthesia risks compared with general anesthesia. This approach is best reserved for patients with straightforward applicator placement; for tumors removed from the periphery of the liver where patient pain may limit the full, planned ablation; and for patients who have contraindications for general anesthesia.

PREPARATION AND PATIENT POSITIONING

For laparoscopic and open surgical tumor ablation, supine positioning is frequently used. Percutaneous tumor ablation is best performed in a position that allows best visualization of the targeted tumor and avoidance of adjacent structures.

For US-guided procedures, left lateral decubitus positioning frequently leads to improved visualization of tumors in the right hepatic lobe, especially those at the dome. A subcostal approach is often possible.

When utilizing US guidance for percutaneous procedures, the patient is positioned and US performed to confirm planned approach prior to sterile field preparation. Performing US-guided percutaneous procedures in a CT suite allows confirmation of needle placement, evaluation of adjacent structures prior to ablation, CT guidance if necessary, and immediate assessment of the ablation zone with contrast-enhanced CT.[29]

PROCEDURAL APPROACH
Adjunctive Maneuvers (if Necessary)

Combination with intra-arterial therapies
The decreased local control of tumors greater than 3 cm with RFA led to the evaluation of multiple synergistic combination therapies. The most widely reported is combining TACE with ablation for HCC. This combined approach can improve local tumor control.[30] There is no consensus as to which procedure should be performed first. There are advantages to each approach, with decreased perfusion to the tumor potentially accentuating the ablation after TACE while the hyperemia induced by ablation can increase local delivery of chemotherapy and embolic material to the treatment site. The authors' practice is to perform TACE approximately 2 weeks prior to ablation procedures to allow tumor response to the embolic and chemotherapy, while taking advantage of the decreased perfusion.[31]

An additional use of intra-arterial therapies is to improve targeting of tumors by CT when they are not visualized on US (**Fig. 2**).

Hydrodissection
Hydrodissection can be performed to displace adjacent structures, such as bowel, pancreas, or gallbladder. This technique can also be used to create artificial ascites to either protect the diaphragm or body wall from burn, thus decreasing postprocedural pain, or to improve visualization of the tumor (**Fig. 3**).[32,33] When utilizing this technique during RFA, 5% dextrose in water should be used because normal saline is an electrical conductor and can propagate the ablation.

Hydrodissection fluid can be difficult to visualize relative to soft tissue density structures, such as bowel on CT. Adding a 2% contrast solution (20 mL of iodinated contrast in a 1-L bag) to the fluid has been shown to improve visualization.[34]

- Connect tubing between bag of sterile fluid and the dissection needle with an intervening 3-way stopcock attached to a 60-mL syringe. Remove any air from the line (if US-guided needle placement is planned).

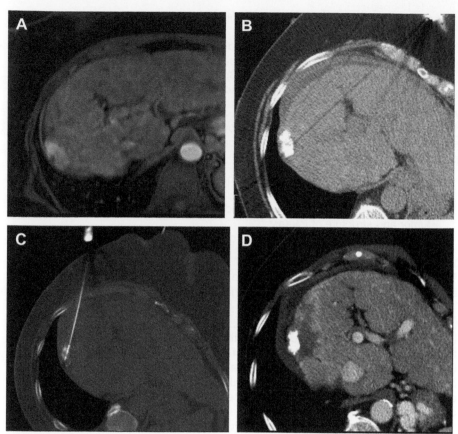

Fig. 2. (*A*) HCC at the lateral hepatic dome, which could not be visualized with US. (*B*) HCC post-TACE is easily visualized on CT for needle guidance. (*C*) MW antenna in place within tumor. (*D*) Immediate post-treatment CT showing nonenhancing ablation zone covering the tumor and an appropriate margin.

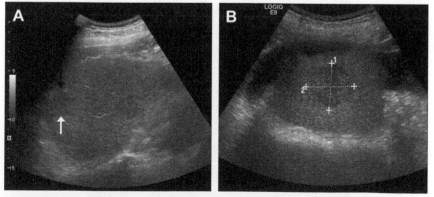

Fig. 3. (*A*) Renal cell carcinoma metastasis at the hepatic dome is incompletely visualized (*arrow*). (*B*) After instillation of 500-mL artificial ascites to protect the diaphragm and improve visualization, the tumor (calipers) is well delineated for US-guided needle placement.

- Place needle into peritoneal cavity for artificial ascites or bowel displacement (**Fig. 4**).
- Place needle into retroperitoneum to displace retroperitoneal structures (**Fig. 5**).
- Place needle through liver into subcapsular space for displacement of gallbladder, pancreas, or stomach (**Fig. 6**).
- Inject fluid with US or CT monitoring to ensure appropriate positioning.

Needle displacement

The needle displacement technique can be performed to displace bowel loops or stomach away from exophytic tumors, typically along the inferior margin of the left hepatic lobe or medial right hepatic lobe.

- Utilize a needle with blunt-tipped cannula and sharp stylet to gain access to the peritoneal cavity.
- Replace needle stylet with blunt-tipped stylet and advance cannula between the tumor and structure of interest.
- Leverage needle to torque structure of interest away from tumor (**Fig. 7**).

Wedge technique

The wedge technique can be performed to treat tumors at the periphery where adequate needle placement to attain margin can be difficult (**Fig. 8**).

Ablation Procedure

Laparoscopic and open procedures will utilize US guidance for needle placement for tumors within the liver, whereas those at the liver surface can be approached by undermining the tumor with the needle via palpation. Percutaneous procedures can be guided with US, CT, MRI, or PET/CT. US and CT are the most common methods of guidance due to availability, resource cost, and ease of access for needle placement.

In the United States, CT (often with CT fluoroscopy) is the most common method of guidance. In the authors' practice, however, they prefer to utilize US for guidance whenever the tumor or appropriate landmarks can be visualized. There are several reasons for this preference, the primary one being the ability to directly visualize the needle during placement into the tumor in real time. This real-time feedback during

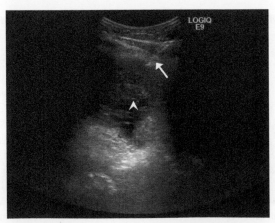

Fig. 4. Needle (*arrow*) in place within peritoneum. Echoes within fluid (*arrowhead*) are created and can be seen moving during injection into the peritoneal space.

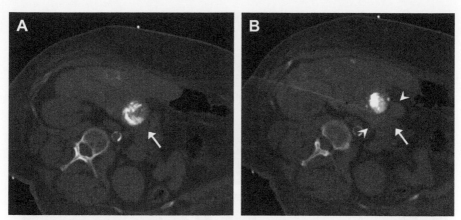

Fig. 5. (*A*) Tumor previously treated with TACE immediately adjacent to the descending duodenum (*arrow*). (*B*) 18-Gauge needle with tip posterior to tumor. Injected contrast contains a 2% contrast solution (20 mL in a 1000-mL bag of 5% dextrose in water) to clearly delineate hydrodissection fluid (*arrowheads*) from adjacent structures, such as bowel (*arrow*).

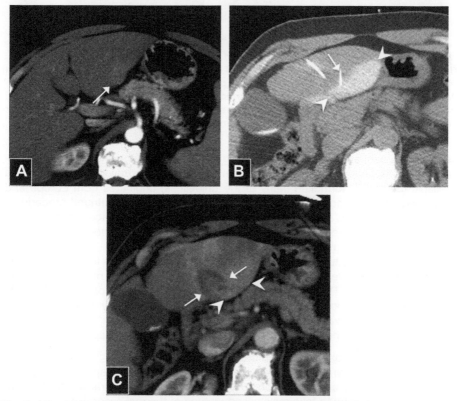

Fig. 6. (*A*) HCC (*arrow*) along the posterior margin of segment III adjacent to pancreas and stomach. (*B*) 20-Gauge needle (*arrow*) placed through liver and hydrodissection with 2% contrast solution (*arrowheads*) performed to displace the pancreas and stomach. (*C*) Ablation zone (*arrows*) encompassing site of tumor with hydrodissection fluid (*arrowheads*) displacing pancreas.

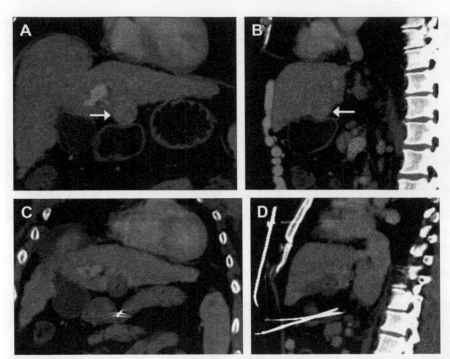

Fig. 7. HCC (*arrows*) exophytic from segment III with mass effect on the stomach on coronal (*A*) and sagittal (*B*) views. Trocar needles were placed between the tumor and stomach under US guidance and blunt tips placed prior to leverage of needle to pull stomach away from the tumor. Coronal (*C*) and sagittal (*D*) images of postablation CT demonstrates trocar needles displacing the stomach and an ablation zone encompassing the HCC.

needle placement allows optimal positioning of the needle within the tumor, which increases the likelihood of adequate ablation. In addition, the majority of patient data available (utilized to formulate many of the guidelines) originates from Europe and Asia where US guidance is overwhelmingly favored.[1,35,36] The authors' procedures are performed in the CT suite to allow for evaluation of needle placement relative to critical structures if needed, and the authors also perform an immediate postprocedure CT scan with intravenous contrast, if patient factors allow.

An important factor to consider when performing the ablation is to ensure that the tumor and an adequate minimal margin of 5 mm for HCC and 10 mm for metastatic foci can be obtained. This may require multiple needle insertions or an ablation with a system capable of powering multiple applicators simultaneously. Multiple antenna ablations offer the advantage of electrical and thermal synergies, which can avoid clefting inherent with multiple needle insertions at the site of overlap.[26]

- Localize the tumor with US and prepare sterile field.
- Place applicator(s) into tumor with US plane parallel to needle approach (Video 1).
- When using multiple applicators, they should be placed parallel with 1 cm to 1.5 cm of spacing to take maximal advantage of thermal synergies.
- Number of applicators used and placement should account for an ablation with at least 5-mm margin for HCC (2-cm tumor requires at least a 3-cm spherical ablation) and a 10-mm margin for metastatic foci (2-cm tumor requires at least a 4-cm spherical ablation).

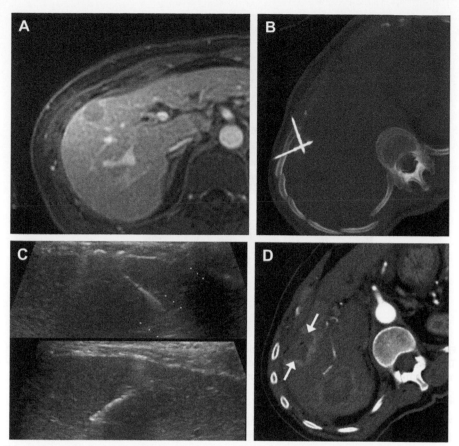

Fig. 8. Wedge technique. (*A*) Peripheral HCC. (*B*) Maximum intensity projection axial image showing wedge placement of needles. (*C*) US images at slightly different levels with needles entering the liver in a wedge fashion. (*D*) Ablation zone (*arrows*) covering the peripheral tumor and a margin.

- If there are dominant vessels near the tumor planned for treatment, applicator placement should be planned so that there is an applicator along the vessel margin to overcome the associated heat sink effects.
- Perform CT (if needed) to evaluate needle positioning and evaluate adjacent structures (**Fig. 9**).
- Perform ablation with real-time US monitoring (Video 2).
  - Monitoring can evaluate if adequate margins are being obtained and evaluate the edge of the ablation zone relative to critical structures (**Figs. 10** and **11**).
  - Utilize full power whenever critical structure is not at risk.
  - When critical structure is at risk, utilize full power at beginning of ablation, then either terminate energy delivery or decrease power as dictated by real-time monitoring.
- Remove applicator(s) with active cautery.
- Perform immediate postprocedure contrast-enhanced CT if patient factors allow.
- Evaluate CT for untreated tumor and inadequate margins. This allows additional treatment in the same session if needed (**Fig. 12**).

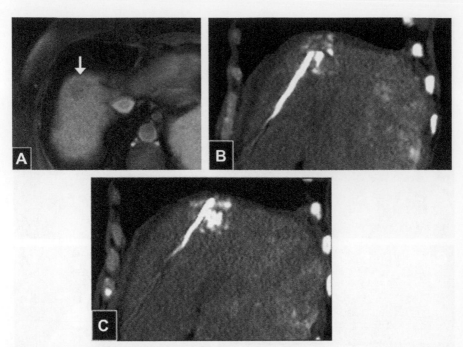

Fig. 9. (*A*) Irregular HCC at the hepatic dome (*arrow*) that was treated with combination TACE and MW ablation. (*B*) Antenna placed under US is short of the dome on needle placement confirmation CT. (*C*) This needle was advanced to the dome prior to ablation.

IMMEDIATE POSTPROCEDURAL CARE

Patients are recovered in a postanesthesia care unit for 1 to 2 hours after the procedure and, in the authors' practice, admitted for overnight observation. Although percutaneous and laparoscopic ablation can be performed on an outpatient basis, admission is the authors' preference to ensure adequate pain control and monitor for complications because many of the patients live in rural areas. When the ablation zone is in close proximity to the diaphragm or body wall, ketorolac at a dose of 15 mg to 30 mg is effective at decreasing pain related to body wall burns for those whose renal function allows administration of this medication. The authors do not routinely perform postprocedure laboratory tests but rather allow patient symptoms to drive any further testing. Patients are discharged the following day with instructions for over-the-counter pain medication use to control pain, with the occasional patient requiring a prescription for a narcotic pain medication. Rarely, in the authors' experience, are narcotic pain medications required for pain control at time of discharge.

REHABILITATION AND RECOVERY

Percutaneous ablation is generally well tolerated and patients can return to normal activity, excluding strenuous exercise, within a few days. Restrictions on activity are rarely necessary beyond 1 week postprocedure.

Imaging Follow-up

Cross-sectional imaging with CT or MRI is the preferred method for follow-up to evaluate both for local tumor progression at the ablation site and new tumors. PET/CT may have a role in metastatic disease, especially when tumor markers rise without an

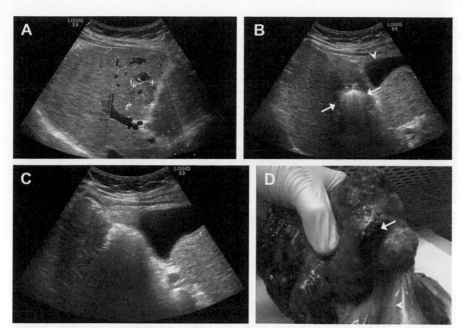

Fig. 10. (*A*) HCC (calipers) abutting cleft extending superiorly from gallbladder. (*B*) Thirty seconds into MW ablation, the gas cloud (*arrows*) has encompassed the tumor and is approaching the gallbladder (*arrowhead*). (*C*) US at completion of ablation with gas cloud abutting the gallbladder, although not involving the gallbladder wall. (*D*) The procedure was performed while the patient was on the transplant waiting list and on postprocedure day 2 the patient underwent transplant. The explant demonstrates burn extending to the hepatic surface (*arrow*) whereas the opposed gallbladder surface (*arrowhead*) is intact.

imaging correlate. Initial follow-up should occur at 1 month to ensure adequate ablation and provide a new baseline examination. After this, imaging should be obtained at 3-month intervals from the time of ablation for the first year, because this is when the risk for local tumor progression and new disease is greatest.

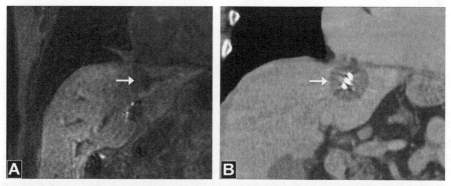

Fig. 11. (*A*) Metastatic colorectal cancer (*arrow*) in the superior left lobe adjacent to the diaphragm. The tumor was treated with cryoablation and the ice ball monitored with CT. (*B*) Ice ball (*arrow*) encompassing the tumor and abutting the diaphragm. The ice ball allows monitoring of the ablation zone, with structures beyond the edge of the ice ball not reaching lethal temperatures.

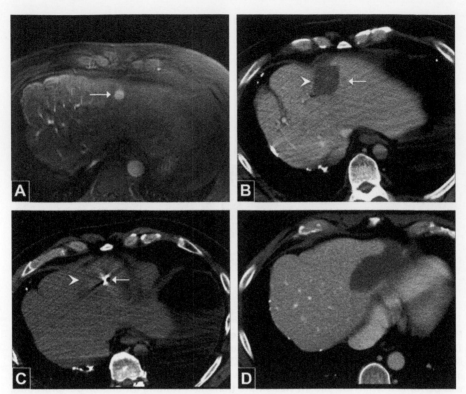

Fig. 12. (*A*) Neuroendocrine tumor (*arrow*) in the remnant left hepatic lobe. (*B*) Hypodense focus (*arrow*) adjacent to the ablation zone (*arrowhead*) concerning for residual tumor postablation. Because the procedure is performed in the CT suite, a repeat ablation was performed in the same session. (*C*) Antenna (*arrow*) in place at the site concerning for residual tumor adjacent to the ablation zone (*arrowhead*). (*D*) One-month follow-up image demonstrating adequate coverage of the tumor.

CLINICAL RESULTS IN THE LITERATURE

The results for tumor ablation can vary significantly based on percutaneous versus surgical approach, guidance method for percutaneous procedures, and tumor type and size, among other factors.

Hepatocellular Carcinoma

The richest data for tumor ablation are available for HCC. The largest experience is with RF ablation (RFA) where 10-year follow-up data are available in some series. RFA has proved superior to percutaneous ethanol injection, particularly for tumors greater than 2 cm.[37] Comparative studies have demonstrated equivalent local tumor control and survival between RF and surgical resection, with lower complication rates for RF.[7,9] The data overall show excellent local control for tumors less than 2 cm in diameter with decreased local tumor control for larger tumor sizes.[35] MW ablation also provides excellent local control for tumors less than 2 cm utilizing modern devices, with improved control of larger tumors up to 5 cm compared with historical RF data.[10,38] Modern internally cooled MW devices lack the long-term follow-up data of RF; however, 5-year follow-up data are available.

Cryoablation has demonstrated success in local tumor control in HCC, although the complication rates are higher in cirrhotic patients, making a heat-based modality best suited for these patients.[27,39] The largest recent series for RF of HCC are listed in **Table 1**. Series reporting modern MW systems that utilize antenna cooling and multi-antenna capability for treatment of HCC are listed in **Table 2**.

Metastatic Colorectal Cancer

The evidence base for treating colorectal liver metastases (CRLMs) with ablation is growing, with 10-year survival data available for RF. No randomized controlled trials exist comparing surgical resection with ablation and the trials available comparing the approaches often do not have matched patient populations. The retrospective comparative studies demonstrate mixed results but often with resection showing greater survival than ablation.[40–43] All of these studies have significant associated biases, however, so drawing conclusions is difficult. Studies evaluating ablation as a first-line treatment of CRLMs show similar survival outcomes to historical controls of resection, particularly for tumors less than 3 cm.[44,45] The largest series of RF for CRLMs are summarized in **Table 3**. Series reporting results with modern MW systems for the treatment of CRLMs are summarized in **Table 4**.

Other Tumors

Almost any primary tumor with isolated metastatic disease in the liver is amenable to tumor ablation. Whether a particular tumor should be treated with ablation, however, should be considered on a case-by-case basis, ideally in a multidisciplinary tumor board. Treatment of neuroendocrine tumors with ablation has shown an ability to prolong overall survival, with 5-year survival rates of 48% to 80% reported, and provides symptom relief in up to 90% of patients for a median of 11 months.[12,13,46] Breast cancer metastatic to the liver treated with ablation has conferred 5-year survival of 30% to 39%.[14,47]

POTENTIAL COMPLICATIONS/MANAGEMENT
Hemorrhage

Clinically significant hemorrhage requiring a transfusion or embolic procedure is rare with RF or MW. Tract cauterization decreases the risk for hemorrhage and ablation can be used to treat active hemorrhage if noted during the procedure (**Fig. 13**). Cryoablation, particularly with large ablations, is at risk for crack in the ice ball, which can lead to catastrophic hemorrhage.

Abscess

Infectious complications are rare due to sterile technique and the administration of intravenous antibiotics at the outset of the procedure. Patients who do have an increased risk of infection are those with a biliary enteric anastomosis or altered bile ducts, although this risk can be significantly reduced by administering antibiotics for 10 days after the ablation procedure.[48]

Postablation Syndrome

Postablation syndrome occurs more frequently with cryoablation, although it can occur with heat-based ablation, particularly when a branch vessel is occluded and there is resultant segmental hepatic infarction. Postablation syndrome presents with malaise and low-grade fevers, often 5 to 7 days postablation, and is best managed with hydration and nonsteroidal anti-inflammatory drugs.

Table 1
Outcomes for radiofrequency ablation of hepatocellular carcinoma

Author, Year	Number of Patients	Patient Population	Approach	Number of Tumors	Average Tumor Diameter	Technique Success/ Complete Ablation	Local Tumor Progression, %			Overall Survival, %					Major Complication Rate, as Defined by Authors	Notes
							1 Year	3 Year	5 Year	1 Year	3 Year	5 Year	7 Year	10 Year		
Lee et al,[50] 2014	162	Child-Pugh A and B Milan criteria	Perc US	182	2.6 cm	96.3	5.9	14.5	14.5	94.4	84.1	67.9	—	—	3.1%	—
Kim et al,[36] 2013	1305	Child-Pugh A and B Milan criteria	Perc US	1502	2.2 cm	94.8	9.7	21.4	27.0	95.5	77.9	54.7	43.2	32.3	2.0%	—
Shiina et al,[51] 2012	1170	Child-Pugh A and B Milan criteria and those deemed curable	Perc US	2982	2.5 cm	99.4	1.4	3.2	3.2	96.6	80.5	60.2	45.1	27.3	1.5%	• Includes combination with TACE for most tumors exceeding 3 cm • Repeat treatments until complete ablation reached
N'Kontchou et al,[52] 2009	235	Child-Pugh A and B Milan criteria	Perc US	307	2.9 cm	94.7	11.5% Overall LTP			—	60	40	—	—	0.9%	Up to 3 RFA sessions to determine success
Livraghi et al,[35] 2008	218	Child-Pugh A All tumors ≤2.0 cm	Perc US	218	—	98.1	0	0.5	0.5	—	76	55	—	—	1.8%	—

Abbreviations: LTP, local tumor progression; Perc, percutaneous.
Data from Refs.[35,36,50–52]

Table 2
Outcomes for microwaves of hepatocellular carcinoma utilizing modern systems

Author, Year	Number of Patients	Patient Population	Approach	Number of Tumors	Average Tumor Diameter	Technique Success/ Complete Ablation	Local Tumor Progression, %	Overall Survival, %			Major Complication Rate, as Defined by Authors	Notes
								1 Year	3 Year	5 Year		
Ziemlewicz et al,[38] 2015	75	Cirrhosis Average MELD 10	Perc US and CT	107	2.5 cm	100	8.2	76% Survival at median 15-mo follow-up			0%	Includes combination with TACE for 22 tumors
Groeschl et al,[53] 2014	139	Not defined	Open 22 Lap 98 Perc CT 19	169	2.6 cm	94.1	12	—	38	19	Not stratified	—
Swan, et al,[54] 2013	54	Child-Pugh A, B, and C	Open Lap	73	2.6 cm	94.4	2.9	72.8	58.8 (2 y)	—	11.5%	Includes combination with TACE in 33%
Liang et al,[10] 2012	1007	Child-Pugh A, B, and C Single tumor <8 cm or ≤3 tumors ≤4 cm	Perc US	1363	2.9 cm	97.1	5.9	91.2	72.8	59.8	2.2%	—

Abbreviations: Lap, laparoscopic; MELD, Model for End-Stage Liver Disease; Perc, percutaneous.
Data from Refs.[10,38,53,54]

Table 3
Outcomes for radiofrequency of colorectal metastasis

Author, Year	Number of Patients	Patient Population	Approach	Number of Tumors	Average Tumor Diameter	Technique Success/ Complete Ablation	Local Tumor Progression, %	Overall Survival, %					Major Complication Rate, as Defined by Authors	Notes
								1 Year	3 Year	5 Year	7 Year	10 Year		
Shady et al,[55] 2015	162	Recurrence after hepatectomy Unresectable disease	Perc CT	233	1.8 cm	94.0	48	90	48	31	—	—	7.0%	LTP decreased to 28% after advent of immediate postablation contrast-enhanced CT.
Agcaoglu et al,[56] 2013	295	Unresectable disease Extrahepatic disease	Lap	885	3.4 cm	—	31	—	—	17	—	—	4%	Comparative trial with resection Improved survival with resection, although ablation patients more comorbid
Solbiati et al,[57] 2012	99	Tumors <4 cm Unresectable	Perc US	202	2.2 cm	88.1	11.9	98.0	69.3	47.8	25.0	18.0	1.3%	—

Study	N	Disease	Approach	Size								Complications	Comments
Van Tilborg et al,[58] 2011	100	Unresectable and resectable disease	Operative 237, US Perc CT	2.4 cm	100	12.7	93	77	36	24 (8 y)	—	6.3%	—
Hammill et al,[44] 2011	64 37	Resectable disease Unresectable disease	Lap 102 130	3.0 cm 4.0 cm	—	8.6% 2.3%	91.7 81.1	59.0 39.8	48.7 18.4	—	—	2.0%	—
Reuter et al,[59] 2009	66	Unresectable disease	Open —	3.2 cm	—	17	—	—	21	—	—	10%	Comparative trial with resection Improved disease control with resection, although survival equivalent
Sorensen et al,[60] 2007	102	Unresectable disease ≤4 Tumors, ≤4 cm	Open 25 Perc US 147 Perc CT 6	2.2 cm	—	—	96	64	44	—	—	6.9%	—

Abbreviations: Lap, laparoscopic; LTP, local tumor progression; Perc, percutaneous.
Data from Refs.[44,55–60]

Table 4
Outcomes for microwaves of colorectal metastasis utilizing modern systems

Author, Year	Number of Patients	Patient Population	Approach	Number of Tumors	Average Tumor Diameter	Technique Success/ Complete Ablation	Local Tumor Progression, %	Overall Survival, %			Major Complication Rate, as Defined by Authors	Notes
								1 Year	3 Year	5 Year		
Eng et al,[61] 2015	33	Unresectable	Open	49	0.5–5.5 cm	—	20.4	80	59	35.2 (4 y)	24.2%	23 Patients had concurrent hepatectomy
Groeschl et al,[53] 2014	198	Unresectable	Open 135 Lap 46 Perc CT 17	403	2.0 cm	98.3	5.2	—	45	17	Not stratified	—
Correa-Gallego et al,[62] 2014	73	Not defined	Open	129	1 cm (median)	—	6	Median overall survival of 55 mo			27%	Comparison with RF Decreased local tumor progression with MW when compared with RF (20%)
Wang et al,[63] 2014	115	<5-cm single tumor <3 cm for 2–3 tumors	Perc US	165	3.1 cm	—	11.3	98.1	78.7	—	4.3%	—

Abbreviations: Lap, laparoscopic; Perc, percutaneous.
Data from Refs.[53,61–63]

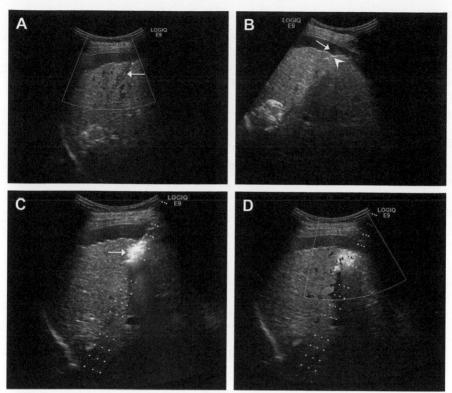

Fig. 13. (A) After needle removal, color Doppler flow is noted along the needle tract (*arrow*) to the liver surface. (B) Echoes (*arrow*) were noted flowing into perihepatic fluid from the hepatic surface at site of needle insertion (*arrowhead*). (C) MW antenna was inserted to the site of bleeding and ablation performed for 1 minute at full power with resultant gas cloud (*arrow*). (D) Final US image with no color Doppler tract or active bleeding noted into perihepatic fluid.

Tumor Seeding

The risk of tumor seeding is low when utilizing needle tract ablation and avoiding direct puncture of peripheral liver tumors by passing through normal liver tissue prior to puncturing the tumor.

Pneumothorax

Treating tumors near the hepatic dome and utilizing an intercostal approach for needle placement both increase the risk of pneumothorax. This risk should not preclude treatment because most pneumothoraces are easily managed. Initially the pneumothorax can be aspirated by placement of a 5-French catheter and aspiration, allowing completion of the procedure. If the pneumothorax persists, a pleural blood patch can be performed by injecting 15 mL to 30 mL of the patients' blood into the pleural space, which has been shown to decrease the risk for chest tube placement during lung biopsies.[49] Chest tubes are generally reserved for symptomatic patients or for those patients in whom aspiration and blood patching are unsuccessful.

SUMMARY

Tumor ablation is a safe and effective treatment option for many cases of early HCC and a subset of hepatic metastases. To achieve optimal outcomes, an understanding of the underlying technology and effect of the various modalities on tissues is necessary. Performing ablation with US guidance is recommended to achieve outcomes that mirror those of the largest series. Physicians performing tumor ablation should be familiar with adjunctive maneuvers that can increase both the efficacy and safety of ablation.

SUPPLEMENTARY DATA

Supplementary data related to this article can be found at http://dx.doi.org/10.1016/j.suc.2015.12.006.

REFERENCES

1. Bruix J, Sherman M, American Association for the Study of Liver Diseases. Management of hepatocellular carcinoma: an update. Hepatology 2011;53(3): 1020–2. Baltimore, MD.
2. Forner A, Llovet JM, Bruix J. Hepatocellular carcinoma. Lancet 2012;379(9822): 1245–55.
3. Lu DS, Yu NC, Raman SS, et al. Percutaneous radiofrequency ablation of hepatocellular carcinoma as a bridge to liver transplantation. Hepatology 2005;41(5): 1130–7.
4. DuBay DA, Sandroussi C, Kachura JR, et al. Radiofrequency ablation of hepatocellular carcinoma as a bridge to liver transplantation. HPB (Oxford) 2011;13(1): 24–32.
5. Gillams A, Goldberg N, Ahmed M, et al. Thermal ablation of colorectal liver metastases: a position paper by an international panel of ablation experts, the interventional oncology sans frontieres meeting 2013. Eur Radiol 2015;25(12): 3438–54.
6. European Association for the Study of the Liver, European Organisation for Research and Treatment of Cancer. EASL–EORTC clinical practice guidelines: management of hepatocellular carcinoma. J Hepatol 2012;56(4):908–43.
7. Chen MS, Li JQ, Zheng Y, et al. A prospective randomized trial comparing percutaneous local ablative therapy and partial hepatectomy for small hepatocellular carcinoma. Ann Surg 2006;243(3):321–8.
8. Huang J, Yan L, Cheng Z, et al. A randomized trial comparing radiofrequency ablation and surgical resection for HCC conforming to the Milan criteria. Ann Surg 2010;252(6):903–12.
9. Feng K, Yan J, Li X, et al. A randomized controlled trial of radiofrequency ablation and surgical resection in the treatment of small hepatocellular carcinoma. J Hepatol 2012;57(4):794–802.
10. Liang P, Yu J, Yu XL, et al. Percutaneous cooled-tip microwave ablation under ultrasound guidance for primary liver cancer: a multicentre analysis of 1363 treatment-naive lesions in 1007 patients in China. Gut 2012;61(7):1100–1.
11. Lubner MG, Brace CL, Hinshaw JL, et al. Microwave tumor ablation: mechanism of action, clinical results, and devices. J Vasc Interv Radiol 2010;21(8 Suppl): S192–203.
12. Mazzaglia PJ, Berber E, Milas M, et al. Laparoscopic radiofrequency ablation of neuroendocrine liver metastases: a 10-year experience evaluating predictors of survival. Surgery 2007;142(1):10–9.

13. Gillams A, Cassoni A, Conway G, et al. Radiofrequency ablation of neuroendo-crine liver metastases: the Middlesex experience. Abdom Imaging 2005;30(4): 435–41.
14. Jakobs TF, Hoffmann RT, Schrader A, et al. CT-guided radiofrequency ablation in patients with hepatic metastases from breast cancer. Cardiovasc Intervent Radiol 2009;32(1):38–46.
15. Doussot A, Nardin C, Takaki H, et al. Liver resection and ablation for metastatic melanoma: a single center experience. J Surg Oncol 2015;111(8):962–8.
16. Pawlik TM, Vauthey JN, Abdalla EK, et al. Results of a single-center experience with resection and ablation for sarcoma metastatic to the liver. Arch Surg 2006; 141(6):537–43 [discussion: 543–4].
17. Gao J, Ke S, Ding XM, et al. Radiofrequency ablation for large hepatic hemangi-omas: initial experience and lessons. Surgery 2013;153(1):78–85.
18. Park SY, Tak WY, Jung MK, et al. Symptomatic-enlarging hepatic hemangiomas are effectively treated by percutaneous ultrasonography-guided radiofrequency ablation. J Hepatol 2011;54(3):559–65.
19. Ziemlewicz TJ, Wells SA, Lubner MA, et al. Microwave ablation of giant hepatic cavernous hemangiomas. Cardiovasc Intervent Radiol 2014;37(5):1299–305.
20. Rhim H, Lim HK, Kim YS, et al. Percutaneous radiofrequency ablation of hepato-cellular adenoma: initial experience in 10 patients. J Gastroenterol Hepatol 2008; 23(8 Pt 2):e422–7.
21. van Vledder MG, van Aalten SM, Terkivatan T, et al. Safety and efficacy of radiofre-quency ablation for hepatocellular adenoma. J Vasc Interv Radiol 2011;22(6):787–93.
22. Hinshaw JL, Lubner MG, Ziemlewicz TJ, et al. Percutaneous tumor ablation tools: microwave, radiofrequency, or cryoablation–what should you use and why? Ra-diographics 2014;34(5):1344–62.
23. Lencioni RA, Allgaier HP, Cioni D, et al. Small hepatocellular carcinoma in cirrhosis: randomized comparison of radio-frequency thermal ablation versus percutaneous ethanol injection. Radiology 2003;228(1):235–40.
24. Huang H, Liang P, Yu XL, et al. Safety assessment and therapeutic efficacy of percutaneous microwave ablation therapy combined with percutaneous ethanol injection for hepatocellular carcinoma adjacent to the gallbladder. Int J Hyper-thermia 2015;31(1):40–7.
25. Lu DS, Raman SS, Limanond P, et al. Influence of large peritumoral vessels on outcome of radiofrequency ablation of liver tumors. J Vasc Interv Radiol 2003; 14(10):1267–74.
26. Harari CM, Magagna M, Bedoya M, et al. Microwave ablation: comparison of simultaneous and sequential activation of multiple antennas in liver model sys-tems. Radiology 2016;278(1):95–103.
27. Seifert JK, Morris DL. World survey on the complications of hepatic and prostate cryotherapy. World J Surg 1999;23(2):109–13 [discussion: 113–4].
28. Faroja M, Ahmed M, Appelbaum L, et al. Irreversible electroporation ablation: is all the damage nonthermal? Radiology 2013;266(2):462–70.
29. Hinshaw JL, Lee FT Jr. Cryoablation for liver cancer. Tech Vasc Interv Radiol 2007;10(1):47–57.
30. Kim JH, Won HJ, Shin YM, et al. Medium-sized (3.1-5.0 cm) hepatocellular carci-noma: transarterial chemoembolization plus radiofrequency ablation versus ra-diofrequency ablation alone. Ann Surg Oncol 2011;18(6):1624–9.
31. Mostafa EM, Ganguli S, Faintuch S, et al. Optimal strategies for combining trans-catheter arterial chemoembolization and radiofrequency ablation in rabbit VX2 hepatic tumors. J Vasc Interv Radiol 2008;19(12):1740–8.

32. Kitchin D, Lubner M, Ziemlewicz T, et al. Microwave ablation of malignant hepatic tumours: intraperitoneal fluid instillation prevents collateral damage and allows more aggressive case selection. Int J Hyperthermia 2014;30(5):299–305.
33. Hinshaw JL, Laeseke PF, Winter TC 3rd, et al. Radiofrequency ablation of peripheral liver tumors: intraperitoneal 5% dextrose in water decreases postprocedural pain. AJR. Am J Roentgenol 2006;186(5 Suppl):S306–10.
34. Patel SR, Hinshaw JL, Lubner MG, et al. Hydrodissection using an iodinated contrast medium during percutaneous renal cryoablation. J Endourol 2012; 26(5):463–6.
35. Livraghi T, Meloni F, Di Stasi M, et al. Sustained complete response and complications rates after radiofrequency ablation of very early hepatocellular carcinoma in cirrhosis: is resection still the treatment of choice? Hepatology 2008;47(1): 82–9. Baltimore, MD.
36. Kim YS, Lim HK, Rhim H, et al. Ten-year outcomes of percutaneous radiofrequency ablation as first-line therapy of early hepatocellular carcinoma: analysis of prognostic factors. J Hepatol 2013;58(1):89–97.
37. Lencioni R. Loco-regional treatment of hepatocellular carcinoma. Hepatology 2010;52(2):762–73.
38. Ziemlewicz TJ, Hinshaw JL, Lubner MG, et al. Percutaneous microwave ablation of hepatocellular carcinoma with a gas-cooled system: initial clinical results with 107 tumors. J Vasc Interv Radiol 2015;26(1):62–8.
39. Rong G, Bai W, Dong Z, et al. Long-term outcomes of percutaneous cryoablation for patients with hepatocellular carcinoma within Milan criteria. PLoS One 2015; 10(4):e0123065.
40. Berber E, Tsinberg M, Tellioglu G, et al. Resection versus laparoscopic radiofrequency thermal ablation of solitary colorectal liver metastasis. J Gastrointest Surg 2008;12(11):1967–72.
41. Oshowo A, Gillams A, Harrison E, et al. Comparison of resection and radiofrequency ablation for treatment of solitary colorectal liver metastases. Br J Surg 2003;90(10):1240–3.
42. Hur H, Ko YT, Min BS, et al. Comparative study of resection and radiofrequency ablation in the treatment of solitary colorectal liver metastases. Am J Surg 2009; 197(6):728–36.
43. Abdalla EK, Vauthey JN, Ellis LM, et al. Recurrence and outcomes following hepatic resection, radiofrequency ablation, and combined resection/ablation for colorectal liver metastases. Ann Surg 2004;239(6):818–25 [discussion: 825–7].
44. Hammill CW, Billingsley KG, Cassera MA, et al. Outcome after laparoscopic radiofrequency ablation of technically resectable colorectal liver metastases. Ann Surg Oncol 2011;18(7):1947–54.
45. Otto G, Düber C, Hoppe-Lotichius M, et al. Radiofrequency ablation as first-line treatment in patients with early colorectal liver metastases amenable to surgery. Ann Surg 2010;251(5):796–803.
46. Taner T, Atwell TD, Zhang L, et al. Adjunctive radiofrequency ablation of metastatic neuroendocrine cancer to the liver complements surgical resection. HPB (Oxford) 2013;15(3):190–5.
47. Sofocleous CT, Nascimento RG, Gonen M, et al. Radiofrequency ablation in the management of liver metastases from breast cancer. AJR Am J Roentgenol 2007;189(4):883–9.
48. Hoffmann R, Rempp H, Schmidt D, et al. Prolonged antibiotic prophylaxis in patients with bilioenteric anastomosis undergoing percutaneous radiofrequency ablation. J Vasc Interv Radiol 2012;23(4):545–51.

49. Wagner JM, Hinshaw JL, Lubner MG, et al. CT-guided lung biopsies: pleural blood patching reduces the rate of chest tube placement for postbiopsy pneumothorax. AJR Am J Roentgenol 2011;197(4):783–8.

50. Lee DH, Lee JM, Lee JY, et al. Radiofrequency ablation of hepatocellular carcinoma as first-line treatment: long-term results and prognostic factors in 162 patients with cirrhosis. Radiology 2014;270(3):900–9.

51. Shiina S, Tateishi R, Arano T, et al. Radiofrequency ablation for hepatocellular carcinoma: 10-year outcome and prognostic factors. Am J Gastroenterol 2012; 107(4):569–77 [quiz: 578].

52. N'Kontchou G, Mahamoudi A, Aout M, et al. Radiofrequency ablation of hepatocellular carcinoma: long-term results and prognostic factors in 235 Western patients with cirrhosis. Hepatology 2009;50(5):1475–83.

53. Groeschl RT, Pilgrim CH, Hanna EM, et al. Microwave ablation for hepatic malignancies: a multiinstitutional analysis. Ann Surg 2014;259(6):1195–200.

54. Swan RZ, Sindram D, Martinie JB, et al. Operative microwave ablation for hepatocellular carcinoma: complications, recurrence, and long-term outcomes. J Gastrointest Surg 2013;17(4):719–29.

55. Shady W, Petre EN, Gonen M, et al. Percutaneous radiofrequency ablation of colorectal cancer liver metastases: factors affecting outcomes-A 10-year experience at a single center. Radiology 2015;142489 [Epub ahead of print].

56. Agcaoglu O, Aliyev S, Karabulut K, et al. Complementary use of resection and radiofrequency ablation for the treatment of colorectal liver metastases: an analysis of 395 patients. World J Surg 2013;37(6):1333–9.

57. Solbiati L, Ahmed M, Cova L, et al. Small liver colorectal metastases treated with percutaneous radiofrequency ablation: local response rate and long-term survival with up to 10-year follow-up. Radiology 2012;265(3):958–68.

58. Van Tilborg AA, Meijerink MR, Sietses C, et al. Long-term results of radiofrequency ablation for unresectable colorectal liver metastases: a potentially curative intervention. Br J Radiol 2011;84(1002):556–65.

59. Reuter NP, Woodall CE, Scoggins CR, et al. Radiofrequency ablation vs. resection for hepatic colorectal metastasis: therapeutically equivalent? J Gastrointest Surg 2009;13(3):486–91.

60. Sorensen SM, Mortensen FV, Nielsen DT. Radiofrequency ablation of colorectal liver metastases: long-term survival. Acta Radiol 2007;48(3):253–8.

61. Eng OS, Tsang AT, Moore D, et al. Outcomes of microwave ablation for colorectal cancer liver metastases: a single center experience. J Surg Oncol 2015;111(4): 410–3.

62. Correa-Gallego C, Fong Y, Gonen M, et al. A retrospective comparison of microwave ablation vs. radiofrequency ablation for colorectal cancer hepatic metastases. Ann Surg Oncol 2014;21(13):4278–83.

63. Wang J, Liang P, Yu J, et al. Clinical outcome of ultrasound-guided percutaneous microwave ablation on colorectal liver metastases. Oncol Lett 2014;8(1):323–6.

Hepatic Artery Infusional Chemotherapy

Heather L. Lewis, MD[a], Mark Bloomston, MD[b],*

KEYWORDS

- Regional therapy • Hepatic metastases • Hepatic artery infusion pump

KEY POINTS

- Hepatic artery infusional chemotherapy is a well-studied, viable option for unresectable colorectal hepatic metastases and as adjuvant therapy after resection for colorectal hepatic metastases.
- When infused intraarterially, 5-fluoro 2-deoxyuridine (FUDR) has high levels of intratumoral concentration and a pharmacokinetic profile that makes it ideal for infusional hepatic therapy.
- Chemotherapeutic agents are best delivered via an implantable hepatic artery pump, which has been demonstrated to be both safe and technically feasible with acceptable morbidity.
- A methodical approach to both arterial isolation and evaluation of anatomy aids in optimizing successful hepatic artery pump insertion.

INTRODUCTION

Colorectal cancer remains the third leading cause of cancer related death in the United States.[1] Hepatic metastases develop in approximately 50% of 150,000 patients who are diagnosed, the majority of whom are not amenable to curative surgical resection. Over the course of the last several decades, advances in treatment regimens for patients with hepatic metastases from colorectal cancer have resulted in a significant improvement in overall survival (OS). Improvements in systemic chemotherapy options along with greater standardization in patient selection for, and the safety profile of, hepatic resection have primarily driven this trend.[2] Still, many patients will present with liver-only or liver-predominant metastatic disease that leads to their demise. It is in these patients where a liver-directed approach to therapy potentially offers a wider

Disclosures: None.
[a] Division of Surgical Oncology, The Ohio State University Wexner Medical Center, N924 Doan Hall, 410 West 10th Avenue, Columbus, OH 43210, USA; [b] Division of Surgical Oncology, 21st Century Oncology, Inc., 4571 Colonial Boulevard, Suite 210, Ft Myers, FL 33966, USA
* Corresponding author.
E-mail address: Mark.bloomston@21co.com

Surg Clin N Am 96 (2016) 341–355
http://dx.doi.org/10.1016/j.suc.2015.11.002
0039-6109/16/$ – see front matter © 2016 Elsevier Inc. All rights reserved.

surgical.theclinics.com

range of treatment options leading to improved disease control and quality of life. Arterial-based treatments such as radioembolization and transarterial chemoembolization are discussed elsewhere. The premise of hepatic artery infusion pump (HAIP) therapy, similar to these other regional therapies, is based on the understanding that hepatic metastases derive their nutritive blood supply from the hepatic artery, in comparison with hepatocytes, whose main blood supply is from the portal circulation.[3] Therefore, local infusion of cytotoxic agents can maximize the direct tumor effects while simultaneously minimizing deleterious systemic effects. However, the biliary tree also relies on arterial blood flow, thus putting it at risk for ischemic injury or direct chemotoxicity.

The use of an implanted catheter for the direct delivery of chemotherapy to the liver in the setting of advanced hepatic neoplastic processes was first studied by Sullivan and colleagues[4] in the late 1950s. The results in 21 patients, 9 of whom had colorectal primary tumors, were published in the *New England Journal of Medicine* in 1964. An objective response to therapy was noted in 10 of the 21 patients who received therapy. Since that time, identification of effective and pharmacologically suitable chemotherapeutic agents for hepatic artery infusion (HAI) therapy, along with the development of a sustainable and safe means of intraarterial delivery of these agents using an implanted pump has allowed for continued study and a better understanding of clinical efficacy and application. HAIP therapy has been studied most broadly in the setting of both resectable and unresectable hepatic colorectal metastases; however, ongoing research is looking at the role of this therapy for primary hepatic tumors, including cholangiocarcinoma and hepatocellular carcinoma.

5-Fluoro 2-deoxyuridine (FUDR) is the deoxyribonucleoside derivative of 5-fluorouracil (5-FU), a pyrimidine antimetabolite, and functions via the inhibition of thymidylate synthetase. Ensminger and colleagues[5] demonstrated that high extraction during the first pass by the liver (94%–99%) followed by rapid clearance occurred with systemic FUDR infusion. Additionally, when hepatic infusion is achieved via an intraarterial route, FUDR has been shown to have tumoral levels that are 15 times greater than if infusion were achieved through the portal vein,[6,7] and 400 times greater than that of systemic administration.[8] FUDR is easily concentrated and has favorable solubility properties, adding to ease of use with an implantable pump. These features collectively make it an optimal drug for HAI therapy. Although other agents have been studied, both individually and in multidrug combinations, FUDR remains the most widely used.

An implantable pump that allowed for the safe and effective continuous hepatic delivery of chemotherapeutic agents was evaluated and reported on by Buchwald and colleagues[9] in 1980. Multiple different manufacturers now offer pump devices that may be used in the setting of HAI therapy. In a recent review of more than 3000 patients who underwent insertion of either a (1) surgically placed catheter, (2) radiographically placed catheter, or (3) fully implanted pump, the lowest rate of complications and highest median number of chemotherapy cycles was associated with use of the fully implanted pump.[10] These devices are typically inserted during an open abdominal operation.[11,12] Minimally invasive techniques such as percutaneous transaxillary insertion of HAI pumps have been studied. However, although the reported duration of hospitalization was decreased with this method, there was a significantly higher rate of catheter-related complications that led to delay or cessation of treatment in the percutaneous group versus the laparotomy group (43% vs 7%; $P = .005$).[13] Laparoscopic placement has been studied by several authors, with comparable results to laparotomy, including management of anomalous arterial vasculature and success of pump placement.[14–16] As noted by Urbach and colleagues,[16] the effective use of this operative strategy necessitates that the surgeon have both advanced laparoscopic skill as well as a thorough understanding of the open pump insertion technique. No randomized comparisons of the open versus laparoscopic technique have yet been published or are planned. Finally, 1 center has reported on robotic insertion of HAI pump using criterion similar to those noted for laparoscopic approach, documenting its feasibility and safety.[17] Suffice it to say, as has been reported in many advanced surgical procedures, that minimally invasive HAIP placement may have a role, but should be undertaken by the most experienced teams in the proper setting.

TECHNIQUE
Preoperative Evaluation

Patients are evaluated in the context of their underlying diagnosis. Thorough evaluation for the presence of extrahepatic disease should be undertaken, although the presence of limited extrahepatic disease is not necessarily an absolute contraindication to liver-directed therapy. We consider the clear presence of metastases to portal nodes preoperatively a relative contraindication to pump placement given the high likelihood of extrahepatic recurrence. Other considerations include:

- Less than 70% replacement of the hepatic parenchyma with tumor burden;
- Preserved hepatic function, including total bilirubin less than 1.5 mg/dL;
- No evidence of portal hypertension or portal vein thrombosis; and
- Good performance status (Eastern Cooperative Oncology Group 0 or 1) and able to tolerate laparotomy.

Patients with chronic hepatitis and/or cirrhosis may be eligible, as long as they are Child-Pugh class A.

Once a patient is deemed to be an appropriate candidate, the technical aspect of HAIP placement is addressed, specifically the hepatic arterial anatomy. This can most often be accomplished by preoperative computed tomography angiogram. The pump catheter is to be inserted into the gastroduodenal artery (GDA); therefore, note should be taken of the caliber of the vessel and its particular anatomic course. The GDA will need to be of adequate caliber to accommodate the 2.3-mm diameter catheter. The presence of aberrant or replaced arterial anatomy, although not an absolute contraindication to HAIP insertion, may greatly increase the technical difficulty of pump placement and/or lead to problems with perfusion in the future. Aberrant or accessory hepatic arterial vasculature may be intraoperatively ligated or embolized postoperatively. Michels[18] described variant hepatic arterial anatomy, estimated to be present in approximately 50% of patients, and categorized 10 different anomalies. Yezhelyev and colleagues have reported on the use of a saphenous vein graft for several different anatomic variants[19]; however, the GDA remains the preferred insertion point unless it is anatomically absent or hepatic arteries are replaced completely. In rare such circumstances, HAIP placement may not be feasible, reserving more complicated/novel placement approaches for the most experienced surgeons and centers.

Pump Preparation

Several pumps have been approved by the Food and Drug Administration for delivery of chemotherapy to the liver. At our institution, we have experience with the Codman 3000 Series constant flow implantable pump (Codman, Johnson & Johnson, Raynham, MA), although this is not an endorsement of 1 pump over another. The general schema of the pump configuration is demonstrated in **Fig. 1**.[20] The device is an

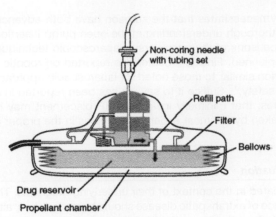

Non-coring needle with tubing set

Refill path

Filter

Bellows

Drug reservoir

Propellant chamber

Fig. 1. Schema of pump configuration. (*Adapted from* Skitzki JJ, Chang AE. Hepatic artery chemotherapy for colorectal liver metastases: technical considerations and review of clinical trials. Surg Oncol 2002;11(3):125; with permission.)

implantable drug delivery device with an attached silicone rubber catheter that infuses at a preset flow rate, ideally suitable for an ambulatory patient. The internal components of the pump are divided into an inner and outer chamber by an accordion-like bellows. The inner chamber contains the drug to be infused, and the outer chamber contains a fluorocarbon propellant permanently sealed inside. The patient's body temperature warms the propellant, which then is able to exert a constant pressure on the bellows to allow the drug to flow out of the inner chamber, through a filter and flow restrictor, and then into the catheter. Some pump systems use an additional programmable, battery-operated mechanism to deliver drug through the catheter. In the operating room, before insertion, the pump is prepared on the back table. This generally entails filling it with heparin saline (30,000 units in 30 mL of saline) and warming it to body temperature, thus verifying flow through the catheter.

Operative Technique

An incision is chosen based on the target anatomy, with consideration given to patient's body habitus and history of prior abdominal procedures. In our experience, a right subcostal incision is typically chosen. Once access to the abdomen has been attained, a retractor system is used to provide adequate exposure of the porta hepatis, duodenum, and lesser curvature of the stomach up to the right crus of the diaphragm. Peritoneal surfaces are examined along with the retroperitoneum to assess for extrahepatic metastatic disease that may preclude pump placement. If a colorectal primary is in place and planning to be resected at the same setting, we typically address this before pump placement. Although we recognize that it is ideal to undertake the cleanest portion of an operation first, undue retraction on the pump and catheter once in place potentially impacts its positioning and function. With proper attention to sterile technique, including removal of previously used instruments before pump placement, contamination is kept to a minimum with secondary infection of the pump being a rarity.

Exposure of the common hepatic artery and adjacent structures is attained in the area of the hepatoduodenal ligament. Any suspicious appearing lymph nodes in the region of the porta hepatis should be sent for further evaluation. Portal lymphatic disease is considered to be a relative contraindication to pump placement because these patients generally have a lower response rate to HAIP.[21] Sampling of nonsuspicious nodes is also undertaken. These data from final hematoxylin and eosin staining are helpful for future planning of systemic therapy, but we do not consider occult portal metastatic disease a contraindication to regional therapy. Isolation and identification of the arterial structures is generally undertaken in a stepwise fashion.

1. The common hepatic artery is isolated circumferentially and any small branches ligated from approximately 2 cm proximal to the origin of the GDA, and distally as far as possible, at a minimum to the branch point of the left and right hepatic arteries.
2. The GDA should then be identified and circumferentially isolated, taking great care to divide any branches that are proximal to the pump insertion site, including the right gastric artery.
3. Any accessory or replaced hepatic arteries are identified and ligated.
4. Any vessels supplying the superior border of the distal stomach and proximal duodenum that arise from the celiac axis should be divided.

The division of these small branch vessels is critical to the success of the procedure to prevent any extrahepatic flow to the gastrointestinal tract, which could result in gastritis, pancreatitis, duodenitis, and ulceration.[22] We typically use an energy device to divide all small vessels and lymphatic tissue up the gastrohepatic ligament all the way to the right crus of the diaphragm, as well behind the portal vein and overlying the inferior vena cava after exposure by a very limited Kocher maneuver. Isolation and ligation of the GDA as distal as possible is generally completed early in the procedure to allow time for any vasospasm that may have occurred during the dissection to abate. Approximately 3 to 4 cm of GDA length is ideal to allow for safe seating of the pump catheter. A cholecystectomy should be completed for all patients who undergo pump insertion to avoid complications related to postoperative chemical/acalculous cholecystitis.[12,23]

Attention is then turned to creating the pump pocket. Our ideal location is in the left lower quadrant of the abdominal wall. This site is marked before incision at the very beginning of the operation as distortion of the abdominal wall related to retraction used for the operation is common. A thick abdominal wall owing to an abundance of subcutaneous fat poses a difficult problem for future pump access. In such cases, our preference is to choose a site on the left lower chest wall just inferior to the inframammary fold to allow easier access. If this is not possible, it is best to limit the size of the pocket to correlate closely with the size of the pump to minimize dead space. Sometimes it is necessary to remove some of the subcutaneous fat that will overly the pump access point to allow for easier palpation and needle insertion. The concern here is that too much dead space can result in fluid accumulation. This allows the pump to float, which eventually leads to erosion of the securing sutures out of the fascia, thus allowing the pump to flip over in the pocket. The dissection is carried down to the anterior fascia with strict attention to hemostasis, because complications related to hematoma could impede the timely delivery of therapy or impair proper pump function in the future. All perforators to the abdominal wall fascia should be obliterated. The pump, which is has been prepared before these steps, should then be placed in the pocket. A tonsil clamp is used to insert the catheter through the anterior abdominal wall by penetrating the peritoneum and advancing through the abdominal wall to the pump pocket. We try to minimize the size of this puncture to avoid bleeding and prevent abdominal fluid, if present, from following the catheter into the pump pocket after surgery. We tend to leave some redundant catheter within the pocket, coiled beneath the base of the pump. We typically orient the catheter/pump junction closest to the liver within the pump pocket (eg, at 12 o'clock when in the lower quadrants and almost at 9 o'clock when over the left lower chest wall).

Insertion of the catheter into the GDA may then commence. The presence of "bumpers" at the end of the catheter allows the catheter to be secured within the lumen of the GDA to prevent proximal or distal migration. The catheter is trimmed with scissors to allow its tip to sit just beyond the origin of the GDA such that at least 1 securing bumper is within the vessel lumen. We typically trim the catheter with a very slight bevel so that the catheter tip is unable to seal flush against the opposing common hepatic artery wall should it migrate proximally. When sizing the catheter, it is important to consider retraction on the liver and stretch on the vessel, both of which will be relieved at the conclusion of the operation. If not already done previously, the distal GDA is ligated with a silk suture at this point. Temporary occlusion of the common and proper hepatic arteries with a bulldog vascular clamp allows for essentially bloodless catheter insertion. A #11 blade scalpel is used to create an arteriotomy on the anterior surface of the distal most aspect of the previously ligated GDA taking great care not to injure the back wall of the vessel. The catheter is then inserted to just distal to the ostium within the GDA (**Fig. 2**). Three-point ligation using #3–0 silk suture is undertaken: one on each side of the securing bumper inside the lumen of the GDA, and one circumferentially around the catheter and GDA at the point of insertion to maintain orientation of the catheter parallel to the vessel (see **Fig. 2**). These should be tied tightly enough to secure the catheter within the lumen of the vessel, but not so tight as to occlude the lumen of the catheter. Patency is verified by flushing the catheter with heparinized saline via the access port or using the bolus needle, depending on which system is being used. Note that spasm in the GDA or hepatic arteries often occurs during portal dissection or catheter insertion. This is self-limiting and rarely a problem for catheter placement, but can be aided by the use of papaverine.

Next, hepatic perfusion and the presence of any extrahepatic flow are assessed by fluorescein dye injection via the catheter while holding an ultraviolet lamp over the right upper quadrant. Baseline fluorescence of the field before the injection of fluorescein, particularly in the fat around the head of the pancreas and lesser curvature of the stomach, should be assessed first. The bowel is retracted away carefully before this step of the procedure so that there is a physical separation between the liver and the rest of the gastrointestinal tract. This step is to minimize any contamination from divided lymphatics, which may obscure visualization of extrahepatic flow. Any free fluid around the field should be suctioned away. Fluorescein (2 mL) is then injected slowly into the catheter. Some spasm is common at this point, so slow injection is important. A flush of 2 mL of heparinized saline should follow the injection of the

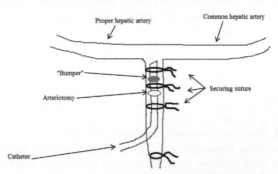

Fig. 2. Catheter insertion to the ostium within the gastroduodenal artery.

fluorescein to clear the catheter. The ultraviolet lamp is again used to assess the operative field after fluorescein injection. Of note, this step is primarily to assess for any extrahepatic flow so that small branch vessels or lymphatics may be ligated. Hepatic perfusion may not seem to be homogenous at this point owing to spasm, but will improve in the days and weeks after the operation. If any points of extrahepatic flow are indeed verified, those areas should be skeletonized and the branches ligated. Finally, the pump is secured to the anterior abdominal wall fascia using 4 points of fixation with permanent suture and the pump pocket is closed in layers including Scarpa's fascia (if possible), dermis, then skin.

Postoperative Care and Imaging

Routine postlaparotomy and/or liver resection care follows the insertion of the HAIP. Before filling the pump with chemotherapeutic agent(s), nuclear imaging using Tc^{99}-labeled macroaggregated albumin through the pump should be completed to evaluate hepatic perfusion and again assess for any evidence of extrahepatic perfusion. We typically complete this study immediately before discharge for patient convenience. If evidence of extrahepatic flow is illustrated, this may be potentially owing to extravasation from the cut edge of the liver if the patient has undergone a resection or from divided lymphatic vessels that have not yet sealed. As such, we repeat the study at first follow-up with a planned refill of heparinized saline. If there is still evidence of extrahepatic flow at this point, then angiography with embolization of any aberrant vessels is undertaken. There must be confirmation of the absence of extrahepatic flow before the initiation of chemotherapy. The most common reported source of anomalous flow is a relatively proximal branch arising from the proper hepatic artery or the right or left hepatic artery.[24] In such cases, extrahepatic flow can be managed successfully using angioembolization in the majority of patients, with surgical intervention rarely being necessary.

MANAGEMENT OF CHEMOTHERAPY

The infusion of FUDR is managed by a multidisciplinary team that consists of a pharmacist, a nurse practitioner, a medical oncologist, and the surgeon. Our institution's practice is to begin the infusion at a rate of 0.1 mg/kg per day (initial dose of 0.12 mg/kg per day is commonly reported). Body weight is calculated using ideal body weight. Aspartate aminotransferase, alkaline phosphatase, and total bilirubin are measured both before and at each 2-week interval while therapy is ongoing. Dose reductions are made based on these values as needed (**Table 1**). Patients are followed with repeat imaging as clinically indicated, typically every 3 months. The use of concomitant systemic therapy is generally safe, the data for which are described elsewhere in this paper.

FUDR is initiated on a cycle of 2 weeks on therapy followed by 2 weeks off of therapy. During off weeks, heparinized saline is placed in the pump reservoir. Given the size of the pump reservoir and the risk of catheter thrombosis if the pump is allowed to completely empty, patients must be compliant with their postoperative visit schedule. The willingness and ability of the patient to be fully compliant should be taken into consideration at the initial evaluation for HAIP therapy. When a patient elects to travel, we prefer that the pump not contain chemotherapy and be as full as possible before departure. Such precautions stem from concerns that the pump flow rate may be impacted by changes in elevation and were issues with the pump to occur during travel, or if the patient had an unanticipated delay in their return, it is undesirable for the patient to be away from the resources necessary to manage these issues with chemotherapy infusing. As such, the pump should be filled with

Table 1			
Management of side effects for patients receiving hepatic artery infusion pump therapy			
Test	Parameter[a]		FUDR Dose
Aspartate aminotransferase	Reference Current value	≤50 U/L 0 to <3 × ref 3 to <4 × ref	>50 U/L 0 to <2 × ref 2 to <3 × ref	— 100% 20% dose reduction
		4 to <5 × ref ≥5 × ref	3 to <4 × ref ≥4 × ref	50% dose reduction Hold
	If held, restart when:	<4 × ref	<3 × ref	50% last dose
Alkaline phosphatase	Reference Current	≤90 U/L 0 to <1.5 × ref 1.5 to <2 × ref	>90 U/L 0 to <1.2 × ref 1.2–1.5 × ref	— 100% 20% dose reduction
		≥2 × ref	≥1.5 × ref	Hold
	If held, restart when:	<1.5 × ref	<1.2 × ref	25% last dose
Total bilirubin	Reference Current	≤1.2 mg/dL 0 to <1.5 × ref 1.5 to <2 × ref	>1.2 mg/dL 0 to <1.2 × ref 1.2 to <1.5 × ref	— 100% 50% dose reduction
		≥2 × ref	≥1.5 × ref	Hold
	If held, restart when:	<1.5 × ref	<1.2 × ref	25% last dose

[a] Reference (ref) is the value at time of last dose of 5-fluoro 2-deoxyuridine (FUDR) and current represents the value at time of pump filling for planned treatment.

Adapted from Power DG, Kemeny NE. The role of floxuridine in metastatic liver disease. Mol Cancer Ther 2009;8(5):1021.

heparinized saline or glycerin when trips longer than the calculated capacity of the pump are planned.

Complications associated with HAIP therapy are largely technical problems with the pump itself (discussed elsewhere in this paper) and the biliary toxicity of FUDR, which is closely monitored during therapy. Elevations in liver enzymes are described collectively as chemical hepatitis, and occur approximately 42% of the time.[20] Additional toxicities include biliary sclerosis, gastritis, peptic ulcer, and diarrhea. Dose reductions may be necessary to mitigate biliary toxicity, and an algorithm for management of side effects is intrinsic to caring for patients receiving HAIP therapy.[23,25,26] Our institution's algorithm has been adopted from other experienced institutions and is outlined in **Table 1**. The addition of dexamethasone during FUDR infusion reduces biliary toxicity and, when evidence of toxicity develops, may be added to the heparinized saline after chemotherapy removal.[27] Mild biliary toxicity is often self-limited and managed by dose reduction and/or temporary cessation of therapy. If hyperbilirubinemia develops and is persistent despite these maneuvers, cholangiography should be undertaken to assess for biliary stricture. Disease progression may also be a cause for apparent biliary toxicity, and so should be considered. Balloon dilation with or without stent placement may be indicated if discrete biliary strictures are identified.

Once patients have completed therapy and/or anticipate an interval off of therapy, the pump may be filled with glycerin. Depending on the concentration of the glycerin used, these injections can last anywhere from 37 to 133 days, thus prolonging the interval necessary for the patient to present to the infusion location. When or if the pump is to be removed, the procedure is straightforward and can be done as an outpatient procedure. The pump pocket is opened, remaining securing sutures to the pump are removed, the pump is elevated out of the pocket, and the catheter is ligated then divided, thus leaving the intraabdominal portion of catheter in situ with redundancy. We prefer to use multiple titanium clips for ligation. The patient may then be discharged home after appropriate recovery from anesthetic.

MANAGEMENT OF TECHNICAL COMPLICATIONS

Complications associated with the use of the implantable pump for HAI have been reported in the range of 12% to 41% of patients.[28] These include issues related directly to the pump, such as seroma or infection of the pocket, wound dehiscence, or a pump that flips in the pocket. Additionally, problems related to the catheter, including erosion, displacement, and thrombosis, have been reported but are rare. Finally, vascular complications such as arterial thrombosis, dissection, and extrahepatic perfusion or incomplete perfusion are additional concerns. In a retrospective review of 15 years of experience at Memorial Sloan-Kettering looking at 544 patients, pump-related complications were identified in 120 patients (22%). The hepatic arterial system was most commonly implicated in 51% of these complications. Catheter-related issues were less common (26%), as well as pocket (16%) and device issues (5%). The majority of complications occurred at greater than 30 days after the implantation of the pump.[28] Similar pump complication rates have been noted by other groups, with a decline over time being noted as greater experience is gained.[10,11,29]

Pump Pocket Complications

Pump pocket–related complications, although uncommon, may result in a delay in the initiation of or timely delivery of scheduled therapy. Seroma formation may typically be managed expectantly; however, needle aspiration may be undertaken should there be failure to resolve in the anticipated timeframe or if access is affected. Hematoma formation is very uncommon. If identified, however, the size of the collection should be quantified using radiographic imaging. Larger collections may require formal evacuation. Hematomas that occur early in the perioperative setting should be taken back to the operating room for evacuation of the clot and identification of the bleeding source. Infection of the pump pocket that is limited to cellulitis is treated with antibiotics, oral or intravenous, depending on the severity of the cellulitis and the patient's clinical condition. When an infected fluid collection within the pump pocket is suspected, attempts at pump salvage should be reserved for those without evidence of systemic infection. In such cases, we have removed the pump from the pocket in the operating room and wrapped it in a betadine-soaked sponge for 10 minutes without dividing the catheter. Concomitantly, the pump pocket is debrided, cultured, and packed with a betadine-soaked sponge. The pump is then reseated and secured in place. The patient is monitored closely in the hospital for signs of systemic infection and continuance of intravenous antibiotics for 24 to 48 hours. If no signs of systemic infection occur, the patient can be discharged on oral antibiotics for the balance of a 2-week course with close outpatient follow-up. Any signs of recurrent infection would result in pump removal. Wound dehiscence that results in a compromise of the integrity of the device would also mandate removal. If the pump were to flip in the pocket, elective operative intervention may be undertaken so as to return the pump to its appropriate position, fixing it in place at 4 points. The pump housing can be replaced as needed with a new pump without the need for laparotomy by dividing the catheter and placement of a new pump using a splicing kit from the manufacturer, assuming that the catheter is not thrombosed.

Vascular and Catheter Complications

Arterial or catheter thrombosis can occur at any time point during which the patient is undergoing treatment; however, it more commonly occurs greater than 30 days after pump insertion. With proper pump refilling, catheter thrombosis is uncommon. Pump flow rates are estimated at each refill by dividing the amount infused (volume of loaded infusate minus residual volume in pump) by the number of days since last refill. A decrease in the infusion rate suggests clot or fibrin formation at the tip of the catheter. This situation can be managed with installation of enough volume of fibrinolytic agent to fill the catheter (see package insert) via the access port or using the bolus needle. This is allowed to dwell and slowly drip through the catheter by being pushed by heparinized saline from the infusion chamber over the next infusion interval. Failure of the flow rate to improve after 1 or 2 attempts should be evaluated radiographically. Erosion of the GDA, displacement of the catheter itself, or the development of a pseudoaneurysm is managed with either direct surgical intervention or with the use of angioembolization, depending on the patient's clinical circumstances. It is important for the patient and any associated providers to be aware that patients with HAI pumps who present with new abdominal pain must be evaluated to exclude bleeding or pseudoaneurysm.

CLINICAL OUTCOMES

Adjuvant Hepatic Artery Infusional Therapy for Resectable Colorectal Hepatic Metastases

The quest for a systemic adjuvant therapy that prolongs survival after resection of colorectal liver metastases (CRLM) has thus far been unsuccessful with only FOLFOX showing some marginal potential. HAI chemotherapy in the adjuvant setting after resection of CRLM, alone or in combination with systemic therapy, is appealing given the high likelihood of intrahepatic recurrence after hepatectomy. The majority of these recurrences will occur within 2 to 3 years after resection.[30,31] Therefore, the use of regional therapy with or without systemic therapy may address both micrometastases in the liver as well as aid in the prevention of extrahepatic spread.

To date, arguably the only data supporting adjuvant therapy after hepatectomy for CRLM stems from a randomized controlled trial of HAI plus systemic chemotherapy by Kemeny and colleagues.[32] In this trial, 156 patients who underwent hepatic resection were assigned to receive either HAI FUDR/dexamethasone (Dex) plus intravenous 5-FU/leucovorin or intravenous 5-FU/Leucovorin alone. Study endpoints included OS, hepatic recurrence-free survival, and disease-free survival (DFS) at 2 years. The median OS was 72.2 months in the dual therapy group compared with 59.3 months in the systemic therapy alone group. The 2-year OS was 86% in the HAI chemotherapy and 74% in the systemic group ($P = .03$), and hepatic recurrence free survival was notably 90% versus 60% ($P \leq .001$) between the HAI chemotherapy and systemic therapy group, respectively. DFS at 2 years was not significant (57% vs 42%; $P = .07$) for the HAI chemotherapy arm and the systemic therapy arm, respectively. The most common site of extrahepatic recurrence was the lung. Toxicity was greater in the combined group and resulted in therapy dose reductions. However, despite an increased number of hospitalizations in these patients, the overall number of deaths during treatment was not different.

Follow-up of this study in 2005, now with a median follow-up time of 10 years, demonstrated DFS in the combined therapy group of 31.3 versus 17.2 months ($P = .02$) in the monotherapy group.[33] The 10-year survival rates were 41.1% for the HAI chemotherapy group and 27.2% in the systemic therapy group.

As understanding of chemotherapy for colorectal cancer has continued to evolve, trials evaluating these more modern agents in conjunction with HAI therapy have been undertaken. Specifically, 2 phase I and II trials have evaluated HAI FUDR/Dex plus FOLFOX and HAI FUDR/Dex plus irinotecan.[34,35] These trials were able to successfully identify the maximum tolerated dose and safety profile for those therapeutic combinations. Continued evaluation with phase III trials remains to be accomplished.

A retrospective review of 125 patients treated between 2000 and 2005 who underwent hepatic resection followed by adjuvant HAI-FUDR/Dex in combination with systemic FOLFOX or FOLFIRI demonstrated on multivariate analysis that HAI-FUDR was independently associated with improved liver recurrence-free survival (hazard ratio, 0.34; $P \leq .01$), overall recurrence-free survival (hazard ratio, 0.65; $P = .01$), and disease-specific survival (hazard ratio, 0.39; $P = .01$).[36] Finally, a recent study by Goere and colleagues[37] looked at patients with 4 or more CRLM who received postoperative HAI combined with either systemic 5-FU or FOLFOX/FOLFIRI versus systemic therapy alone. In this patient population, with a median follow-up of 60 months, the 3-year DFS was significantly higher with HAI therapy compared with systemic therapy alone (33% vs 5%; $P<.0001$). However, the 3-year OS was only slightly higher in the HAI group and did not attain statistical significance.

Although there remains a paucity of large randomized phase III trials of HAI in the adjuvant setting for resected CRLM, the data to date point to a clear improvement in DFS as well as hepatic recurrence-free survival, with evidence suggesting an advantage in OS.

Hepatic Artery Infusional Therapy for Unresectable Colorectal Hepatic Metastases

Multiple randomized controlled trials evaluating HAI therapy in the setting of unresectable CRLM have been undertaken, three of which have been completed since 2000.[38–40]

The German Cooperative group studied 168 patients who were enrolled into 1 of 3 treatment arms: (1) 5-FU/leucovorin via HAI, (2) 5-FU/leucovorin systemic therapy, and (3) HAI FUDR. They observed a median time to progression of 9.2, 6.6 and, 5.9 months and median survival of 18.7, 17.6, and 12.7 months, respectively. Although differences in OS were not significant, the time to progression significantly favored HAI 5-FU/leucovorin over HAI FUDR ($P = .033$).[40] Subsequently, in 2003, Kerr and colleagues[39] published their results of 290 patients randomized to either HAI 5-FU/leucovorin versus systemic 5-FU/leucovorin. No difference was noted in median OS between groups (14.7 vs 14.8 months; $P = .79$), and no differences were noted in progression-free survival.[39] Most recently, the CALGB 9481 trial, which was published in 2006, randomized 135 patients to receive either HAI FUDR/leucovorin/Dex or systemic 5-FU/leucovorin. Unlike other studies preceding it, crossover between arms was not allowed. OS was significantly improved in the HAI therapy group as compared with the systemic treatment group, with a median of 24.4 versus 20 months ($P = .0034$). Additionally, response rates were notably different at 47% in the HAI group versus 24% in the systemic therapy group. Of note, this trial was the first to document a significant difference in OS with HAI chemotherapy for unresectable CRLM.

The ability to convert patients with unresectable disease to resectable has been found to be between 25% and 47% in recent studies using HAI in combination with systemic chemotherapy suggesting that, for a specific group of patients, even further benefit may be dervived,[41,42] because surgery remains the only potentially curative treatment for CRLM. In 1 group of patients with advanced CRLM, HAI was used as an adjunct along with systemic chemotherapy and 2-stage hepatic resection. The median overall disease-specific survival was 52 months, with 88% of patients able to undergo both stages of hepatic resection.[43] These studies emphasize the role that HAI may play in bridging patients to surgical resection.

Combination therapy using HAI along with systemic chemotherapy has been evaluated in the setting of second-line therapy for those patients who have failed first-line chemotherapy. Using modern chemotherapy agents, several phase I trials have evaluated the inclusion of HAI. A phase I trial using HAI FUDR plus systemic irinotecan in 46 patients who had previously received systemic therapy showed no adverse increase in toxicity when the therapies were combined; median OS was 17.2 months.[44] A second phase I study looked at the use of HAI FUDR and either systemic oxaliplatin/irinotecan or systemic FOLFOX.[45] Response rates were noted to be 87% in the HAI plus oxaliplatin/irinotecan group and 90% in the HAI plus FOLFOX group. These promising results demonstrate significant potential benefit from HAI chemotherapy in conjunction with modern systemic chemotherapy in patients with unresectable CRLM who fail first-line therapy.

Primary Liver Tumors and Hepatic Artery Infusional Therapy

An evolving new target for HAI therapy is primary cancer of the liver, including intrahepatic cholangiocarcinoma (ICC) and hepatocellular carcinoma. Although there is only a small body of literature to date, initial results demonstrate that the therapy is feasible and safe. Jarnagin and colleagues[46] reported a phase II trial in 2009 using HAI FUDR/Dex in 34 patients with unresectable primary liver cancer, including both ICC and hepatocellular carcinoma. Partial response was seen in almost one-half of the patients treated (47%), and median survival was 29.5 months.[46] A recent update to these data looked at 44 patients with ICC treated with HAI FUDR/Dex or HAI FUDR/Dex plus bevacizumab, which again demonstrated a partial response in approximately one-half of the patients (48%) and a median OS of approximately 28 months.[47] It is important to note that the addition of bevacizumab significantly increased toxicity. Ongoing clinical trials will aim to better address what role HAI will have in unresectable ICC and hepatocellular carcinoma in the future.

SUMMARY

HAI therapy represents a well-studied and viable regional therapy for patients with hepatic metastases, as well as an evolving role for primary liver cancers. Implantable pump devices may be safely placed intraarterially with minimal morbidity in experienced hands. Like other regional therapies, HAI treatments can be used as an adjunct to systemic therapy, not a replacement. Future trials may address the sequencing of therapies, alternating between systemic and regional approaches, and the combination thereof. These treatments, however, are not without their complications. Thus, they require close monitoring and attention to detail. When used properly and followed appropriately, HAI therapy offers reasonable control of liver tumor burden with high levels of patient satisfaction. As such, they are ideally managed in concert between medical and surgical oncologists dedicated to a successful program.

REFERENCES

1. Siegel RL, Miller KD, Jemal A. Cancer statistics, 2015. CA Cancer J Clin 2015; 65(1):5–29.
2. Kopetz S, Chang GJ, Overman MJ, et al. Improved survival in metastatic colorectal cancer is associated with adoption of hepatic resection and improved chemotherapy. J Clin Oncol 2009;27(22):3677–83.

3. Breedis C, Young G. The blood supply of neoplasms in the liver. Am J Pathol 1954;30(5):969–77.
4. Sullivan RD, Norcross JW, Watkins E Jr. Chemotherapy of metastatic liver cancer by prolonged hepatic-artery infusion. N Engl J Med 1964;270:321–7.
5. Ensminger WD, Rosowsky A, Raso V, et al. A clinical-pharmacological evaluation of hepatic arterial infusions of 5-fluoro-2'-deoxyuridine and 5-fluorouracil. Cancer Res 1978;38(11 Pt 1):3784–92.
6. Sigurdson ER, Ridge JA, Kemeny N, et al. Tumor and liver drug uptake following hepatic artery and portal vein infusion. J Clin Oncol 1987;5(11):1836–40.
7. Daly JM, Kemeny N, Sigurdson E, et al. Regional infusion for colorectal hepatic metastases. A randomized trial comparing the hepatic artery with the portal vein. Arch Surg 1987;122(11):1273–7.
8. Dizon DS, Schwartz J, Kemeny N. Regional chemotherapy: a focus on hepatic artery infusion for colorectal cancer liver metastases. Surg Oncol Clin N Am 2008;17(4):759–71, viii.
9. Buchwald H, Grage TB, Vassilopoulos PP, et al. Intraarterial infusion chemotherapy for hepatic carcinoma using a totally implantable infusion pump. Cancer 1980;45(5):866–9.
10. Bacchetti S, Pasqual E, Crozzolo E, et al. Intra-arterial hepatic chemotherapy for unresectable colorectal liver metastases: a review of medical devices complications in 3172 patients. Med Devices (Auckl) 2009;2:31–40.
11. Curley SA, Chase JL, Roh MS, et al. Technical considerations and complications associated with the placement of 180 implantable hepatic arterial infusion devices. Surgery 1993;114(5):928–35.
12. Kemeny MM. The surgical aspects of the totally implantable hepatic artery infusion pump. Arch Surg 2001;136(3):348–52.
13. Arru M, Aldrighetti L, Gremmo F, et al. Arterial devices for regional hepatic chemotherapy: transaxillary versus laparotomic access. J Vasc Access 2000;1(3):93–9.
14. Cheng J, Hong D, Zhu G, et al. Laparoscopic placement of hepatic artery infusion pumps: technical considerations and early results. Ann Surg Oncol 2004; 11(6):589–97.
15. Feliciotti F, Paganini A, Guerrieri M, et al. Laparoscopic intra-arterial catheter implantation for regional chemotherapy of liver metastasis. Surg Endosc 1996; 10(4):449–52.
16. Urbach DR, Herron DM, Khajanchee YS, et al. Laparoscopic hepatic artery infusion pump placement. Arch Surg 2001;136(6):700–4.
17. Hellan M, Pigazzi A. Robotic-assisted placement of a hepatic artery infusion catheter for regional chemotherapy. Surg Endosc 2008;22(2):548–51.
18. Michels NA. Newer anatomy of the liver and its variant blood supply and collateral circulation. Am J Surg 1966;112(3):337–47.
19. Yezhelyev M, Osgood M, Egnatashvili V, et al. Saphenous vein graft conduits for insertion of hepatic arterial infusion pumps in patients with abnormal hepatic arterial anatomy. J Surg Oncol 2008;97(1):85–9.
20. Skitzki JJ, Chang AE. Hepatic artery chemotherapy for colorectal liver metastases: technical considerations and review of clinical trials. Surg Oncol 2002;11(3):123–35.
21. Ammori JB, D'Angelica MI, Fong Y, et al. Hepatic artery infusional chemotherapy in patients with unresectable colorectal liver metastases and extrahepatic disease. J Surg Oncol 2012;106(8):953–8.
22. Hohn DC, Stagg RJ, Price DC, et al. Avoidance of gastroduodenal toxicity in patients receiving hepatic arterial 5-fluoro-2'-deoxyuridine. J Clin Oncol 1985;3(9): 1257–60.

23. Kemeny MM, Battifora H, Blayney DW, et al. Sclerosing cholangitis after continuous hepatic artery infusion of FUDR. Ann Surg 1985;202(2):176–81.
24. Perez DR, Kemeny NE, Brown KT, et al. Angiographic identification of extrahepatic perfusion after hepatic arterial pump placement: implications for surgical prevention. HPB (Oxford) 2014;16(8):744–8.
25. Power DG, Kemeny NE. The role of floxuridine in metastatic liver disease. Mol Cancer Ther 2009;8(5):1015–25.
26. Ito K, Ito H, Kemeny NE, et al. Biliary sclerosis after hepatic arterial infusion pump chemotherapy for patients with colorectal cancer liver metastasis: incidence, clinical features, and risk factors. Ann Surg Oncol 2012;19(5):1609–17.
27. Kemeny N, Seiter K, Niedzwiecki D, et al. A randomized trial of intrahepatic infusion of fluorodeoxyuridine with dexamethasone versus fluorodeoxyuridine alone in the treatment of metastatic colorectal cancer. Cancer 1992;69(2):327–34.
28. Allen PJ, Nissan A, Picon AI, et al. Technical complications and durability of hepatic artery infusion pumps for unresectable colorectal liver metastases: an institutional experience of 544 consecutive cases. J Am Coll Surg 2005;201(1):57–65.
29. Scaife CL, Curley SA, Izzo F, et al. Feasibility of adjuvant hepatic arterial infusion of chemotherapy after radiofrequency ablation with or without resection in patients with hepatic metastases from colorectal cancer. Ann Surg Oncol 2003;10(4):348–54.
30. Vigano L, Ferrero A, Lo Tesoriere R, et al. Liver surgery for colorectal metastases: results after 10 years of follow-up. Long-term survivors, late recurrences, and prognostic role of morbidity. Ann Surg Oncol 2008;15(9):2458–64.
31. Fong Y, Cohen AM, Fortner JG, et al. Liver resection for colorectal metastases. J Clin Oncol 1997;15(3):938–46.
32. Kemeny N, Huang Y, Cohen AM, et al. Hepatic arterial infusion of chemotherapy after resection of hepatic metastases from colorectal cancer. N Engl J Med 1999;341(27):2039–48.
33. Kemeny NE, Gonen M. Hepatic arterial infusion after liver resection. N Engl J Med 2005;352(7):734–5.
34. Kemeny N, Jarnagin W, Gonen M, et al. Phase I/II study of hepatic arterial therapy with floxuridine and dexamethasone in combination with intravenous irinotecan as adjuvant treatment after resection of hepatic metastases from colorectal cancer. J Clin Oncol 2003;21(17):3303–9.
35. Kemeny N, Capanu M, D'Angelica M, et al. Phase I trial of adjuvant hepatic arterial infusion (HAI) with floxuridine (FUDR) and dexamethasone plus systemic oxaliplatin, 5-fluorouracil and leucovorin in patients with resected liver metastases from colorectal cancer. Ann Oncol 2009;20(7):1236–41.
36. House MG, Kemeny NE, Gonen M, et al. Comparison of adjuvant systemic chemotherapy with or without hepatic arterial infusional chemotherapy after hepatic resection for metastatic colorectal cancer. Ann Surg 2011;254(6):851–6.
37. Goere D, Benhaim L, Bonnet S, et al. Adjuvant chemotherapy after resection of colorectal liver metastases in patients at high risk of hepatic recurrence: a comparative study between hepatic arterial infusion of oxaliplatin and modern systemic chemotherapy. Ann Surg 2013;257(1):114–20.
38. Kemeny NE, Niedzwiecki D, Hollis DR, et al. Hepatic arterial infusion versus systemic therapy for hepatic metastases from colorectal cancer: a randomized trial of efficacy, quality of life, and molecular markers (CALGB 9481). J Clin Oncol 2006;24(9):1395–403.

39. Kerr DJ, McArdle CS, Ledermann J, et al. Intrahepatic arterial versus intravenous fluorouracil and folinic acid for colorectal cancer liver metastases: a multicentre randomised trial. Lancet 2003;361(9355):368–73.
40. Lorenz M, Muller HH. Randomized, multicenter trial of fluorouracil plus leucovorin administered either via hepatic arterial or intravenous infusion versus fluorodeoxyuridine administered via hepatic arterial infusion in patients with nonresectable liver metastases from colorectal carcinoma. J Clin Oncol 2000;18(2):243–54.
41. Ammori JB, Kemeny NE, Fong Y, et al. Conversion to complete resection and/or ablation using hepatic artery infusional chemotherapy in patients with unresectable liver metastases from colorectal cancer: a decade of experience at a single institution. Ann Surg Oncol 2013;20(9):2901–7.
42. Power DG, Kemeny NE. Chemotherapy for the conversion of unresectable colorectal cancer liver metastases to resection. Crit Rev Oncol Hematol 2011;79(3): 251–64.
43. Cardona K, Donataccio D, Kingham TP, et al. Treatment of extensive metastatic colorectal cancer to the liver with systemic and hepatic arterial infusion chemotherapy and two-stage hepatic resection: the role of salvage therapy for recurrent disease. Ann Surg Oncol 2014;21(3):815–21.
44. Kemeny N, Gonen M, Sullivan D, et al. Phase I study of hepatic arterial infusion of floxuridine and dexamethasone with systemic irinotecan for unresectable hepatic metastases from colorectal cancer. J Clin Oncol 2001;19(10):2687–95.
45. Kemeny N, Jarnagin W, Paty P, et al. Phase I trial of systemic oxaliplatin combination chemotherapy with hepatic arterial infusion in patients with unresectable liver metastases from colorectal cancer. J Clin Oncol 2005;23(22):4888–96.
46. Jarnagin WR, Schwartz LH, Gultekin DH, et al. Regional chemotherapy for unresectable primary liver cancer: results of a phase II clinical trial and assessment of DCE-MRI as a biomarker of survival. Ann Oncol 2009;20(9):1589–95.
47. Konstantinidis IT, Do RK, Gultekin DH, et al. Regional chemotherapy for unresectable intrahepatic cholangiocarcinoma: a potential role for dynamic magnetic resonance imaging as an imaging biomarker and a survival update from two prospective clinical trials. Ann Surg Oncol 2014;21(8):2675–83.

Hepatic Perfusion Therapy

Rahul Rajeev, MBBS, T. Clark Gamblin, MD, MS,
Kiran K. Turaga, MD, MPH*

KEYWORDS

- Isolated hepatic perfusion • Hepatocellular carcinoma • Melanoma
- Colorectal cancer • Hepatic metastases • Regional therapies
- Percutaneous hepatic perfusion

KEY POINTS

- Isolated hepatic perfusion (IHP) depends on the unique vascular structure of the liver to deliver cytotoxic chemotherapies to liver malignancies. Cytotoxic chemotherapy is delivered via the hepatic artery and extracted from the retrohepatic inferior vena cava to reduce systemic leakage.
- Hepatic perfusion has been used with oncologic efficacy in patients with metastatic ocular melanoma, hepatocellular carcinoma, and colorectal cancer liver metastases, among other histologies.
- Advances in techniques of chemosaturation with percutaneous hepatic perfusion may offer novel minimally invasive avenues of treating patients with metastatic disease.

 Video content accompanies this article at http://www.surgical.theclinics.com

INTRODUCTION

Although curative surgical resection is the optimal treatment of primary and metastatic malignancies of the liver, few patients are eligible because of the unique biology of liver disease. Regional therapies of the liver use the hepatic arterial-dominant supply of tumors to deliver high concentrations of chemotherapy, embolic particles, and radiation. Perfusion, as opposed to infusion, relies on the flow of cytotoxic therapy through the liver with extraction of the drug via the venous outflow. The anatomic reliance on the vascular supply of the liver is paramount in the ability to perform an isolated hepatic perfusion.

SURGICAL TECHNIQUE AND SELECTION OF PATIENTS

Hepatic perfusion has been performed for numerous histologic subtypes, but the largest body of evidence exists for its use in patients with metastatic ocular

Disclosure: The authors have nothing to disclose.
Division of Surgical Oncology, Medical College of Wisconsin, 9200 West Wisconsin Avenue, Milwaukee, WI 53226, USA
* Corresponding author.
E-mail address: kturaga@mcw.edu

Surg Clin N Am 96 (2016) 357–368
http://dx.doi.org/10.1016/j.suc.2015.12.005
0039-6109/16/$ – see front matter © 2016 Elsevier Inc. All rights reserved.

melanoma, colorectal liver metastases, neuroendocrine tumors, and primary liver tumors including hepatocellular carcinoma and cholangiocarcinoma. There are three broad methods of performing a hepatic perfusion: (1) isolated hepatic perfusion (IHP), (2) percutaneous hepatic perfusion (PHP; a misnomer because it indicates chemosaturation), and (3) liver perfusional chemotherapy (which is primarily infusional).

Selection of Patients

Before a liver perfusion, it is important to consider a few additional factors related to general oncologic surgical principles. Hepatic arterial anatomy can vary at least 20% of the time with the commonest anatomic variations shown in **Fig. 1**.

Although hepatic perfusion can be considered in patients with variants in anatomy, it is important to understand the hepatic arterial anatomy in great detail before attempting a perfusion. In addition, it is critically important to select patients who are robust enough to undergo the procedure and can tolerate any complications. Because up to 22% of patients can develop veno-occlusive disease and a few patients develop vanishing bile duct syndrome (more commonly seen with hepatic artery infusion [HAI] pumps), it is important to select patients with intact synthetic and excretory function of the liver.[1,2] Although pretreatment with chemotherapy is not a contraindication

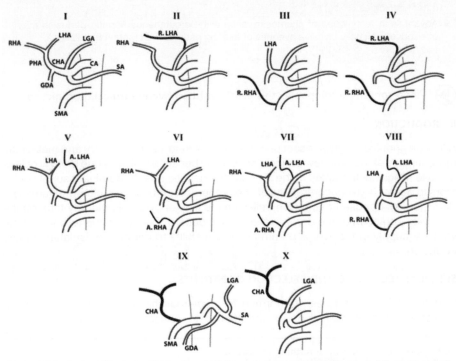

Fig. 1. Michels classification of hepatic arterial anatomy. A. LHA, accessory left hepatic artery; A. RHA, accessory right hepatic artery; CA, celiac artery; CHA, common hepatic artery; GDA, gastroduodenal artery; LGA, left gastric artery; LHA, left hepatic artery; PHA, proper hepatic artery; R. LHA, replaced left hepatic artery; R. RHA, replaced right hepatic artery; RHA, right hepatic artery; SA, splenic artery; SMA, superior mesenteric artery. (*From* Caserta MP, Sakala M, Shen P, et al. Presurgical planning for hepatobiliary malignancies: clinical and imaging considerations. Magn Reson Imaging Clin N Am 2014;22(3):447–65; with permission.)

to the procedure, it is important to note hematologic parameters of patients before planning the procedure.

Technical Details of an Isolated Hepatic Pesrfusion

Modern techniques of hepatic perfusion have significantly advanced since its original advent by Ausman[3] and subsequent refinement by Skibba and Quebbeman[4] at the Medical College of Wisconsin. A hybrid technique of an IHP has been adopted by many centers, which combines advances in percutaneous and open surgery. Anesthetic considerations for an IHP include the ability to place the patient on venovenous bypass, and need for systemic heparinization during the case. An epidural is generally discouraged because of the risk of an epidural hematoma, and preoperative assessment of neck and femoral veins is often undertaken to ensure successful placement of the cannulas. Fluid management is essential to ensure easy mobilization of the liver, but extreme fluid restriction is not necessary as needed in hepatic resection.

The procedure often begins with the placement of a 17F to 19F catheter cannula in the right internal jugular vein and an 8F catheter central venous line in the left internal jugular vein for access (Video 1). A diagnostic laparoscopy is undertaken to rule out extrahepatic disease. Wide exposure is gained by a right subcostal incision with a midline extension. A cholecystectomy is not always necessary but routinely performed to reduce the risk of cholecystistis. Complete mobilization of the liver and the inferior vena cava (IVC) are essential for this procedure. The right adrenal vein is usually ligated and divided, and occasionally the phrenic veins also need to be dissected and divided. Control of the infrahepatic IVC is gained by encircling it with a Rummel tourniquet and the suprahepatic IVC is controlled with the angled vascular clamp. The portal dissection includes dissecting at least 2 cm of the gastroduodenal artery (GDA) and identifying the common hepatic artery to clamp it. The portal triad is not completely dissected and an angled clamp is chosen to create complete portal occlusion. Wires are then placed through bilateral femoral vein access into the IVC and systemic heparinization is reached with a target activated clotting time greater than 300. At this point, a 17F to 19F catheter is placed via the left femoral vein and is positioned by palpation of the distal IVC/common iliac vein. A 14F catheter cannula is also threaded through the right femoral vein and is placed in the retrohepatic IVC. The Rummel tourniquet is clamped around the retrohepatic cannula and the venovenous bypass circuit is begun from the left femoral vein access to the internal jugular access (**Fig. 2**). At this point, the GDA is cannulated with a 5F catheter cannula and the proximal common hepatic artery is clamped. The porta hepatis is also clamped, as is the suprahepatic IVC, and an oxygenated pH balanced perfusion is begun through the GDA into the liver with a retrohepatic drainage. Flow rates of 400 to 700 mL/min are achieved and the inline arterial pressures are kept less than 150 mm Hg. Temperature probes are used to monitor the temperature of the liver, which is increased to 40°C. The perfusate leakage can often be detected by stability of the reservoir volume. Although historically perfusate leakage was documented using radiolabelled tracers, this method seems to be quite effective without adding extra logistic steps.[5] The reservoir volume can fluctuate minimally because of expansion of the liver or leakage from the capsule but this should be completely stable before adding the chemotherapy drug. Cytotoxic chemotherapy (usually melphalan) is added and constant adjustment of the milieu is necessary to maintain a pH of 7.20 during the perfusion. Following a 60-minute perfusion, washout of the liver with crystalloid, and colloid and replacement of plasma with fresh frozen plasma occurs. Decannulation of the hepatic perfusion occurs, with either ligation of the GDA or subsequent preparation of the artery for placement of HAI pump. The venovenous circuit is decannulated and the heparinization is reversed. Some

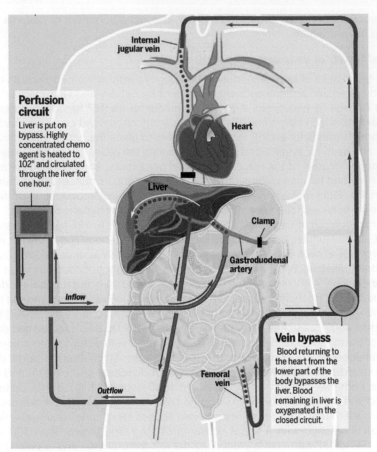

Internal jugular vein

Perfusion circuit
Liver is put on bypass. Highly concentrated chemo agent is heated to 102° and circulated through the liver for one hour.

Heart

Liver

Clamp

Gastroduodenal artery

Inflow

Vein bypass
Blood returning to the heart from the lower part of the body bypasses the liver. Blood remaining in liver is oxygenated in the closed circuit.

Femoral vein

Outflow

Fig. 2. Technique of isolated hepatic perfusion. (*From* Fauber J. Froedtert doctors try using heat, chemo to halt liver cancer. Milwaukee Journal Sentinel 2011; with permission. Available at: http://www.jsonline.com/news/health/froedtert-doctors-try-using-heat-chemo-to-halt-liver-cancer-id2qg37-134220898.html. Accessed November 21, 2011.)

techniques with variant arterial anatomy described by some authors are shown in **Fig. 3**.

Special attention should be paid to massive hepatocyte injury, loss of synthetic function, and hematologic derangements during perioperative recovery. Occurrence of veno-occlusive disease and disappearing bile ducts are subacute toxicities of the perfusion.[1,2] Experienced critical care staff is necessary during the early postoperative period of the patient's care.

Variants of the Perfusion

1. Choice of venovenous circuit access: As with cardiac surgery, venovenous access is easily obtained via the axillary vein, the saphenous vein, or other similar venous access structures.
2. Orthograde versus retrograde portal flow: Current techniques use portal occlusion, which leads to orthograde flow. This has been shown to have up to a 55% leakage of perfusate in some studies.[6] Retrograde flow has been proposed to reverse the

portal flow and allow the portal vein to drain the blood from the liver.[7,8] Leakage occurs with both techniques.

3. Hypoxic perfusion: Some authors have suggested the use of hypoxia to augment the cytotoxic effects of the drug. The rate of severe systemic toxicity of hypoxic perfusions is 0% to 4% and the outcomes in two papers are similar to reported outcomes of classical IHP.[6,8]

4. Tumor necrosis factor (TNF)-α in the perfusion: The use of immunomodulating drugs, such as TNF, has been proposed in early studies of the IHP. Early results, although promising, have not been substantiated, and toxicity remains high.[9,10]

Percutaneous Hepatic Perfusion (Chemosaturation)

PHP achieves vascular isolation and chemosaturation with cytotoxic chemotherapy. Unlike the normal IHP circuit where cytotoxic chemotherapy is extracted before leakage or absorption into the circulation, the PHP circuit relies on extracorporeal hemofiltration to remove the chemotherapy[11,12] (**Fig. 4**). This leads to two unintended consequences (delivering higher concentrations of drug with a shorter duration, and filtration of catecholamines), leading to profound hemodynamic alterations.[13] Regardless, this is a minimally invasive procedure that can be repeated with minimal risk to the patient. Contrast allergy is a relative contraindication for this procedure, although CO_2 angiography and premedication could be used as an alternative. The procedure uses the Delcath catheter to create isolation of the hepatic venous outflow (Delcath Systems, Inc, New York, NY). A balloon is usually inflated to 20 to 35 mL after systemic heparinization and is used to snag the cavoatrial junction under fluoroscopy. The distal IVC balloon is used to flatten out the IVC in a suprarenal position and confirmation of vascular isolation is achieved by a contrast venogram. The hepatic artery is cannulated percutaneously. Occasionally, the GDA is coil embolized to reduce leakage via the artery. Nitroglycerin and papaverine are often used to reduce vasospasm.[14] Chemosaturation then occurs for 30 minutes during which significant hemodynamic support is required because of catecholamine losses. Although veno-occlusive disease and vanishing bile duct syndrome can occur, the commonest toxicity is hematologic. The usual hospital length of stay is 3 to 5 days after such a procedure.[14]

LIVER PERFUSIONAL CHEMOTHERAPY

The technique of liver perfusional chemotherapy has been popularized in Japan, and although termed perfusional chemotherapy, this is best classified as an infusional chemotherapy. This technique uses two catheters placed at the time of surgery into the hepatic artery and the portal vein (via the middle colic vein) through which chemotherapy is administered for 28 days after resection.[15,16] This has been used in the adjuvant/prophylactic setting with demonstrable feasibility, although oncologic durability is unknown. Regardless, the lack of extraction of chemotherapy other than by bioavailability makes this more of an infusion akin to hepatic arterial infusional therapies.[16]

OCULAR MELANOMA

Metastatic ocular melanoma has poor overall survival and liver metastases are no exception. Trials of MAP-kinase inhibitors against standard dacarbazine/temozolomide chemotherapy have shown improved progression-free survival (15.9 vs 7 weeks) and objective response rates (14% vs 0%).[17] Despite advances in

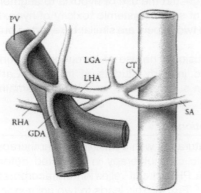

A

ANATOMY BEFORE PERFUSION

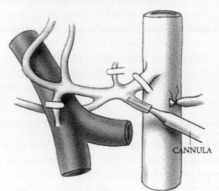

ARTERIAL CANNULATION

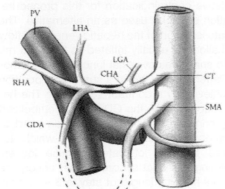

B

ANATOMY BEFORE PERFUSION

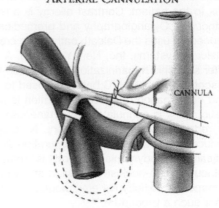

ARTERIAL CANNULATION

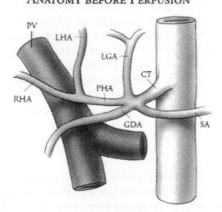

C

ANATOMY BEFORE PERFUSION

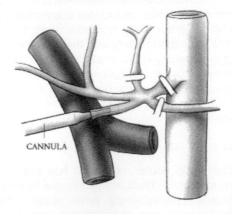

ARTERIAL CANNULATION

anti-BRAF therapy, such as vemurafenib, the utility is limited for patients with ocular melanoma metastases who do not harbor such mutations.[18] Immunotherapy trials including checkpoint inhibitors do not usually include patients with ocular melanoma, and such drugs as selumetinib have shown only marginal benefit.[17,19] IHP has been shown to have significant survival benefit in patients with ocular melanoma (**Table 1**). However, PHP has been tested in a phase III trial against the best available care, which suggested an improvement in disease-free survival. Unfortunately, the data were not published because of concerns regarding data management during the trial.[20] An ongoing trial (SCANDIUM) is currently investigating the role of IHP in the management of metastatic ocular melanoma. The trial is a phase III randomized controlled trial with an expected accrual of 78 patients.[21]

HEPATOCELLULAR CARCINOMA

Although curative resection offers 5-year overall survival rates of 40%, only 10% to 30% of patients are potential resection candidates because hepatocellular carcinoma commonly develops in the backdrop of chronic liver disease, diminishing the salvage-able functional liver reserve.[22,23] Feldman and colleagues[24] investigated the efficacy of hyperthermic ILP using mephalan with or without TNF on primary hepatic malignancies (hepatocellular carcinoma and intrahepatic cholangiocarcinoma). Patients had advanced disease (average of 13 hepatic lesions per patient with a mean lesion size of 10 cm) and four out of nine patients had failed prior therapy. Partial radiographic response was observed in 67% of patients and toxicities were self-limited (**Table 2**). After promising results on an initial prospective study of reductive surgery followed by percutaneous IHP, Fukumoto and colleagues[25] reported results of the same treatment in more aggressive hepatocellular carcinoma (portal vein invasion, median tumor size of 8.3 cm, BCLC stage B or C) with background liver dysfunction (cirrhosis in 33.8%, chronic hepatitis in 60.3%) and achieved an objective response rate of 70.6% and median overall survival of 25 months.

LIVER METASTASES FROM COLORECTAL CANCER

Studies have shown that IHP in combination with systemic or hepatic arterial chemotherapy improves response rates and overall survival in patients with colorectal liver metastases (**Table 3**). Melphalan alone or in combination with TNF was the most commonly used drug, although recent trials have used oxaliplatin after favorable toxicity profiles in HAI trials.[26] Alexander and colleagues[27] looked at the use of IHP as a second-line therapy in patients who failed first-line chemotherapy with irinotecan, and the response rate was 60% with a median survival

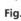

Fig. 3. (*A*) Vascular anatomy and technique of arterial cannulation when the left and right hepatic arteries and the splenic artery originate from celiac trunk. (*B*) Vascular anatomy and technique of arterial cannulation in cases of stenosis of common hepatic artery. (*C*) Vascular anatomy and technique of arterial cannulation when left hepatic artery originates from left gastric artery and gastroduodenal artery arises from the celiac trunk. CHA, common hepatic artery; CT, celiac trunk; GDA, gastroduodenal artery; LGA, left gastric artery; LHA, left hepatic artery; PHA, proper hepatic artery; PV, portal vein; RHA, right hepatic artery; SA, splenic artery; SMA, superior mesenteric artery. (*From* Oldhafer KJ, Lang H, Frerker M, et al. First experience and technical aspects of isolated liver perfusion for extensive liver metastasis. Surgery 1998;123(6):625; with permission.)

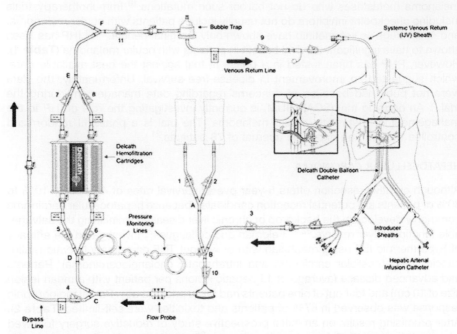

Fig. 4. Technique of percutaneous isolated hepatic perfusion. (*From* Yamamoto M, Zager JS. Isolated hepatic perfusion for metastatic melanoma. J Surg Oncol 2014;109(4):385; with permission.)

of 12 months. The role of IHP in the setting of evolving chemotherapy is still undefined. Sequencing of treatment of patients with unresectable metastatic disease with systemic chemotherapy could include liver perfusion after 2 to 3 months of systemic therapy with concurrent floxuridine and oxaliplatin in the postoperative setting. Alternatively, liver perfusion can be used in a salvage setting after completing first-line therapy.

Table 1
Selected studies of isolated hepatic perfusion in hepatic metastases of ocular melanoma

Author, Year	N	IHP Agent	ORR	Median OS (mo)
Alexander et al,[10] 2000	22	Melphalan with or without TNF	62%	11
Noter et al,[28] 2004	8	Melphalan with or without TNF	50%	9.9
Rizell et al,[29] 2008	27	Melphalan	70%	7.5
van Etten et al,[7] 2009	8	Melphalan (hypoxic IHP)	37%	11
Varghese et al,[30] 2010	17	Melphalan	50%	11.6
Pingpank et al,[20] 2010	93	Melphalan (percutaneous IHP)	34%	Not reported
Olofsson et al,[31] 2014	34	Melphalan	68%	24
Forster et al,[32] 2014	10	Melphalan (percutaneous IHP)	50%	12.6

Abbreviations: ORR, objective response rate; OS, overall survival.
   Data from Refs.[7,10,20,28–32]

Table 2
Selected studies of isolated hepatic perfusion in primary hepatocellular carcinoma

Author, Year	N	Patients	Cirrhosis	Treatment Received	ORR	Median OS
Fukumoto et al,[25] 2014	68	Multiple bilobar HCC	33.8%	Reductive hepatectomy + sequential PIHP with doxorubicin with or without mitomycin C	70.6%	25
Feldman et al,[24] 2004	9	Primary HCC and intrahepatic cholangiocarcinoma	0%	Hyperthermic IHP (melphalan with or without TNF)	67%	16.3 (mean)

Abbreviations: HCC, hepatocellular carcinoma; OS, overall survival; PIHP, percutaneous isolated hepatic perfusion.

Data from Feldman ED, Wu PC, Beresneva T, et al. Treatment of patients with unresectable primary hepatic malignancies using hyperthermic isolated hepatic perfusion. J Gastrointest Surg 2004;8(2):200–7; and Fukumoto T, Tominaga M, Kido M, et al. Long-term outcomes and prognostic factors with reductive hepatectomy and sequential percutaneous isolated hepatic perfusion for multiple bilobar hepatocellular carcinoma. Ann Surg Oncol 2014;21(3):971–8.

Table 3
Selected studies of isolated hepatic perfusion in liver metastases of colorectal origin

Author, Year	N	Study Details	IHP Agent	ORR	Median OS (mo)
Marinelli et al,[33] 1996	9	Phase 1 trial	Mitomycin C	22%	17
Vahrmeijer et al,[34] 2000	24	Phase 1 trial	Melphalan	29%	19
Alexander et al,[35] 2002	7	Failed systemic and HAI therapy	Hyperthermia Melphalan/TNF/both	71%	19.7
Rothbarth et al,[36] 2003	73	27% underwent adjuvant therapy after primary resection	High-dose melphalan	59%	28.8
Alexander et al,[27] 2005	25	Failed first-line irinotecan therapy	Hyperthermia Melphalan	60%	12
van Iersel et al,[37] 2007	30	53% received prior chemotherapy	Melphalan (IHP + HAI)	50%	27.8
van Iersel et al,[38] 2008	105	48% patients had pre-IHP chemotherapy	Melphalan	50%	24.8
Zeh et al,[39] 2009	13	Phase 1 trial for patients scheduled for HAI	Hyperthermia Oxaliplatin	66%	25
Alexander et al,[40] 2009	120	80% received prior chemotherapy	Hyperthermia Melphalan/TNF/both	61%	17.4
Magge et al,[41] 2013	12	Patients scheduled for HAI and with prior chemotherapy	Oxaliplatin + 5-FU	82%	Not reached[a]

Abbreviation: OS, overall survival.
[a] Median survival not reached at a median follow-up of 24 months.
Data from Refs.[27,33–41]

SUMMARY

IHP relies on vascular isolation of the liver to deliver cytotoxic therapy with limited systemic leakage. Although promising results have been seen in the management of ocular melanoma and colorectal liver metastases, its morbidity and the need for specialized expertise have limited widespread use of the therapy. Advances in perfusion techniques including PHP (or chemosaturation) and prophylactic perfusion may provide exciting new avenues.

SUPPLEMENTARY DATA

Supplementary data related to this article can be found at http://dx.doi.org/10.1016/j.suc.2015.12.005.

REFERENCES

1. Cercek A, D'Angelica M, Power D, et al. Floxuridine hepatic arterial infusion associated biliary toxicity is increased by concurrent administration of systemic bevacizumab. Ann Surg Oncol 2014;21(2):479–86.
2. van Iersel LB, Hoekman EJ, Gelderblom H, et al. Isolated hepatic perfusion with 200 mg melphalan for advanced noncolorectal liver metastases. Ann Surg Oncol 2008;15(7):1891–8.
3. Ausman RK. Development of a technic for isolated perfusion of the liver. N Y State J Med 1961;61:3993–7.
4. Skibba JL, Quebbeman EJ. Tumoricidal effects and patient survival after hyperthermic liver perfusion. Arch Surg 1986;121(11):1266–71.
5. Runia RD, de Brauw LM, Kothuis BJ, et al. Continuous measurement of leakage during isolated liver perfusion with a radiotracer. Int J Rad Appl Instrum B 1987; 14(2):113–8.
6. van Etten B, Brunstein F, van IMG, et al. Isolated hypoxic hepatic perfusion with orthograde or retrograde flow in patients with irresectable liver metastases using percutaneous balloon catheter techniques: a phase I and II study. Ann Surg Oncol 2004;11(6):598–605.
7. van Etten B, de Wilt JH, Brunstein F, et al. Isolated hypoxic hepatic perfusion with melphalan in patients with irresectable ocular melanoma metastases. Eur J Surg Oncol 2009;35(5):539–45.
8. Verhoef C, de Wilt JH, Brunstein F, et al. Isolated hypoxic hepatic perfusion with retrograde outflow in patients with irresectable liver metastases; a new simplified technique in isolated hepatic perfusion. Ann Surg Oncol 2008;15(5):1367–74.
9. Alexander HR Jr, Bartlett DL, Libutti SK, et al. Isolated hepatic perfusion with tumor necrosis factor and melphalan for unresectable cancers confined to the liver. J Clin Oncol 1998;16(4):1479–89.
10. Alexander HR, Libutti SK, Bartlett DL, et al. A phase I-II study of isolated hepatic perfusion using melphalan with or without tumor necrosis factor for patients with ocular melanoma metastatic to liver. Clin Cancer Res 2000;6(8):3062–70.
11. Yamamoto M, Zager JS. Isolated hepatic perfusion for metastatic melanoma. J Surg Oncol 2014;109(4):383–8.
12. Deneve JL, Choi J, Gonzalez RJ, et al. Chemosaturation with percutaneous hepatic perfusion for unresectable isolated hepatic metastases from sarcoma. Cardiovasc Intervent Radiol 2012;35(6):1480–7.
13. Reddy SK, Kesmodel SB, Alexander HR Jr. Isolated hepatic perfusion for patients with liver metastases. Ther Adv Med Oncol 2014;6(4):180–94.

14. Heather A, Lillemoe HRA Jr. Current status of percutaneous hepatic perfusion as regional treatment for patients with unresectable hepatic metastases: a review. Am Oncology and Hematology Rev 2014;15–23.
15. Kurosaki I, Kawachi Y, Nihei K, et al. Liver perfusion chemotherapy with 5-fluorouracil followed by systemic gemcitabine administration for resected pancreatic cancer: preliminary results of a prospective phase 2 study. Pancreas 2009; 38(2):161–7.
16. Ishikawa O, Ohigashi H, Sasaki Y, et al. Liver perfusion chemotherapy via both the hepatic artery and portal vein to prevent hepatic metastasis after extended pancreatectomy for adenocarcinoma of the pancreas. Am J Surg 1994;168(4): 361–4.
17. Carvajal RD, Sosman JA, Quevedo JF, et al. Effect of selumetinib vs chemotherapy on progression-free survival in uveal melanoma: a randomized clinical trial. JAMA 2014;311(23):2397–405.
18. Chapman PB, Hauschild A, Robert C, et al. Improved survival with vemurafenib in melanoma with BRAF V600E mutation. N Engl J Med 2011;364(26):2507–16.
19. Robert C, Dummer R, Gutzmer R, et al. Selumetinib plus dacarbazine versus placebo plus dacarbazine as first-line treatment for BRAF-mutant metastatic melanoma: a phase 2 double-blind randomised study. Lancet Oncol 2013;14(8): 733–40.
20. Pingpank JF, Faries MB, Zager JS, et al. A phase III random assignment trial comparing percutaneous hepatic perfusion with melphalan (PHP-mel) to standard of care for patients with hepatic metastases from metastatic ocular or cutaneous melanoma. 2010 ASCO Annual Meeting. June 4–8, 2010.
21. Olofsson R, Ny L, Eilard MS, et al. Isolated hepatic perfusion as a treatment for uveal melanoma liver metastases (the SCANDIUM trial): study protocol for a randomized controlled trial. Trials 2014;15:317.
22. Llovet JM, Schwartz M, Mazzaferro V. Resection and liver transplantation for hepatocellular carcinoma. Semin Liver Dis 2005;25(2):181–200.
23. Schwartz M, Roayaie S, Konstadoulakis M. Strategies for the management of hepatocellular carcinoma. Nat Clin Pract Oncol 2007;4(7):424–32.
24. Feldman ED, Wu PC, Beresneva T, et al. Treatment of patients with unresectable primary hepatic malignancies using hyperthermic isolated hepatic perfusion. J Gastrointest Surg 2004;8(2):200–7.
25. Fukumoto T, Tominaga M, Kido M, et al. Long-term outcomes and prognostic factors with reductive hepatectomy and sequential percutaneous isolated hepatic perfusion for multiple bilobar hepatocellular carcinoma. Ann Surg Oncol 2014; 21(3):971–8.
26. Bartlett DL, Libutti SK, Figg WD, et al. Isolated hepatic perfusion for unresectable hepatic metastases from colorectal cancer. Surgery 2001;129(2):176–87.
27. Alexander HR Jr, Libutti SK, Pingpank JF, et al. Isolated hepatic perfusion for the treatment of patients with colorectal cancer liver metastases after irinotecan-based therapy. Ann Surg Oncol 2005;12(2):138–44.
28. Noter SL, Rothbarth J, Pijl ME, et al. Isolated hepatic perfusion with high-dose melphalan for the treatment of uveal melanoma metastases confined to the liver. Melanoma Res 2004;14(1):67–72.
29. Rizell M, Mattson J, Cahlin C, et al. Isolated hepatic perfusion for liver metastases of malignant melanoma. Melanoma Res 2008;18(2):120–6.
30. Varghese S, Xu H, Bartlett D, et al. Isolated hepatic perfusion with high-dose melphalan results in immediate alterations in tumor gene expression in patients with metastatic ocular melanoma. Ann Surg Oncol 2010;17(7):1870–7.

31. Olofsson R, Cahlin C, All-Ericsson C, et al. Isolated hepatic perfusion for ocular melanoma metastasis: registry data suggests a survival benefit. Ann Surg Oncol 2014;21(2):466–72.
32. Forster MR, Rashid OM, Perez MC, et al. Chemosaturation with percutaneous hepatic perfusion for unresectable metastatic melanoma or sarcoma to the liver: a single institution experience. J Surg Oncol 2014;109(5):434–9.
33. Marinelli A, de Brauw LM, Beerman H, et al. Isolated liver perfusion with mitomycin C in the treatment of colorectal cancer metastases confined to the liver. Jpn J Clin Oncol 1996;26(5):341–50.
34. Vahrmeijer AL, van Dierendonck JH, Keizer HJ, et al. Increased local cytostatic drug exposure by isolated hepatic perfusion: a phase I clinical and pharmacologic evaluation of treatment with high dose melphalan in patients with colorectal cancer confined to the liver. Br J Cancer 2000;82(9):1539–46.
35. Alexander HR Jr, Libutti SK, Bartlett DL, et al. Hepatic vascular isolation and perfusion for patients with progressive unresectable liver metastases from colorectal carcinoma refractory to previous systemic and regional chemotherapy. Cancer 2002;95(4):730–6.
36. Rothbarth J, Pijl ME, Vahrmeijer AL, et al. Isolated hepatic perfusion with highdose melphalan for the treatment of colorectal metastasis confined to the liver. Br J Surg 2003;90(11):1391–7.
37. van Iersel LB, Verlaan MR, Vahrmeijer AL, et al. Hepatic artery infusion of highdose melphalan at reduced flow during isolated hepatic perfusion for the treatment of colorectal metastases confined to the liver: a clinical and pharmacologic evaluation. Eur J Surg Oncol 2007;33(7):874–81.
38. van Iersel LB, Gelderblom H, Vahrmeijer AL, et al. Isolated hepatic melphalan perfusion of colorectal liver metastases: outcome and prognostic factors in 154 patients. Ann Oncol 2008;19(6):1127–34.
39. Zeh HJ 3rd, Brown CK, Holtzman MP, et al. A phase I study of hyperthermic isolated hepatic perfusion with oxaliplatin in the treatment of unresectable liver metastases from colorectal cancer. Ann Surg Oncol 2009;16(2):385–94.
40. Alexander HR Jr, Bartlett DL, Libutti SK, et al. Analysis of factors associated with outcome in patients undergoing isolated hepatic perfusion for unresectable liver metastases from colorectal center. Ann Surg Oncol 2009;16(7):1852–9.
41. Magge D, Zureikat AH, Bartlett DL, et al. A phase I trial of isolated hepatic perfusion (IHP) using 5-FU and oxaliplatin in patients with unresectable isolated liver metastases from colorectal cancer. Ann Surg Oncol 2013;20(7):2180–7.

Transarterial Therapy for Colorectal Liver Metastases

Neal Bhutiani, MD[a], Robert C.G. Martin II, MD, PhD[a,b],*

KEYWORDS

- Hepatic arterial therapy (HAT) • Chemoembolization • Hepatic artery infusion (HAI)
- Colorectal liver metastases • Surgical resection • Yttrium-90
- Drug-eluting beads (DEB)

KEY POINTS

- Hepatic arterial therapy (HAT) represents a minimally invasive fluoroscopy-guided trans-arterial catheter-directed therapy that has been used for the treatment of colorectal liver metastases; its primary goal is high-dose local regional drug delivery. Therapy-associated complication rates are low.
- New HAT-drug-eluting bead (DEB) technologies lead to significantly increased cytotoxic drug concentrations in the target liver metastases with lower systemic toxicity than systemic treatments.
- Repeat HAT-DEB procedures augment tumor response to treatment. Repeat Yttrium-90 treatments should be performed with the understanding that repeat treatments increase the possibility of producing durable refractory radiation-induced liver dysfunction.
- HAT may augment the results of first-line systemic chemotherapy in the treatment of patients with unresectable colorectal liver metastases. It may represent a valuable tool in the preoperative management of potential surgical candidates as a method for downsizing and for early conversion to resectability without adverse effects associated with systemic chemotherapy.
- HAT could potentially be used after surgery or ablative therapy to prevent local recurrence with the aim of improving overall survival without major side effects.

BACKGROUND

Colorectal liver metastases (CLM) represent the fourth most common malignancy, and the second most common cause of cancer-related death in Western countries. The presence and extent of liver metastases are major prognostic factors with respect

Disclosures: The authors have no disclosures or conflicts of interest.
[a] Division of Surgical Oncology, Department of Surgery, University of Louisville, Louisville, KY, USA; [b] Division of Surgical Oncology, Upper Gastrointestinal and Hepato-Pancreatico-Biliary Clinic, 315 East Broadway, #311, Louisville, KY 40202, USA
* Corresponding author.
E-mail address: Robert.Martin@louisville.edu

to overall survival (OS). At the time of diagnosis of colorectal cancer, 25% to 50% of patients exhibit liver metastases. Furthermore, up to 80% of patients diagnosed with colorectal cancer will develop liver metastases on follow-up evaluation. Because the microstructure of the liver is an effective tumor cell barrier, early distant metastasis due to hematogenous spread is rare. A variety of therapies exist for the treatment of CLM—surgical resection, systemic chemotherapy (CTx), molecular substances, and local ablative treatments. What constitutes the optimal treatment strategy for a given patient depends on tumor stage, mutation status, sequence and pattern of metastases, performance status, and patient preference.[1,2]

Surgical resection is currently accepted as optimal first-line treatment. Resectability with curative intent can be characterized by 5 isolated metastases per liver lobe or less, at least 2 tumor-free adjacent liver segments, and a volume of the liver remnant greater than 20% by reference to the initial liver volume.[3,4] At the time of diagnosis, less than 20% of patients have resectable CLM,[3,4] and 60% to 80% of those undergoing resection will develop recurrent colorectal metastases at follow-up, of which half have a recurrence within the liver.[5,6]

The greater than 80% of patients who do not qualify for CLM resection at the time of diagnosis receive CTx and/or biologic therapy according to the current available European guidelines.[1] Currently, 5-fluorouracil (5-FU) -based regimens consisting of 5-FU, irinotecan, and/or oxaliplatin (eg, FOLFOX, FOLFIRI, and FOLFOXIRI) result in response rates and median OS of 40% to 57% and 15 to 20 months, respectively, but reported 5-year OS rates are still close to 0%.[1,2,7–12] On average, the median OS of patients with stage IV colorectal cancer approximates 21 months with multiagent chemotherapy (intravenous 5-FU plus irinotecan/oxaliplatin). The introduction of molecular substances such as antiepidermal growth factor receptor (EGFR) and anti-vascular endothelial growth factor (VEGF) antibodies have further improved outcomes after administration of systemic therapies. Controlled trials showed that the addition of a monoclonal antibody to CTx regimens increased OS to more than 24 months.[1,13]

Current evidence suggests that CTx with or without the use of biologic agents followed by liver resection is safe and effective for selected patients with initially unresectable CLM.[14–18] Use of hepatic arterial therapy (HAT) toward the same end represents an enticing concept, because it allows for markedly higher concentration of drugs or radiation therapy within target liver area, while decreasing the systemic toxicity and adverse effects of CTx or external beam radiation therapy.[19]

TRANSARTERIAL HEPATIC THERAPY
Rationale

Although normal liver parenchyma is largely supplied by the portal vein, malignant liver tumors derive their blood supply from hepatic arterial branches.[20] Thus, transarterial drug delivery into the liver allows a considerably increased local drug concentration/radiation dosage compared with CTx/external beam radiation therapy. At the same time, healthy nonaffected liver parenchyma can be spared, and the liver toxicity that is observed after systemic applications is avoided or at least minimized. Chemotherapy-associated liver injury (CALI; eg, sinusoidal obstruction syndrome [SOS] and nonalcoholic steatohepatitis [NASH])—are relevant limitations to cytotoxic therapy that impact preoperative treatment plans. Hepatic steatosis without inflammation (simple steatosis) may occur with chemotherapy. SOS may occur with oxaliplatin treatment, with increased severity associated with prolonged treatments (>6 cycles). Bevacizumab can be used safely in the preoperative setting when discontinued at least 5 weeks before liver resection and seems to decrease the incidence and severity of sinusoidal injury after oxaliplatin therapy.[21]

For patients with unresectable liver-only metastases, a response to chemotherapy/ radiotherapy could enable resection and should be considered an initial treatment goal. For such patients, oxaliplatin- or irinotecan-based combinatorial regimens represent first-line systemic treatment. The addition of bevacizumab may increase response rates and possibly reduce the risk of CALI.[2] In KRAS wild-type tumors, anti-EGFR antibodies may also augment response rates and improve survival.[2,22]

Unlike systemic administration of chemotherapy, transarterial administration does not force drugs to undergo first-pass metabolism by hepatocytes before reaching their targets. As a result, lower volumes of drugs can result in higher drug concentration within target liver lesions while resulting in less systemic toxicity.[19]

Because angiogenesis is integral to hematogenous spread of primary tumors as well as growth of distant metastases, epidermal growth factor, VEGF, angiopoietin, and cyclo-oxygenase all represent potential targets to modulate the arterial blood supply of CLM. The exact role of these pathways and targeted biologic therapies with respect to treatment of colorectal cancer remains nebulous. Although cetuximab and bevacizumab have been used in the treatment of ependymoma and glioblastoma, respectively, no groups have reported transarterial use of biologic agents in treatment of CLM.[23,24]

Reported Techniques

Because of the lack of an evidence-based treatment standard, multiple chemotherapeutics and embolic agents are used in different combinations and doses.[25–27] Historically, transarterial therapies have been classified as (1) conventional transarterial chemoembolization (cTACE), (2) degradable starch microscophere chemoembolization (DSM-TACE), and (3) hepatic arterial drug-eluting bead therapy (HAT-DEB). Currently, the latter two modalities comprise the majority of the transarterial treatments for CLM.

cTACE involves direct injection of chemotherapeutics into the hepatic arterial system followed by infusion of a vascular occlusive agent such as gelfoam to induce embolization. For DSM-TACE, one or more chemotherapeutics (eg, mitomycin C, gemcitabine, and/or irinotecan) are mixed with DSMs (allowing both to be infused simultaneously), or DSMs are used after treatment to induce embolization.[28,29] In both methods, solutions are injected directly into the right and left hepatic arteries after gaining access to the arterial circulation via the femoral artery. The solution is injected into target areas over a period of approximately 10 minutes. Preinfusion embolization of gastric or duodenal arterial branches is performed in situations whereby there is concern for infusion overflow into these vessels. In cTACE, infusion of a solution containing a vascular occlusive agent is then performed; that agent is a DSM in DSM-TACE. cTACE results in permanent arterial embolization, whereas DSM-TACE induces only temporary vascular occusion because human serum amylase dissolves the DSMs. In Europe, available DSMs (EmboCept S; PharmaCept, Berlin, Germany) have a mean microsphere diameter of 50 μm and a recanalization time of about 60 minutes. **Table 1** lists various published studies examining the safety and efficacy of various different cTACE and DSM-TACE regimens.

Recently, HAT-DEB has become an increasingly popular embolization technique. The concept is based on loading permanent microspheres with a cytotoxic drug such as irinotecan and doxorubicin. After intra-arterial injection of DEBs, a controlled drug release occurs over a period of hours to days within the target tissue.[38] Because the type and dose of the chemotherapeutic can be selected individually and combined

Table 1
Original studies of safety and efficacy of conventional transarterial chemoembolization and degradable starch microsphere for colorectal liver metastases

Reference	Patients (n)	Therapy Stage (1st Line, 2nd Line, 3rd Line, Beyond 3rd Line)	Chemoembolics (Embolic Agents + Chemotherapeutics)	Median Follow-Up (mo)	Progression-free Survival (mo)	Median OS (mo)
Ceelen et al,[30] 1996	14 9	NR	Lipiodol and gelfoam + cisplatin + surgery Surgery alone	15.5 17.5	NR	NR
Tellez et al,[31] 1998	30	NR	Bovine collagen material + cisplatin, doxorubicin, and mitomycin C	NR	NR	8.6
Leichman et al,[32] 1999	31	NR	Collagen suspension + doxorubicin, mitomycin C, and cisplatin	NR	8	14
Müller et al,[33] 2001	103 —	Beyond 2nd line	Group A: HAI 5-FU × 4 d; HAI granulocyte-macrophage colony-stimulating factor (GM-CSF) × 2 d; cTACE lipiodol, gelfoam, melphalan × 1 d Group B: HAI 5-FU/leucovorin/GM-CSF × 2 d; cTACE lipiodol, gelfoam, melphalan × 1 d	42 —	7 8	17 28
Salman et al,[34] 2002	26 24	2nd line	Polyvinyl alcohol (PVA) PVA AND 5-FU + IFN	NR	4 3	10 15
Tsuchiya et al,[29] 2007	27	NR	DSMs + irinotecan and mitomycin C	NR	NR	NR
Vogl et al,[35] 2009	463	2nd line	Lipiodol and DSMs + mitomycin C alone (52.5%), mitomycin C, and gemcitabine (33.0%) or mitomycin C and irinotecan (14.5%)	NR	NR	14
Albert et al,[36] 2011	121	Beyond 2nd line	Lipiodol and PVA + mitomycin C, doxorubicin, cisplatin	NR	3	9
Nishiofuku et al,[28] 2013	24	Beyond 2nd line	DSMs + cisplatin powder	17.4	8.8	21.1
Gruber-Roth et al,[37] 2014	564	NR	Lipiodol AND mitomycin C OR mitomycin C + irinotecan OR mitomycin C + irinotecan + cisplatin	NR	NR	14.3

Data from Refs.[28–37]

with a particular microsphere size and volume, HAT-DEB is gaining significant popularity among HATs in the treatment of CLM.

Tables 2 and **3** provide an overview of (1) chemotherapeutics and biologic agents available for transarterial use and (2) embolic agents used for HAT. With respect to tumor response, it remains unclear which specific combination of drug and embolic agent should be used for an optimal treatment result. The predefined calibration of microsphere size allows an exact control of the embolization depth, whereby the occluded vessel diameters correspond to the nominal diameter of the microsphere. Only randomized controlled studies can determine which chemoembolics result in the best tumor response rates. In contrast to permanent embolic agents, DSMs result in reduced ischemic effects and, therefore, less neoangiogenesis. Future studies examining the use of angiogenesis inhibitors such as bevacizumab in conjunction with HAT are warranted to further address the issue of neoangiogenesis in the setting of HAT.

HEPATIC ARTERIAL DRUG-ELUTING BEAD THERAPY
Rationale

HAT-DEB is a minimally invasive image-guided transarterial liver-directed therapy. After lobar, selective, or superselective injection of one or more chemotherapeutic drugs and one or more embolic agents into the arterial blood supply to liver metastases, combined antitumoral effects (chemotoxicity and ischemia) are observed. The use of an embolic agent before and/or after transarterial drug application results in a reduction of the arterial flow, combining reduced chemotherapeutic clearance with decreased tumor perfusion; however, this can lead to great toxicity and worse adverse effects.[19,58] Some investigators think that achieving stasis for metastatic colorectal disease can lead to enhanced outcomes; however, the degree of stasis has never proven to be a predictor of outcomes.[4,30,58–61] According to the current guidelines, and in contrast to hepatocellular carcinoma, HAT-DEB is still *not* recommended as a standard therapy for CLM. Nevertheless, use of this technology for treatment of CLM is increasing, and recent studies have shown efficacy of repetitive HAT-DEB in patients with liver-dominant colorectal metastases after failure of surgical, ablative, and/or systemic therapies.

Technique

HAT-DEB is indicated for patients with a life expectancy greater than 3 months and an appropriate health status (Eastern Cooperative Oncology Group status $\leq$2).[20,25] Patients must have adequate liver function: bilirubin less than 3 mg/dL, albumin greater than 3 g/dL, and international normalized ratio >1.6. Preinterventional staging (ie, <1 month from treatment) with high-quality thin-cut triphasic contrast-enhanced computed tomography (CT) or dynamic MRI before conventional catheter angiographies are necessary to adequately assess the biology of the disease and to ensure liver-only or liver-dominant disease. Peri-interventional medications include analgesics and antiemetics. In cases of large tumor volumes, intravenous corticosteroids (eg, dexamethasone 250 mg) can effectively treat the tumor edema after HAT-DEB. Prophylactic antibiotics to prevent bloodstream and/or intrahepatic infections are recommended only in high-risk patients.[62]

The correct choice of the catheter position for drug delivery as well as the DEB endpoint are key factors for safe and effective treatments, and both must consider the amount of drug to be delivered (ie, number of vials of beads), size, location, and vascularization of the liver metastases. Treatment via the right or left hepatic artery

Table 2
Chemotherapeutics (including molecular substances) available for transarterial use

Type	Maximum Single Dose	Major Indications	Major Toxicity and Side Effects	Reference Study for Transarterial Use	Reference Study for Colorectal Liver Metastases
Bevacizumab	15 mg/kg body weight	Colorectal cancer, lung cancer, breast cancer, ovarian cancer, renal cancer	Hypertension, fatigue, diarrhea, proteinuria, thromboemboli, hemorrhage, bowel perforation	Burkhardt et al,[24] 2012	Glimelius et al,[39] 2012
Carboplatin	300 mg/m[2] body surface	Lung cancer, breast cancer, ovarian cancer, testicular cancer	Nausea and vomitus, tinnitus, allergy, abdominal pain, diarrhea, constipation, neurotoxicity, bone marrow suppression	Barletta et al,[40] 2006	Shimonov et al,[41] 2005
Caelyx (liposomal doxorubicin)	30 mg/m[2] body surface	See doxorubicin	See doxorubicin	Gonzalez Cao et al,[42] 2006	Moroney et al,[43] 2012
Cetuximab	100 mg/m[2] body surface	Colorectal cancer, head and neck cancer	Acnelike skin reaction, pruritus, hypomagnesemia, fever, shivering, vertigo, dyspnea	Rajappa et al,[23] 2010	Glimelius et al,[39] 2012
Cisplatin	100 mg/m[2] body surface	Head and neck cancer, lung cancer, ovarian cancer, cervix carcinoma, chorion carcinoma, testicular cancer, bladder cancer	Bone marrow suppression, anemia, hyperuremia, fever, heart arrhythmia, dyspnea, pneumonia, allergy	Mancini et al,[44] 2003	Gruber-Routh et al,[37] 2014
Doxorubicin	50 mg/m[2] body surface	Lung cancer, breast cancer, ovarian cancer, lymphoma	Bone marrow suppression, nephrotoxicity, cardiotoxicity,[a] skin ulceration	Liu et al,[45] 2015	Albert et al,[36] 2011
Docetaxel	75 mg/m[2] body surface	Head and neck cancer, lung cancer, breast cancer, ovarian cancer, prostate cancer, gastric cancer	Bone marrow suppression, fever, neurotoxicity, diarrhea, alopecia, hepatotoxicity, heart arrhythmia	Nakanishi et al,[46] 2012	Seki & Hori,[47] 2011

Drug	Dose	Cancer types	Side effects	Reference	Reference
Epirubicin	75 mg/m² body surface	Lung cancer, breast cancer, ovarian cancer, gastric cancer, bladder cancer, lymphoma, sarcoma	Bone marrow suppression, alopecia, stomatitis, abdominal pain, nausea, and vomitus, diarrhea, anorexia	Tawada et al,[48] 2015	Fiorentini et al,[49] 2004
Fotemustin	100 mg/m² body surface	Melanoma, lymphoma	Bone marrow suppression, fatigue, nausea, vomitus, and alopecia	Edelhauser et al,[50] 2012	Hartmann et al,[51] 1997
Gemcitabine	1000 mg/m² body surface	Lung cancer breast cancer, ovarian cancer, pancreatic cancer, cholangiocellular carcinoma, sarcoma	Bone marrow suppression skin reaction, alopecia, stomatitis, hepatotoxicity, neurotoxicity, nephrotoxicity	Vogl et al,[52] 2008	Gruber-Routh et al,[37] 2014
Irinotecan	200 mg/m² body surface	Lung cancer, cervix carcinoma, esophagus cancer, gastric cancer, pancreatic cancer, cholangiocellular carcinoma, sarcoma	Bradycardia, lacrimation flush, diarrhea, hyperhidrosis, bone marrow suppression alopecia, nephrotoxicity, hepatotoxicity	Tsuchiya et al,[29] 2007	Gruber-Routh et al,[37] 2014
Mitomycin C	10 mg/m² body surface	Colorectal cancer, head and neck cancer, lung cancer, breast cancer, cervix carcinoma, esophagus cancer, gastric cancer, pancreatic cancer, hepatocellular carcinoma, bladder cancer	Skin necrosis, lung fibrosis, nephrotoxicity, bone marrow suppression, skin reaction, nausea and vomitus, cardiotoxicity	Vogl et al,[52] 2008	—
Mitoxantrone	14 mg/m² body surface	Breast cancer, prostate cancer, lymphoma, multiple sclerosis	Nausea and vomitus, anorexia, alopecia, stomatitis, bone	Boulin et al,[53] 2011	Link et al,[54] 2001

(continued on next page)

Table 2
(continued)

Type	Maximum Single Dose	Major Indications	Major Toxicity and Side Effects	Reference Study for Transarterial Use	Reference Study for Colorectal Liver Metastases
			marrow suppression, cardiotoxicity		
Oxaliplatin	660–80 mg/m² body surface	Colorectal cancer	Diarrhea, nausea and vomitus, bone marrow suppression, stomatitis, nephrotoxicity, neurotoxicity	Chen et al,[55] 2014	Nordlinger et al,[15] 2008
Paclitaxel	175 mg/m² body surface	Lung cancer (non-small cell lung cancer), breast cancer, ovarian cancer, prostate cancer	Bone marrow suppression, neurotoxicity, myalgia, alopecia, diarrhea nausea and vomitus	Koga et al,[56] 2003	Tsimberidou et al,[57] 2011

According to the guidelines, chemotherapeutic standards in the different lines for CLM include FOLFOX (1. folin acid [=leucovorin], 2. 5-FU, and 3. Oxaliplatin), FOLFIRI (1. folin acid [=leucovorin], 2. 5-FU, and 3. irinotecan), FOLFOXIRI (1. folin acid [=leucovorin], 2. 5-FU, 3. oxaliplatin, and 4. Irinotecan), FOLFIRINOX (1. folin acid [=leucovorin], 2. 5-FU, 3. irinotecan, and 4. oxaliplatin), Xelox (1. capectitabine [Xeloda; Roche, Basel, Switzerland] and 2. Oxaliplatin) and XELIRI (1. capecitabine [Xeloda; Roche] and 2. irinotecan); molecular substances are frequently used; the anti-EGFR antibodies Cetuximab (Erbitux; Imclone Systems, Bristol-Meyers Squibb, New York, NY, USA) and panitumumab (Vectibix; Amgen, Thousand Oaks, CA, USA) to block the growth receptor cascade as well as the anti-VEGF antibodies bevacizumab (Avastin; Roche) and regorafenib (Stivarga; Bayer, Berlin, Germany) to block neoangiogenes. For CLM, all relevant chemotherapeutics and molecular substances are available either for transarterial use (Oxaliplatin and irinotecan as well as Cetuximab [Erbitux; Imclone Systems, Bristol-Meyers Squibb]) and antibodies bevacizumab (Avastin; Roche) or for oral use (leucovorin, 5-FU, capecitabine (Xeloda; Roche) and the anti-VEGF antibody regorafenib (Stivarga; Bayer) (see also **Tables 4 and 5**).

a Dexrazoxane can used as cardioprotective medication in palliative patients.

Data from Refs.[15,23,24,29,36,37,39–57]

Table 3
Embolic agents used for hepatic arterial therapy

Product	Material	Type of HAT (cTACE, DSM-TACE, DEB-TACE, Y-90)	Sizes (μm)
Bead block (BTG, London, UK)	PVA	cTACE	100–300 or 300–500
Contour-SE (Boston Scientific, Marlborough, MA, USA)	PVA	cTACE	45–15, 150–250, or 250–355
DC Bead (BTG)	PVA loaded with irinotecan or doxocubicin	HAT-DEB	≈75, 100–300, 30–500
EmboCept S (PharmaCept)	Starch	DSM-DEB	≈50
EmboSphere (Merit Medical, South Jordan, UT, USA)	Tris-acryl gelatin	cTACE	40–120,100–300, or 300–500
Embozene Microspheres (CeloNova BioSciences, San Antonio, TX, USA)	Hydrogel core with a biocompatible nonocoat consisting of Polyzene-F	cTACE	40, 785, 100, 250, or 500
Gelatine sponge (Spongostan; Johnson & Johnson, New Brunswick, NJ, USA)	Gelatin	cTACE	Dependent on its formulation (pieces of ≈500 m, ≈1000, or ≈2000)
Gelfoam (Pfizer, New York, NY, USA)	Gelatin powder	cTACE	≈50
HepaSphere (Merit Medical)	PVA loaded with irinotecan or doxocubicin	HAT-DEB	30–60, 50–100, 100–150, or 150–200
Lipiodol (Laboratoire Guerbet, Aulnay-sous-Bois, France)	Iodized poppy seed oil	cTACE	Dependent on its formulation (droplets of 15–200)
LifePearl (Terumo, Tokyo, Japan)	Polyethylene glycol with sulfonide bonding loaded with irinotecan or doxocubicin	HAT-DEB	100, 200, or 300
PVA (Cook, Bloomington, IN, USA)	PVA	cTACE	90–180, 180–300, or 300–500
Spherex (Pharmacia AB, Stockholm, Sweden)	Starch	DSM-TACE	≈40
TANDEM (CeloNova BioSciences)	Hydrogel core with a biocompatible nonocoat consisting of Polyzene-F loaded with irinotecan or doxocubicin	HAT-DEB	40, 75, or 100
TheraSphere (Biocompatibles UK, Surrey, UK)	Y-90 impregnated glass	Y-90 radioembolization	20–30
SIR-Spheres (Sirtex Medical, Woburn, MA, USA)	Y-90 impregnated resin	Y-90 Radioembolization	20–60

is used for selective targeting of either the right or the left lobe of the liver.[60,61,63] Diagnostic angiography and intraprocedural cone-beam CT can help delineate the anatomy of all tumor-feeding arteries and allow operators to navigate the microcatheter accordingly. Catheter location is confirmed intraprocedurally using fluoroscopy. The selection of the adequate chemoembolics is another key and depends on several parameters (see later discussion).

After HAT-DEB, patients are monitored for treatment effect and disease recurrence through the use of clinical examination, blood tests, and contrast-enhanced imaging. Subsequent HAT-DEB treatments are commonly required and should be scheduled in conjunction with the off-week of the patient's systemic therapy, usually 4 to 6 weeks, with exact timing based on patient tolerance to combined therapy. Commonly, the right lobe is treated twice and the left lobe is treated once (over a 10- to 12-week time interval) before repeat response imaging is obtained. Official recommendations such as the Standards of Practice Guidelines of the Cardiovascular and Interventional Radiological Society of Europe can help to further standardize HAT-DEB for CLM.[64]

Technical Success, Complications, and Adverse Effects

In key studies of HAT-DEB for CLM, technical success—successful catheterization with subsequent selective/superselective deposition of chemoembolic agents within the target region—is close to 100%. Dissection or thrombosis of the hepatic artery is extremely rare.[20] Temporary vasospasm during catheterization is common but can be treated effectively with vasodilators (eg, repetitive transarterial bolus injections of 0.25 mg nitroglycerin). Arterioportal and arteriovenous shunts should be occluded to avoid the risk for nontarget embolization. After one or more HAT-DEB cycles, the chemoembolics can alter the larger tumor-feeding arteries. Very small microspheres (eg, irinotecan-loaded microspheres with a diameter of 40 ± 10 µm) can then be used to embolize the diffuse tumor vasculature together with protective temporary embolization of the nontarget liver tissue using DSMs if necessary.[65]

The "post-embolization syndrome," a relatively frequent side effect of HAT-DEB, comprises one or more of the following: fatigue, nausea, vomiting, mild fever, and laboratory values indicative of tumor necrosis. A recent review compared relevant toxicities of HAT-DEB, cTACE, CTx, and hepatic artery infusion (HAI).[20] For HAT-DEB, cited toxicities were nausea/vomiting (2%–55%), hypertension (4%–80%), liver dysfunction/failure (6%), cholecystitis (1%), gastritis (1%), anorexia (3%), abdominal pain (0%–57%), hematologic toxicity (9%–90%), fatigue (60%), and alopecia (5%–35%). For cTACE, toxicities comprised nausea/vomiting (18%–83%), fever (13%–83%), fatigue (24%–60%), abdominal pain (82%–100%), liver dysfunction/failure (13%–33%), gastritis (17%), neurotoxicity (45%), diarrhea (9%–31%), hematologic toxicity (13%–33%), and renal failure (4%). Finally, for CTx and HAI, cited toxicities were chemical hepatitis (7%–15% and 4%–79%, respectively), biliary sclerosis (not reported [NR] and 4% to 21%, respectively), peptic/duodenal ulceration (0%–3% and 0%–17%, respectively), gastritis/duodenitis (1%–7% and 1%–21%, respectively), diarrhea (16%–70% and 1%–44%, respectively), nausea/vomitus (35%–46% and 21%–61%, respectively), and stomatitis (14%–87% and 0%–76%, respectively).

Major complications of HAT-DEB such as liver abscess and tumor rupture are rare. Results of nontarget embolization (eg, pancreatitis or cholecystitis) can be avoided by sufficient evaluation of the arterial anatomy (eg, by using high-resolution angiography or intraprocedural cone-beam CT) and by using accepted hepatic embolization techniques (eg, flow-mediated embolization or balloon protection).[25,58] In experienced centers, the overall major and minor complication rates during and after HAT-DEB are generally very low.[25–27,58] The procedure can be regarded as safe and well-tolerated provided standard catheterization and modern imaging techniques are used and the appropriate perioperative supporting medications are consistently administered.

Oncologic Outcomes

To assess the reported outcomes of HAT in patients with CLM, the authors reviewed articles describing HAT-DEB for CLM (search strategy: MEDLINE = database, "drug eluting beads + colorectal liver metastases" = search term for primary selections, cross references for additional selections). The original studies identified along with their relevant characteristics and disease-free and OS figures are detailed in **Table 4**. In summary, HAT-DEB for CLM is usually performed after failure of at least one and, more often, more systemic and/or surgical therapies. Otherwise, it is performed concomitantly with systemic therapy or in the perioperative period after hepatic resection. HAT-DEB regimens can produce a tumor response rate of 89%, a progression-free survival (PFS) rate of 13.6 months, and an OS of greater than 28 months.

Since 2011, several review articles addressing HAT-DEB for CLM have been published.[13,20,26,27,78–81] Some investigators emphasize an increased survival benefit and conclude that HAT-DEB should be implemented earlier in treatment algorithms for CLM, namely, after patients fail first- and second-line systemic therapy.[13] Others, however, state that the use of HAT-DEB cannot be definitively recommended for unresectable CLM because of the lack of prospective, randomized trials that would allow fair comparison with systemic regimens.[26] Regardless of their recommendations, all investigators acknowledge the appeal of evolving HAT-DEB techniques but recognize the lack of prospective clinical data from randomized trials.[4,10,26–29,38,58] They also agree that the safety and toxicity profile of HAT-DEB are comparable to or better than that of salvage CTx.

In terms of oncologic long-term outcomes, however, the optimal timing and utilization of HAT-DEB remain unclear. Thus, physicians should work toward standardization of HAT-DEB methodology. Finally, further investigations should examine the effect of earlier implementation of HAT-DEB in treatment algorithms as opposed to using such therapy only after failure of multiple surgical or systemic therapies.

Hepatic Arterial Therapy in Combination with Systemic Chemotherapy and/or Surgery

Few studies have reported outcomes of patients with CLM after HAT-DEB in combination with surgical resection. In the 1990s, Ceelen and colleagues[30] performed the only controlled trial with cTACE before resection. Fourteen patients underwent preoperative cTACE, whereas 9 patients were treated with partial hepatectomy alone. Reported OS and tumor recurrence rates were 93% and 8% (mean follow-up 15.5 months) versus 67% and 67% (mean follow-up 17.5 months), respectively. In this context, cTACE was *not* associated with increased operating time, transfusion requirement, or perioperative complication rates. The investigators concluded that preoperative cTACE reduces 12-month recurrence rates after curative liver resection and may improve OS.

Jones and colleagues[82] published 2 studies examining the radiologic-pathologic correlation of resection specimens in patients who underwent HAT-DEB before surgical resection. In the first study, a case-control series, 3 patients were treated with HAT-DEB (DEBIRI; 200 mg irinotecan loaded in a particle volume of 2 mL [particle size of 100–300 μm; DC Bead; BTG, London, UK]). Pathologic analysis of the surgical specimen demonstrated 0% tumor viability for all targeted liver metastases.

Table 4
Original studies of safety and efficacy of hepatic arterial drug-eluting bead therapy for colorectal liver metastases

Reference	Patients (n)	Therapy Stage (1st Line, 2nd Line, 3rd Line, Beyond 3rd Line)	Chemoembolics (Embolic Agents + Chemotherapeutics)	Median Follow-Up (mo)	Progression-free Survival (mo)	Median OS (mo)
Aliberti et al,[66] 2006	10	NR	DEBIRI (100 mg irinotecan) every 3 wk	NR	NR	NR
Martin et al,[60] 2009	30	2nd line	DEBs (100–700 μm)	9	NR	NR
Martin et al,[61] 2009	55	2nd line	DEBs (100–900 μm)	18	6.5	11.3
Martin et al,[58] 2010	84	2nd line	DEBs (100–700 μm)	NR	NR	NR
Martin et al,[67] 2011	55	2nd line	DEBs (100–700 μm)	18	11	19
Aliberti et al,[68] 2011	82	2nd line	DEBIRI	29	8	25
Fiorentini et al,[69] 2012	36 / 38[a]	NR	DEBIRI / FOLFIRI	NR	7 / 4	22 / 15
Martin et al,[70] 2012	10	During the off week of FOLFOX	DEBIRI (100 mg irinotecan, 100–300 μm)	NR	NR	15.2
Jones et al,[71] 2013	22	Easily resectable CLM were treated with TACE 4 wk before resection	DEBIRI	22	13.6	NR
Eichler et al,[72] 2012	11	2nd line	DEBIRI (100–500 μm)	2.7	5.1	NR
Jones et al,[73] 2013	10	NR	DEBIRI (200 mg irinotecan) as part of PARAGON II	NR	NR	NR
Narayanan et al,[74] 2013	28	NR	DEBIRI	6.9	4	13.3
Huppert et al,[75] 2014	29	Beyond 2nd line	DEBIRI (35–400 mg irinotecan)	8	5	8
Akinwande et al,[76] 2014	22 / 149[b]	NR	DEBIRI + capecitabine / DEBIRI only	10 / —	7 / 9	22 / 13
Martin et al,[77] 2015	70	1st line	FOLFOX + DEBIRI / FOLFOX alone	NR	17 / 15	13.7 / 16

[a] TACE versus systemic therapy.
[b] TACE 1 capecitabine versus TACE only.
Data from Refs.[58,60,61,66–77]

Nontargeted liver metastases as well as those detected at the time of operation also showed a response: 2 in the nontreated contralateral liver lobe (30% and 45% tumor viability, respectively) as well as 3 in the ipsilateral liver lobe (0%, 0%, and 60% tumor viability, respectively). Such data support the hypothesis that HAT-DEB has the potential to treat nontargeted liver metastases as well as micrometastases. In the second study, 22 patients were treated with HAT-DEB for 4 weeks before liver resection.[71] Disease-free survival was 13.6 months. However, the investigators noted that the Response Evaluation Criteria in Solid Tumors (RECIST) poorly predicted both pathologic response and clinical outcome. Accordingly, clinicians have discussed the use of different modalities for response assessment—cone-beam CT, angio-CT, hybrid-imaging, and biomarkers.

The use of systemic therapy in the preoperative setting to downstage CLM has been well established. The reported response rate and rate of conversion to resectability after CTx (FOLFOX, FOLFIRI, or FOLFOXIRI) range from 30% to 84% and 4% to 22%, respectively.[14,17,18,81,83] Patient selection and timing, dose, and type of the systemic therapy are relevant predictors of outcome. Kemeny and colleagues[84] recently demonstrated the potential of a strategy combining transarterial and systemic therapies. Fifty-three patients with primarily unresectable CLM (defined as at least one of the following: >5 liver metastases, bilobar disease, ≥6 involved segments) were treated with transarterial 5-fluoro-deoxyuridine and dexamethasone as HAI as well as systemic oxaliplatin and irinotecan. Tumor response rate was 92%, with 47% converting to resectability.

Akinwande and colleagues[76] subsequently described the combined use of HAT-DEB and oral systemic therapies. They showed that HAT-DEB plus Xeloda conferred a survival advantage (although not statistically significant) without additional toxicity compared with patients undergoing HAT-DEB only (22 vs 13 months). Their findings suggest that further studies should be undertaken to examine the effects of combining other oral agents for use in treatment of CLM (**Table 5**) with HAT-DEB.

Recently, Martin and colleagues[77] published the results of a randomized controlled trial assessing the safety and efficacy of DEBIRI with FOLFOX and bevacizumab versus FOLFOX and bevacizumab alone. They demonstrated no difference in toxicity between the FOLFOX-DEBIRI versus FOLFOX/bevacizumab treatment arms, a 6-month overall response rate of 76% versus 60% ($P = .05$), a conversion to resectability of 35% versus 16% ($P = .05$), and a median PFS of 15.3 versus 7.6 months. These findings suggest that DEBIRI represents a powerful adjunct to first-line CTx in patients with unresectable CLM.

YTTRIUM-90 RADIOEMBOLIZATION
Rationale and Patient Selection

Initially described in the 1980s, radioembolization represents another locoregional modality for the treatment of CLM.[85] Targeted arterial injection of Yttrium-90 (Y-90) microspheres results in embolization (and stasis) of tumor blood supply and the brachytherapy (localized delivery of radiation to hepatic tumors). As with patients being considered for HAT-DEB, candidates for Y-90 therapy should have greater than 3 months life expectancy and metastatic colorectal cancer with liver-predominant tumor burden. Absolute contraindications including the potential of greater than 30 Gy of radiation to the lung or the gastrointestinal tract can be avoided by manipulation of catheters. These possibilities are determined by a pretreatment macroaggregated albumin scan. Relative contraindications include poor baseline liver function, persistently elevated serum bilirubin, portal vein compromise, and prior hepatic radiation

Table 5
Original studies of safety and efficacy of Yttrium-90 radioembolization for colorectal liver metastases

Reference	Patients (n)	Therapy Stage (1st Line, 2nd Line, 3rd Line, >3rd Line)	Radioembolic Agent	Median Follow-Up (mo)	Median PFS (mo)	Median OS (mo)
Mantravadi et al,[85] 1982	15	NR	TheraSpheres	NR	NR	NR
Herba et al,[86] 2002	37	2nd line or beyond	TheraSpheres	8	NR	NR
Murthy et al,[87] 2007	10	3rd line or beyond	SIR-Spheres	5	NR	5.8
Sharma et al,[88] 2007	22	1st line	SIR-Spheres (+FOLFOX4)	NR	9.3	NR
Jakobs et al,[89] 2008	36	2nd line or beyond	SIR-Spheres	7.9	NR	10.5
Mulcahy et al,[90] 2009	72	2nd line or beyond	TheraSpheres	26.2	15.4	14.5
Nace et al,[91] 2011	51	3rd line	SIR-Spheres	NR	NR	10.2
Lam et al,[92] 2013	8	1st line or beyond	TheraSpheres SIR-Spheres	24.7	NR	3.1
Gunduz et al,[93] 2014	78	NR	SIR-Spheres	NR	4.4	10.1
Kalva et al,[94] 2014	45	2nd line or beyond	SIR-Spheres	4.9	NR	6.1
Abbott et al,[95] 2015	68	1st line or beyond	TheraSpheres	NR	NR	11.6

Data from Refs.[85–95]

therapy. As with HAT-DEB, pretreatment planning should also include CT or MRI, tumor markers, and serum chemistries. Furthermore, hepatic arterial flow characteristics should be carefully delineated using both preprocedural hepatic angiogram and intraprocedural fluoroscopy via percutaneously inserted intra-arterial catheters. Care should be taken to protect the gastrointestinal tract from inadvertent delivery of Y-90 by protective embolization of feeding blood vessels before radioembolization of the target hepatic lesions.[96,97]

Treatment and Toxicity

Y-90 treatments can be performed in 1 of 3 ways: whole liver, sequential (treating one hepatic lobe followed by the other), and lobar (treating only a single lobe of the liver). The optimal treatment varies based on disease burden and distribution, baseline hepatic function, and the patient's overall performance status. Projecting Y-90 microsphere activity is performed using either the (recommended) body surface area method or the empiric method. Dosing can be reduced by as much as 30% to account for impaired hepatic function or marginal hepatic reserve.[96,97]

Toxicity and complications of Y-90 treatment, much like DEBIRI, derive from the treatment itself (radiation), destruction of normal hepatocytes, and aberrant delivery of Y-90 microspheres. An analogue of post-embolization syndrome, post-radioembolization syndrome, consists of fatigue, nausea/vomiting, cachexia, and/or abdominal pain. Reported rates range from 20% to 70% and are rarely severe enough to require hospitalization.[98,99] In addition, although hepatic dysfunction occurs with 40% to 60% of Y-90 treatments, the vast majority is mild (grade I or II) and resolves within 30 days of treatment. Factors associated with persistent hepatic dysfunction are repeated radioembolization, prior external radiation therapy to the liver, and elevated pretreatment serum bilirubin and/or transaminases.[92,98] Other sequelae include biliary complications such as cholecystitis and cholangitis (more likely in patients with previous biliary procedures or surgeries), pancreatitis, and gastroenteritis.[100–102] These complications are infrequent (<5%–10%) and stem from aberrant deposition of microspheres into arterial communications with biliary, pancreatic, and/or enteric structures. They can be prevented through careful preprocedural assessment of each patient's arterial anatomy and prudent utilization of protective embolization before deposition of Y-90 beads.[98]

Efficacy and Response Evaluation

The safety and efficacy of Y-90 therapy have been demonstrated by several groups for treatment of chemotherapy-refractory CLM.[86,89,90,94,95,103–105] Specifically, Jakobs and colleagues[89] showed a median OS of 10.5 months with an adverse event rate of approximately 8%. The group also demonstrated an increased survival benefit in patients experiencing a decrease in carcinoembryonic antigen (CEA) level as well as a response on posttreatment imaging. More recently, Abbott and colleagues[95] assessed response in patients with varying hepatic burdens of disease and differing number of prior chemotherapy regimens. They showed a median OS of 11.6 months, with significantly greater median OS (19.6 months vs 3.4 months, $P<.001$) for patients with less than 25% hepatic disease burden (HBD) compared with those with greater than 25% HBD. On multivariate analysis, factors associated with decreased OS were age, 3 or more lines of prior chemotherapy, HBD greater than 25%, and higher CEA level.

As with DEBIRI, several groups have investigated the optimal means of assessing response to Y-90. In a 2007 report, Miller and colleagues[106] reviewed the imaging responses of CLM to Y-90 therapy using CT with various response criteria (World Health

Organization, RECIST, necrosis) as well as PET. They found that use of combined necrosis and RECIST criteria resulted in the highest response rate and also detected responses earlier than size criteria alone. PET also allowed for greater detection of treatment response than CT using RECIST or combined criteria. Finally, their statement that the use of PET in conjunction with CT imaging to detect recurrence earlier after treatment has been supported elsewhere in the literature, and PET should be considered a useful tool in posttreatment follow-up of patients treated with Y-90 therapy for CLM.[107]

Concomitant Use with Systemic Chemotherapy, Surgery

As with HAT-DEB, several investigators have examined the use of Y-90 with CTx.[88,108–110] Sharma and colleagues[88] combined Y-90 therapy with systemic FOLFOX4 in the treatment of 22 patients with CLM. Median PFS was 9.3 months, with a median hepatic-specific PFS of 12.3 months. In addition, 2 patients underwent conversion to resectability after treatment. De Souza and Daly[109] recently authored a case report describing the use of aflibercept (Aylea, Regeneron Pharmaceuticals, Tarrytown, NY, USA) with FOLFIRI and Y-90 radioembolization. The patient underwent 2 discrete Y-90 treatments, first targeting the largest right lobe tumor and then targeting the left lobe tumor with re-treatment of the right lobe tumor. Based on the modified RECIST criteria, she demonstrated a partial response on CT and also experienced a decrease in her CEA levels. Currently, Gibbs and colleagues[108] and Dutton and colleagues[110] are conducting two randomized controlled trials assessing Y-90 therapy combined with FOLFOX6 ± bevacizumab versus FOLFOX6 ± bevacizumab alone and OxMdG with or without Y-90 therapy for treatment of unresectable CLM. Gibbs and colleagues[108] project an increase in median PFS from 9.4 to 12.5 months, similar to the data described by Sharma and colleagues.[88]

Several groups have also investigated the safety of hepatic resection after administration of Y-90. Whitney and colleagues[111] described 4 patients who underwent Y-90 therapy with good response and subsequently underwent hepatic resection with or without concomitant hepatic ablation. No patients demonstrated hepatic dysfunction or hepatic-specific recurrence after hepatectomy, and median survival was 2 years. Importantly, the investigators noted that the utility of preoperative Y-90 therapy lies not only in downstaging patients but also in assessing tumor biology, informing prognosis, and guiding therapy.

SUMMARY

The last several years have witnessed a significant increase in the use of HAT in patients with therapy-refractory CLM. The emergence of calibrated microspheres, together with improvements in DEB technology, has enabled physicians to perform both HAT-DEB and Y-90 embolization in a highly standardized and effective fashion. In most published studies, HAT-DEB and Y-90 are used either in the setting of controlled trials with patients who had failed first- or second-line chemotherapy or as salvage therapy for patients who had failed multiple previous surgical, ablative, and/or systemic therapies. The results of a randomized trial demonstrating the benefit of adding HAT-DEB to first-line CTx for unresectable CLM has recently been published. Currently, two similarly oriented trials for Y-90 are underway. Preoperatively, HAT may be used for tumor downsizing and conversion to resectability of CLM with minimal systemic toxicity and fewer adverse effects compared with systemic therapy. In addition, postoperatively, it can be used to prevent recurrence and improve OS. In nonsurgical candidates with liver-dominant metastases, palliative HAT in combination with systemic therapy (chemotherapeutics and/or biologic agents) should be evaluated. Further randomized trials are required to better characterize the efficacy of HAT technologies for patients with CLM in the first, second, and third line and beyond.

REFERENCES

1. Zhao Z, Pelletier E, Barber B, et al. Patterns of treatment with chemotherapy and monoclonal antibodies for metastatic colorectal cancer in Western Europe. Curr Med Res Opin 2012;28(2):221–9.
2. Schwarz RE, Berlin JD, Lenz HJ, et al. Systemic cytotoxic and biological therapies of colorectal liver metastases: expert consensus statement. HPB 2013; 15(2):106–15.
3. Bentrem DJ, Dematteo RP, Blumgart LH. Surgical therapy for metastatic disease to the liver. Annu Rev Med 2005;56:139–56.
4. Folprecht G. Treatment of colorectal liver metastases. Dtsch Med Wochenschr 2013;138(41):2098–103 [in German].
5. Goere D, Benhaim L, Bonnet S, et al. Adjuvant chemotherapy after resection of colorectal liver metastases in patients at high risk of hepatic recurrence: a comparative study between hepatic arterial infusion of oxaliplatin and modern systemic chemotherapy. Ann Surg 2013;257(1):114–20.
6. Bozzetti F, Doci R, Bignami P, et al. Patterns of failure following surgical resection of colorectal cancer liver metastases. Rationale for a multimodal approach. Ann Surg 1987;205(3):264–70.
7. Hind D, Tappenden P, Tumur I, et al. The use of irinotecan, oxaliplatin and raltitrexed for the treatment of advanced colorectal cancer: systematic review and economic evaluation. Health Technology Assess (Winchester, England) 2008; 12(15):iii–ix. xi-162.
8. Hochster HS, Hart LL, Ramanathan RK, et al. Safety and efficacy of oxaliplatin and fluoropyrimidine regimens with or without bevacizumab as first-line treatment of metastatic colorectal cancer: results of the TREE Study. J Clin Oncol 2008;26(21):3523–9.
9. Thirion P, Michiels S, Pignon JP, et al. Modulation of fluorouracil by leucovorin in patients with advanced colorectal cancer: an updated meta-analysis. J Clin Oncol 2004;22(18):3766–75.
10. Tournigand C, Andre T, Achille E, et al. FOLFIRI followed by FOLFOX6 or the reverse sequence in advanced colorectal cancer: a randomized GERCOR study. J Clin Oncol 2004;22(2):229–37.
11. Van Cutsem E, Kohne CH, Hitre E, et al. Cetuximab and chemotherapy as initial treatment for metastatic colorectal cancer. N Engl J Med 2009;360(14):1408–17.
12. Ychou M, Viret F, Kramar A, et al. Tritherapy with fluorouracil/leucovorin, irinotecan and oxaliplatin (FOLFIRINOX): a phase II study in colorectal cancer patients with non-resectable liver metastases. Cancer Chemother Pharmacol 2008; 62(2):195–201.
13. Foubert F, Matysiak-Budnik T, Touchefeu Y. Options for metastatic colorectal cancer beyond the second line of treatment. Dig Liver Dis 2014;46(2):105–12.
14. Alberts SR, Horvath WL, Sternfeld WC, et al. Oxaliplatin, fluorouracil, and leucovorin for patients with unresectable liver-only metastases from colorectal cancer: a North Central Cancer Treatment Group phase II study. J Clin Oncol 2005; 23(36):9243–9.
15. Nordlinger B, Sorbye H, Glimelius B, et al. Perioperative chemotherapy with FOLFOX4 and surgery versus surgery alone for resectable liver metastases

from colorectal cancer (EORTC Intergroup trial 40983): a randomised controlled trial. Lancet (London, England) 2008;371(9617):1007–16.

16. Haraldsdottir S, Wu C, Bloomston M, et al. What is the optimal neo-adjuvant treatment for liver metastasis? Ther Adv Med Oncol 2013;5(4):221–34.

17. Lam VW, Spiro C, Laurence JM, et al. A systematic review of clinical response and survival outcomes of downsizing systemic chemotherapy and rescue liver surgery in patients with initially unresectable colorectal liver metastases. Ann Surg Oncol 2012;19(4):1292–301.

18. Malik H, Khan AZ, Berry DP, et al. Liver resection rate following downsizing chemotherapy with cetuximab in metastatic colorectal cancer: UK retrospective observational study. Eur J Surg Oncol 2015;41(4):499–505.

19. Collins JM. Pharmacologic rationale for regional drug delivery. J Clin Oncol 1984;2(5):498–504.

20. Lewandowski RJ, Geschwind JF, Liapi E, et al. Transcatheter intraarterial therapies: rationale and overview. Radiology 2011;259(3):641–57.

21. Abdalla EK, Vauthey JN. Chemotherapy prior to hepatic resection for colorectal liver metastases: helpful until harmful? Dig Surg 2008;25(6):421–9.

22. Amado RG, Wolf M, Peeters M, et al. Wild-type KRAS is required for panitumumab efficacy in patients with metastatic colorectal cancer. J Clin Oncol 2008; 26(10):1626–34.

23. Rajappa P, Krass J, Riina HA, et al. Super-selective basilar artery infusion of bevacizumab and cetuximab for multiply recurrent pediatric ependymoma. Interv Neuroradiol 2011;17(4):459–65.

24. Burkhardt JK, Riina H, Shin BJ, et al. Intra-arterial delivery of bevacizumab after blood-brain barrier disruption for the treatment of recurrent glioblastoma: progression-free survival and overall survival. World Neurosurg 2012;77(1):130–4.

25. Pellerin O, Geschwind JF. Intra-arterial treatment of liver metastases from colorectal carcinoma. J Radiol 2011;92(9):835–41 [in French].

26. Xing M, Kooby DA, El-Rayes BF, et al. Locoregional therapies for metastatic colorectal carcinoma to the liver–an evidence-based review. J Surg Oncol 2014;110(2):182–96.

27. Alberts SR. Update on the optimal management of patients with colorectal liver metastases. Crit Rev Oncol Hematol 2012;84(1):59–70.

28. Nishiofuku H, Tanaka T, Matsuoka M, et al. Transcatheter arterial chemoembolization using cisplatin powder mixed with degradable starch microspheres for colorectal liver metastases after FOLFOX failure: results of a phase I/II study. J Vasc Interv Radiol 2013;24(1):56–65.

29. Tsuchiya M, Watanabe M, Otsuka Y, et al. Transarterial chemoembolization with irinotecan (CPT-11) and degradable starch microspheres (DSM) in patients with liver metastases from colorectal cancer. Gan To Kagaku Ryoho 2007;34(12): 2038–40 [in Japanese].

30. Ceelen W, Praet M, Villeirs G, et al. Initial experience with the use of preoperative transarterial chemoembolization in the treatment of liver metastasis. Acta Chir Belg 1996;96(1):37–40.

31. Tellez C, Benson AB 3rd, Lyster MT, et al. Phase II trial of chemoembolization for the treatment of metastatic colorectal carcinoma to the liver and review of the literature. Cancer 1998;82(7):1250–9.

32. Leichman CG, Jacobson JR, Modiano M, et al. Hepatic chemoembolization combined with systemic infusion of 5-fluorouracil and bolus leucovorin for patients with metastatic colorectal carcinoma: a Southwest Oncology Group pilot trial. Cancer 1999;86(5):775–81.

33. Muller H, Nakchbandi W, Chatzissavvidis I, et al. Intra-arterial infusion of 5-fluorouracil plus granulocyte-macrophage colony-stimulating factor (GM-CSF) and chemoembolization with melphalan in the treatment of disseminated colorectal liver metastases. Eur J Surg Oncol 2001;27(7):652–61.

34. Salman HS, Cynamon J, Jagust M, et al. Randomized phase II trial of embolization therapy versus chemoembolization therapy in previously treated patients with colorectal carcinoma metastatic to the liver. Clin Colorectal Cancer 2002; 2(3):173–9.

35. Vogl TJ, Gruber T, Balzer JO, et al. Repeated transarterial chemoembolization in the treatment of liver metastases of colorectal cancer: prospective study. Radiology 2009;250(1):281–9.

36. Albert M, Kiefer MV, Sun W, et al. Chemoembolization of colorectal liver metastases with cisplatin, doxorubicin, mitomycin C, ethiodol, and polyvinyl alcohol. Cancer 2011;117(2):343–52.

37. Gruber-Rouh T, Naguib NN, Eichler K, et al. Transarterial chemoembolization of unresectable systemic chemotherapy-refractory liver metastases from colorectal cancer: long-term results over a 10-year period. Int J Cancer 2014; 134(5):1225–31.

38. Gnutzmann DM, Mechel J, Schmitz A, et al. Evaluation of the plasmatic and parenchymal elution kinetics of two different irinotecan-loaded drug-eluting embolics in a pig model. J Vasc Interv Radiol 2015;26(5):746–54.

39. Glimelius B, Cavalli-Bjorkman N. Metastatic colorectal cancer: current treatment and future options for improved survival. Medical approach–present status. Scand J Gastroenterol 2012;47(3):296–314.

40. Barletta E, Fiore F, Daniele B, et al. Second-line intra-arterial chemotherapy in advanced pancreatic adenocarcinoma. Front Biosci 2006;11:782–7.

41. Shimonov M, Hayat H, Chaitchik S, et al. Combined systemic chronotherapy and hepatic artery infusion for the treatment of metastatic colorectal cancer confined to the liver. Chemotherapy 2005;51(2–3):111–5.

42. Gonzalez Cao M, Bastarrika G, Garcia-Foncillas J, et al. Ileal carcinoid tumor with liver metastases and cardiac involvement treated with intraarterial liposomal doxorubicin and valve replacement. Clin Transl Oncol 2006;8(5): 369–71.

43. Moroney J, Fu S, Moulder S, et al. Phase I study of the antiangiogenic antibody bevacizumab and the mTOR/hypoxia-inducible factor inhibitor temsirolimus combined with liposomal doxorubicin: tolerance and biological activity. Clin Cancer Res 2012;18(20):5796–805.

44. Mancini R, Tedesco M, Garufi C, et al. Hepatic arterial infusion (HAI) of cisplatin and systemic fluorouracil in the treatment of unresectable colorectal liver metastases. Anticancer Res 2003;23(2c):1837–41.

45. Liu B, Huang JW, Li Y, et al. Single-agent versus combination doxorubicin-based transarterial chemoembolization in the treatment of hepatocellular carcinoma: a single-blind, randomized, phase II trial. Oncology 2015;89(1): 23–30.

46. Nakanishi M, Yoshida Y, Natazuka T. Prospective study of transarterial infusion of docetaxel and cisplatin to treat non-small-cell lung cancer in patients contraindicated for standard chemotherapy. Lung Cancer (Amsterdam, Netherlands) 2012;77(2):353–8.

47. Seki A, Hori S. Transcatheter arterial chemoembolization with docetaxel-loaded microspheres controls heavily pretreated unresectable liver metastases from colorectal cancer: a case study. Int J Clin Oncol 2011;16(5):613–6.

48. Tawada A, Chiba T, Ooka Y, et al. Transarterial chemoembolization with miriplatin plus epirubicin in patients with hepatocellular carcinoma. Anticancer Res 2015;35(1):549–54.
49. Fiorentini G, Poddie DB, Cantore M, et al. Hepatic intra-arterial chemotherapy (HIAC) of high dose mitomycin and epirubicin combined with caval chemofiltration versus prolonged low doses in liver metastases from colorectal cancer: a prospective randomized clinical study. J Chemother (Florence, Italy) 2004; 16(Suppl 5):51–4.
50. Edelhauser G, Schicher N, Berzaczy D, et al. Fotemustine chemoembolization of hepatic metastases from uveal melanoma: a retrospective single-center analysis. AJR Am J Roentgenol 2012;199(6):1387–92.
51. Hartmann J, Schmoll E, Bokemeyer C, et al. Hepatic arterial infusion of the nitrosourea derivate fotemustine for the treatment of liver metastases from colorectal carcinoma. Oncol Rep 1997;4(1):167–72.
52. Vogl TJ, Zangos S, Eichler K, et al. Palliative hepatic intraarterial chemotherapy (HIC) using a novel combination of gemcitabine and mitomycin C: results in hepatic metastases. Eur Radiol 2008;18(3):468–76.
53. Boulin M, Guiu S, Chauffert B, et al. Screening of anticancer drugs for chemoembolization of hepatocellular carcinoma. Anticancer Drugs 2011;22(8): 741–8.
54. Link KH, Sunelaitis E, Kornmann M, et al. Regional chemotherapy of nonresectable colorectal liver metastases with mitoxantrone, 5-fluorouracil, folinic acid, and mitomycin C may prolong survival. Cancer 2001;92(11):2746–53.
55. Chen Y, Wang XL, Wang JH, et al. Transarterial infusion with gemcitabine and oxaliplatin for the treatment of unresectable pancreatic cancer. Anticancer Drugs 2014;25(8):958–63.
56. Koga Y, Ohchi T, Kudo S, et al. Effective transarterial neoadjuvant chemotherapy with paclitaxel (TXL) in a case of locally advanced breast cancer. Gan To Kagaku Ryoho 2003;30(2):255–8.
57. Tsimberidou AM, Letourneau K, Fu S, et al. Phase I clinical trial of hepatic arterial infusion of paclitaxel in patients with advanced cancer and dominant liver involvement. Cancer Chemother Pharmacol 2011;68(1):247–53.
58. Martin RC, Howard J, Tomalty D, et al. Toxicity of irinotecan-eluting beads in the treatment of hepatic malignancies: results of a multi-institutional registry. Cardiovasc Interv Radiol 2010;33(5):960–6.
59. Cohen AD, Kemeny NE. An update on hepatic arterial infusion chemotherapy for colorectal cancer. Oncologist 2003;8(6):553–66.
60. Martin RC, Joshi J, Robbins K, et al. Transarterial chemoembolization of metastatic colorectal carcinoma with drug-eluting beads, irinotecan (DEBIRI): multi-institutional registry. J Oncol 2009;2009:539795.
61. Martin RC, Robbins K, Tomalty D, et al. Transarterial chemoembolisation (TACE) using irinotecan-loaded beads for the treatment of unresectable metastases to the liver in patients with colorectal cancer: an interim report. World J Surg Oncol 2009;7:80.
62. Geschwind JF, Kaushik S, Ramsey DE, et al. Influence of a new prophylactic antibiotic therapy on the incidence of liver abscesses after chemoembolization treatment of liver tumors. J Vasc Interv Radiol 2002;13(11):1163–6.
63. Liu DM, Thakor AS, Baerlocher M, et al. A review of conventional and drug-eluting chemoembolization in the treatment of colorectal liver metastases: principles and proof. Future Oncol (London, England) 2015;11(9):1421–8.

64. Basile A, Carrafiello G, Ierardi AM, et al. Quality-improvement guidelines for hepatic transarterial chemoembolization. Cardiovasc Intervent Radiol 2012;35(4): 765–74.
65. Meyer C, Pieper CC, Ezziddin S, et al. Feasibility of temporary protective embolization of normal liver tissue using degradable starch microspheres during radioembolization of liver tumours. Eur J Nucl Med Mol Imaging 2014;41(2):231–7.
66. Aliberti C, Tilli M, Benea G, et al. Trans-arterial chemoembolization (TACE) of liver metastases from colorectal cancer using irinotecan-eluting beads: preliminary results. Anticancer Res 2006;26(5b):3793–5.
67. Martin RC, Joshi J, Robbins K, et al. Hepatic intra-arterial injection of drug-eluting bead, irinotecan (DEBIRI) in unresectable colorectal liver metastases refractory to systemic chemotherapy: results of multi-institutional study. Ann Surg Oncol 2011;18(1):192–8.
68. Aliberti C, Fiorentini G, Muzzio PC, et al. Trans-arterial chemoembolization of metastatic colorectal carcinoma to the liver adopting DC Bead(R), drug-eluting bead loaded with irinotecan: results of a phase II clinical study. Anticancer Res 2011;31(12):4581–7.
69. Fiorentini G, Aliberti C, Tilli M, et al. Intra-arterial infusion of irinotecan-loaded drug-eluting beads (DEBIRI) versus intravenous therapy (FOLFIRI) for hepatic metastases from colorectal cancer: final results of a phase III study. Anticancer Res 2012;32(4):1387–95.
70. Martin RC 2nd, Scoggins CR, Tomalty D, et al. Irinotecan drug-eluting beads in the treatment of chemo-naive unresectable colorectal liver metastasis with concomitant systemic fluorouracil and oxaliplatin: results of pharmacokinetics and phase I trial. J Gastrointest Surg 2012;16(8):1531–8.
71. Jones RP, Stattner S, Dunne DF, et al. Radiological assessment of response to neoadjuvant transcatheter hepatic therapy with irinotecan-eluting beads (DEBIRI((R))) for colorectal liver metastases does not predict tumour destruction or long-term outcome. Eur J Surg Oncol 2013;39(10):1122–8.
72. Eichler K, Zangos S, Mack MG, et al. First human study in treatment of unresectable liver metastases from colorectal cancer with irinotecan-loaded beads (DEBIRI). Int J Oncol 2012;41(4):1213–20.
73. Jones RP, Sutton P, Greensmith RM, et al. Hepatic activation of irinotecan predicts tumour response in patients with colorectal liver metastases treated with DEBIRI: exploratory findings from a phase II study. Cancer Chemother Pharmacol 2013;72(2):359–68.
74. Narayanan G, Barbery K, Suthar R, et al. Transarterial chemoembolization using DEBIRI for treatment of hepatic metastases from colorectal cancer. Anticancer Res 2013;33(5):2077–83.
75. Huppert P, Wenzel T, Wietholtz H. Transcatheter arterial chemoembolization (TACE) of colorectal cancer liver metastases by irinotecan-eluting microspheres in a salvage patient population. Cardiovasc Intervent Radiol 2014;37(1):154–64.
76. Akinwande O, Miller A, Hayes D, et al. Concomitant capecitabine with hepatic delivery of drug eluting beads in metastatic colorectal cancer. Anticancer Res 2014;34(12):7239–45.
77. Martin RC 2nd, Scoggins CR, Schreeder M, et al. Randomized controlled trial of irinotecan drug-eluting beads with simultaneous FOLFOX and bevacizumab for patients with unresectable colorectal liver-limited metastasis. Cancer 2015; 121(20):3649–58.

78. Chan DL, Alzahrani NA, Morris DL, et al. Systematic review and meta-analysis of hepatic arterial infusion chemotherapy as bridging therapy for colorectal liver metastases. Surg Oncol 2015;24(3):162–71.
79. Fiorentini G, Aliberti C, Mulazzani L, et al. Chemoembolization in colorectal liver metastases: the rebirth. Anticancer Res 2014;34(2):575–84.
80. Richardson AJ, Laurence JM, Lam VW. Transarterial chemoembolization with irinotecan beads in the treatment of colorectal liver metastases: systematic review. J Vasc Interv Radiol 2013;24(8):1209–17.
81. Cai GX, Cai SJ. Multi-modality treatment of colorectal liver metastases. World J Gastroenterol 2012;18(1):16–24.
82. Jones RP, Dunne D, Sutton P, et al. Segmental and lobar administration of drug-eluting beads delivering irinotecan leads to tumour destruction: a case-control series. HPB 2013;15(1):71–7.
83. Ho WM, Ma B, Mok T, et al. Liver resection after irinotecan, 5-fluorouracil, and folinic acid for patients with unresectable colorectal liver metastases: a multicenter phase II study by the Cancer Therapeutic Research Group. Med Oncol (Northwood, London, England) 2005;22(3):303–12.
84. Kemeny NE, Melendez FD, Capanu M, et al. Conversion to resectability using hepatic artery infusion plus systemic chemotherapy for the treatment of unresectable liver metastases from colorectal carcinoma. J Clin Oncol 2009; 27(21):3465–71.
85. Mantravadi RV, Spigos DG, Tan WS, et al. Intraarterial yttrium 90 in the treatment of hepatic malignancy. Radiology 1982;142(3):783–6.
86. Herba MJ, Thirlwell MP. Radioembolization for hepatic metastases. Semin Oncol 2002;29(2):152–9.
87. Murthy R, Eng C, Krishnan S, et al. Hepatic yttrium-90 radioembolotherapy in metastatic colorectal cancer treated with cetuximab or bevacizumab. J Vasc Interv Radiol 2007;18(12):1588–91.
88. Sharma RA, Van Hazel GA, Morgan B, et al. Radioembolization of liver metastases from colorectal cancer using yttrium-90 microspheres with concomitant systemic oxaliplatin, fluorouracil, and leucovorin chemotherapy. J Clin Oncol 2007; 25(9):1099–106.
89. Jakobs TF, Hoffmann RT, Dehm K, et al. Hepatic yttrium-90 radioembolization of chemotherapy-refractory colorectal cancer liver metastases. J Vasc Interv Radiol 2008;19(8):1187–95.
90. Mulcahy MF, Lewandowski RJ, Ibrahim SM, et al. Radioembolization of colorectal hepatic metastases using yttrium-90 microspheres. Cancer 2009; 115(9):1849–58.
91. Nace GW, Steel JL, Amesur N, et al. Yttrium-90 radioembolization for colorectal cancer liver metastases: a single institution experience. Int J Surg Oncol 2011; 2011:571261.
92. Lam MG, Louie JD, Iagaru AH, et al. Safety of repeated yttrium-90 radioembolization. Cardiovasc Intervent Radiol 2013;36(5):1320–8.
93. Gunduz S, Ozgur O, Bozcuk H, et al. Yttrium-90 radioembolization in patients with unresectable liver metastases: determining the factors that lead to treatment efficacy. Hepato Gastroenterol 2014;61(134):1529–34.
94. Kalva SP, Rana RS, Liu R, et al. Yttrium-90 radioembolization as salvage therapy for liver metastases from colorectal cancer. Am J Clin Oncol 2014;11(3): 195–9.
95. Abbott AM, Kim R, Hoffe SE, et al. Outcomes of therasphere radioembolization for colorectal metastases. Clin Colorectal Cancer 2015;14(3):146–53.

96. Kennedy A, Nag S, Salem R, et al. Recommendations for radioembolization of hepatic malignancies using yttrium-90 microsphere brachytherapy: a consensus panel report from the radioembolization brachytherapy oncology consortium. Int J Radiat Oncol Biol Phys 2007;68(1):13–23.

97. Lau WY, Kennedy AS, Kim YH, et al. Patient selection and activity planning guide for selective internal radiotherapy with yttrium-90 resin microspheres. Int J Radiat Oncol Biol Phys 2012;82(1):401–7.

98. Riaz A, Awais R, Salem R. Side effects of yttrium-90 radioembolization. Front Oncol 2014;4:198.

99. Peterson JL, Vallow LA, Johnson DW, et al. Complications after 90Y microsphere radioembolization for unresectable hepatic tumors: an evaluation of 112 patients. Brachytherapy 2013;12(6):573–9.

100. Atassi B, Bangash AK, Lewandowski RJ, et al. Biliary sequelae following radioembolization with Yttrium-90 microspheres. J Vasc Interv Radiol 2008;19(5):691–7.

101. Murthy R, Brown DB, Salem R, et al. Gastrointestinal complications associated with hepatic arterial Yttrium-90 microsphere therapy. J Vasc Interv Radiol 2007; 18(4):553–61 [quiz: 562].

102. Hoffmann RT, Jakobs TF, Kubisch CH, et al. Radiofrequency ablation after selective internal radiation therapy with Yttrium90 microspheres in metastatic liver disease-Is it feasible? Eur J Radiol 2010;74(1):199–205.

103. Gulec SA, Mesoloras G, Dezarn WA, et al. Safety and efficacy of Y-90 microsphere treatment in patients with primary and metastatic liver cancer: the tumor selectivity of the treatment as a function of tumor to liver flow ratio. J Transl Med 2007;5:15.

104. Padia SA, Kwan SW, Roudsari B, et al. Superselective yttrium-90 radioembolization for hepatocellular carcinoma yields high response rates with minimal toxicity. J Vasc Interv Radiol 2014;25(7):1067–73.

105. Deleporte A, Flamen P, Hendlisz A. State of the art: radiolabeled microspheres treatment for liver malignancies. Expert Opin Pharmacother 2010;11(4):579–86.

106. Miller FH, Keppke AL, Reddy D, et al. Response of liver metastases after treatment with yttrium-90 microspheres: role of size, necrosis, and PET. AJR Am J Roentgenol 2007;188(3):776–83.

107. Annunziata S, Treglia G, Caldarella C. The role of 18F-FDG-PET and PET/CT in patients with colorectal liver metastases undergoing selective internal radiation therapy with yttrium-90: a first evidence-based review. ScientificWorldJournal 2014;2014:879469.

108. Gibbs P, Gebski V, Van Buskirk M, et al. Selective Internal Radiation Therapy (SIRT) with yttrium-90 resin microspheres plus standard systemic chemotherapy regimen of FOLFOX versus FOLFOX alone as first-line treatment of non-resectable liver metastases from colorectal cancer: the SIRFLOX study. BMC Cancer 2014;14:897.

109. De Souza A, Daly KP. Safety and efficacy of combined yttrium 90 resin radioembolization with aflibercept and FOLFIRI in a patient with metastatic colorectal cancer. Case Rep Oncol Med 2015;2015:461823.

110. Dutton SJ, Kenealy N, Love SB, et al. FOXFIRE protocol: an open-label, randomised, phase III trial of 5-fluorouracil, oxaliplatin and folinic acid (OxMdG) with or without interventional Selective Internal Radiation Therapy (SIRT) as first-line treatment for patients with unresectable liver-only or liver-dominant metastatic colorectal cancer. BMC Cancer 2014;14:497.

111. Whitney R, Tatum C, Hahl M, et al. Safety of hepatic resection in metastatic disease to the liver after yttrium-90 therapy. J Surg Res 2011;166(2):236–40.

Index

Note: Page numbers of article titles are in **boldface** type.

Surg Clin N Am 96 (2016) 393–405
http://dx.doi.org/10.1016/S0039-6109(16)00031-1
0039-6109/16/$ – see front matter © 2016 Elsevier Inc. All rights reserved.

surgical.theclinics.com

Moving?

Make sure your subscription moves with you!

To notify us of your new address, find your **Clinics Account Number** (located on your mailing label above your name), and contact customer service at:

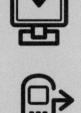

Email: journalscustomerservice-usa@elsevier.com

800-654-2452 (subscribers in the U.S. & Canada)
314-447-8871 (subscribers outside of the U.S. & Canada)

Fax number: 314-447-8029

Elsevier Health Sciences Division
Subscription Customer Service
3251 Riverport Lane
Maryland Heights, MO 63043

*To ensure uninterrupted delivery of your subscription, please notify us at least 4 weeks in advance of move.

ELSEVIER

Printed and bound by CPI Group (UK) Ltd, Croydon, CR0 4YY

03/10/2024

01040391-0005